Recent Advances in Geriatrics

Recent Advances in Geriatrics

Edited by

Mario Barbagallo and
Giuseppe Licata

University of Palermo
Palermo, Italy

and

James R. Sowers

Wayne State University
School of Medicine
Detroit, Michigan

Plenum Press • New York and London

Library of Congress Cataloging-in-Publication Data

Recent advances in geriatrics / edited by Mario Barbagallo, Giuseppe Licata, and James R. Sowers.
p. cm.
"Proceedings of the eighth course of the Internationnal School of Gerontology and Geriatrics on advances in geriatrics: cardiovascular system, arterial hypertension, and osteoporois"--T.p. verso.
Includes bibliographical references and index.
ISBN 0-306-45779-2
1. Aged--Diseases--Congresses. 2. Cardiovascular diseases in old age--Congresses. 3. Aging--Physiological aspects--Congresses. I. Barbagallo, Mario. II. Licata, Giuseppe. III. Sowers, James R. (James Russell), 1942- . IV. Universitià di Palermo. International School of Gerontology and Geriatrics.
[DNLM: 1. Geriatrics--congresses. 2. Cardiovascular Diseases--in old age--congresses. 3. Hypertension--in old age--congresses. 4. Osteoporosis, Postmenopausal--congresses. WT 100 R295 1997]
RC952.A2R43 1997
618.97--dc21
DNLM/DLC
for Library of Congress 97-46470
CIP

Proceedings of the Eighth Course of the International School of Gerontology and Geriatrics on Advances in Geriatrics: Cardiovascular System, Arterial Hypertension, and Osteoporosis, held March 20–25, 1997, in Erice, Italy

ISBN 0-306-45779-2

A Division of Plenum Publishing Corporation
233 Spring Street, New York, N.Y. 10013

http://www.plenum.com

10 9 8 7 6 5 4 3 2 1

Printed in the United States of America

PREFACE

This book, *Recent Advances in Geriatrics*, is based on the proceedings of the 8th Course of the School of Gerontology and Geriatrics held in Erice (Trapani, Italy) at the International Centre for Scientific Culture "Ettore Majorana" on March 20–25, 1997. This international effort was organized jointly by professors from the University of Palermo (Italy) and from Wayne State University (Michigan, USA) as a result of a cross-cultural collaboration of several years.

The increasing average age of the populations in industrialized countries has resulted in increased interest in the different biological, medical, psychological, and economic aspects related to the health and social care of the elderly. Physicians and health care practitioners are realizing the need for a revised approach to geriatric care.

Comprising contributions of clinicians and scientists from Italy and North America, the present volume provides a multidisciplinary approach to many gerontological and geriatric problems, examined from a scientific and a practical point of view. Several of the most important aspects of the aging process — the genetics of aging, body composition modification, immunological, endocrinological, and renal physiology changes — have been addressed. Data from a multi-center Italian study on centenarians is reported, together with an update on clinical and pharmacological approaches to dementia syndromes and economic and social aspects related to the care of the elderly.

Particular attention has been given to aspects related to the aging of the cardiovascular system: senile anatomic and functional modifications, the physiopathology of ischemic events, the peculiar aspects of cardiac insufficiency in the elderly, endothelial and cellular aspects of hypertension, and therapeutic approachs.

The last part of the book is devoted to the changes in calcium metabolism in the elderly and to senile osteoporosis. This is an increasingly important public health concern, due to the extremely frequent and dangerous complications that can arise, such as fractures and immobilization. The most recent advances in the physiology, diagnosis, and therapy of the disease are examined and discussed.

Thus, this volume intends to be a useful and up-to-date review of the problems associated with human aging, from a scientific and practical point of view. We trust it may be helpful to all physicians and professionals interested in providing quality health care to the elderly.

Mario Barbagallo, MD
Giuseppe Licata, MD
James R. Sowers, MD

CONTENTS

1

RECENT ADVANCES IN GERONTOLOGY AND GERIATRICS IN ITALY

P. U. Carbonin

Cattedra di Gerontologia e Geriatria
Università Cattolica del Sacro Cuore
Rome, Italy

The whole Italian health care system has currently reached a critical point; indeed, similar situations can be found in all westernized countries. Nevertheless, many sound results from Italian geriatricians testify a reassuring vitality of Geriatrics in Italy. In fact, the recent advances in research in both gerontological and geriatric fields have been developing in a multidisciplinary context, including clinical, biological, and socio-behavioral settings.

The first work that I would like to mention is the atlas on the aging of the Italian population which has been published in 1995 by Professor Golini and coworkers.[1] This book, which provides detailed information about all Italian regions, is a precious tool for every geriatrician, and yields a picture of the forthcoming demographics in the next 30 years. The impressive increase in life expectancy over the last century (as depicted in Table 1) should be first outlined. The most interesting data refer to the 80+ age segment, which includes most geriatric patients. At present, life expectancy among Italian 80-year-old subjects has reached 6.4 years for males and 8 years for females, respectively. Given this prolonged lifespan, persons aged 80+ deserve all the care that may be necessary to gain the best quality of life. Currently, Italian subjects aged 80+ exceed 1,700,000 units, and a two-fold increase in their number is expected over the next 20 years (Table 2). Such a forecast could become true only if the current socio-economical situation in Italy will keep constant. Noteworthy, data from UNICEF show an impressive decline in life expectancy among Russian populations following the fall of the Berlin wall (Table 3).[2] Thus, those who manage economical resources should be aware that financial straits may yield devastating effects on a population's health status, mainly among the most frail segments, such as older persons. In this setting, it should be outlined that low-income subjects are the main determinants of health expenditure, since they are at higher risk of disease.[3] Now I will compare such demographic data with some results from the ILSA Study of the Progetto Finalizzato Invecchiamento of the CNR, in which many geriatricians have been involved.[4] The ILSA is the only Italian study which examined a homogeneous sample of all the national population. According to data from ILSA (Figures 1 and 2) and to demographic data (Table 2) two important conclusions can be derived. First, the prevalence of functional impairment—evaluated as ADLs and IADLs—progressively increases among older age segments, so that beyond the

Recent Advances in Geriatrics, edited by Barbagallo, Licata, and Sowers.
Plenum Press, New York, 1998.

Table 1. Life expectancy at 60 and 80 years (from Lori et al.[1])

	Age (years)			
	≥ 60		≥ 80	
Years	M	F	M	F
1899–1902	13.5	13.6	4.0	4.0
1950–1953	16.0	17.5	5.0	5.5
1970–1972	16.7	20.2	5.8	6.7
1990	18.4	23.0	6.4	8.0

Table 2. Total and older population in Italy, 1990–2020 (from Lori et al.[1])

	Number (thousands)				% of total population			
Age groups	1990	2000	2010	2020	1990	2000	2010	2020
Total population	57,633	57,863	56,516	53,674	100.0	100.0	100.0	100.0
60+ years	11,422	13,240	14,536	15,705	19.8	22.9	25.7	29.3
60–79 years	9,719	11,230	11,803	12,456	16.9	19.4	20.9	23.2
65+ years	8,136	9,894	11,016	11,982	14.1	17.1	19.5	22.3
80+ years	1,703	2,010	2,733	3,249	3.0	3.5	4.8	6.1

Table 3. Life expectancy in Russia over 1989–1993 (UNICEF[2])

	1989	1993	Variation
Men	64.2	59.0	–5.2 years
Women	74.5	72.7	–1.8 years

age of 80 more than 50% of subjects suffer from moderate to severe loss of dependency. In this age group, at least 700,000 persons need continuous care in Italy. These subjects will double over the next 20 years if no extraordinary advances occur for the treatment of some conditions, such as Alzheimer's disease. This problem is so pressing that a thorough reorganization of continuous care systems, which lie in precarious conditions in most Italian regions, should not be delayed. With no doubts, the future of the welfare status will mainly depend upon a successful resolution of the problems related to the care of dependent elderly. Second, the remarkable quote of older persons who are free of functional deficits deserves

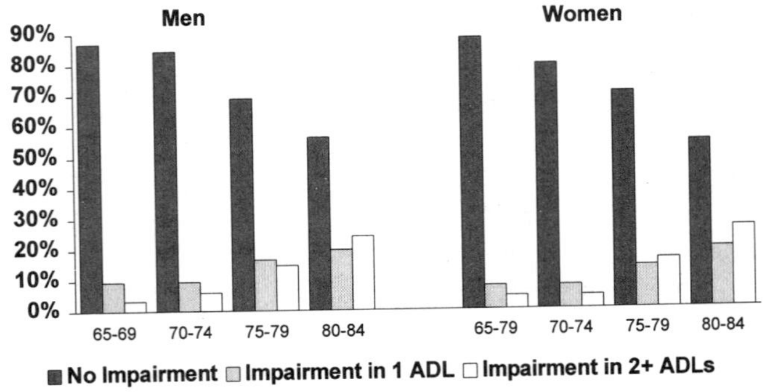

Figure 1. Prevalence of functional impairment (IADLs) according to age and gender in Italy, 1993–1995.[4]

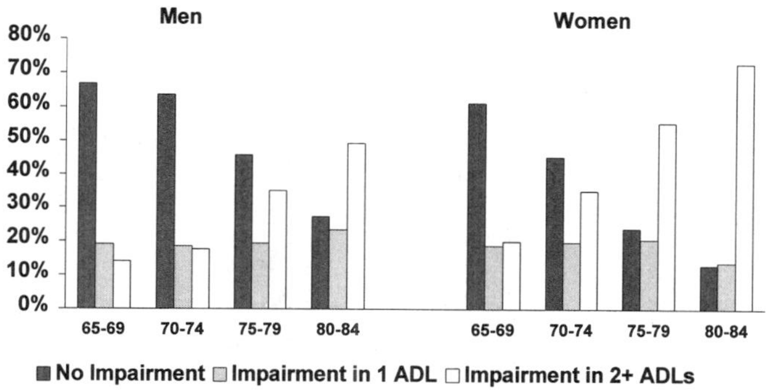

Figure 2. Prevalence of functional impairment (ADLs) according to age groups in Italy, 1993–1995.[4]

attention. The potential for an effective geriatric and gerontological prevention should allow the current 20% prevalence of "oldest olds" in good health conditions to significantly increase. A 10 to 20 percent increase would result in a 300,000–600,000-unit reduction of dependent elderly who need to be assisted. An effective gerontological and geriatric prevention must therefore be considered a major target for our society in the forthcoming years.

Pharmacoepidemiology is a field in which the Italian Geriatric Society has yielded excellent results. Such results have been obtained by the full cooperation (from 1987) of many of our fellows working in more than 50 hospital or university geriatric and medicine divisions all over the national territory. The Gruppo Italiano di Farmacoepidemiologia nell'Anziano (GIFA) has so far published many papers, often in excellent international journals, and has been acknowledged internationally, e.g. in the Merk Manual of Geriatrics.[5] The GIFA has anticipated the changes in hospital stays following the introduction of the DRG-ROD service funding system.[6] Implementation of the DRG-ROD has considerably reduced the length of hospital stays during 1995 (Figure 3), but with a simultaneous decrease of in-hospital mortality (Figure 4) and increased incidence of patients who were discharged in unstable conditions (Figure 5). Thus, the decrease in length of hospital stays may have been obtained at the expense of the quality of hospital care of terminally ill and dependent patients. Such results indicate that services in the territory must be potentiated in order to avoid both a fall in quality of care and an excess expenditure due to hospital readmissions (Figure 6). In a more general sense, hospital readmissions derive from a baseline issue: the outcome of the new health organization will depend upon the ability to yield a rational dis-

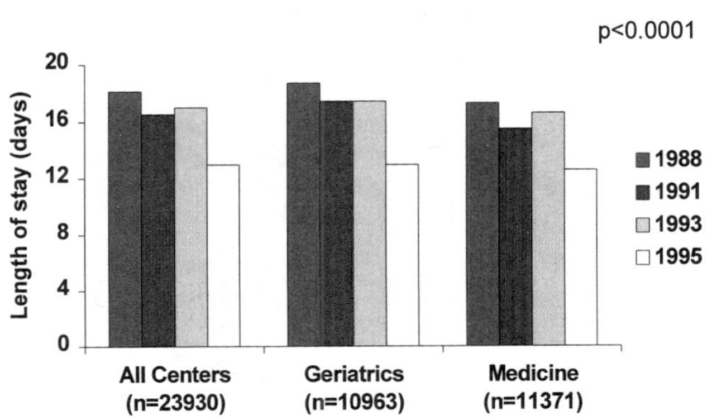

Figure 3. Variations in length of hospital stays in Italy from 1988 to 1995.[6]

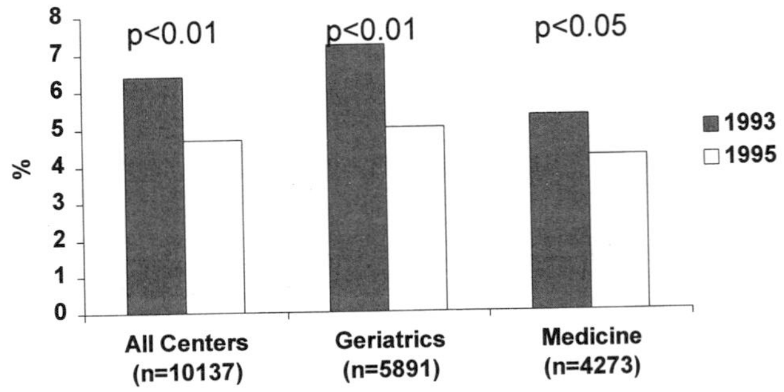

Figure 4. Comparison between mortality rates in Italian geriatric and general medicine divisions during the 1993 and 1995 GIFA surveys.[6]

tribution of available resources. In this setting, a good example is offered by another GIFA analysis on the days of unnecessary hospital stay (Figure 7), which account for 14% of all hospitalization days in the participating divisions.[6] Should this result apply to the whole national territory, eradication of such 14% unwarranted stays would result in a 5.000–7.000 billion I£ saving, which is nearly enough to implement an efficient integrated home care service in most regions. In fact, optimizing health expenses implies eradication of any resources wasting. As the current budgets probably will not increase, effective answers to

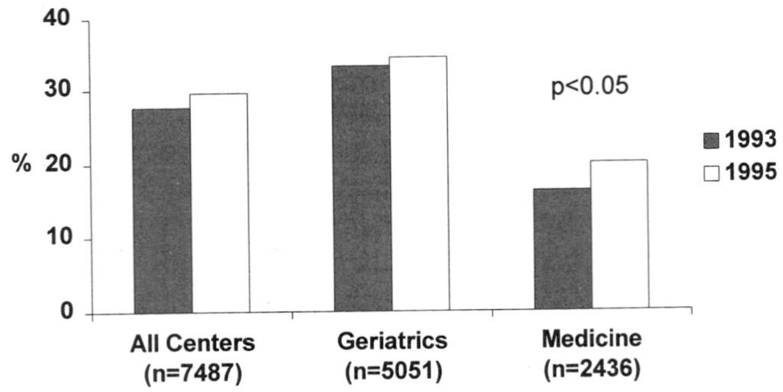

Figure 5. Comparison of prevalences in 1+ ADLs at discharge from Italian general medicine and geriatric divisions during the 1993 and 1995 GIFA surveys.[6]

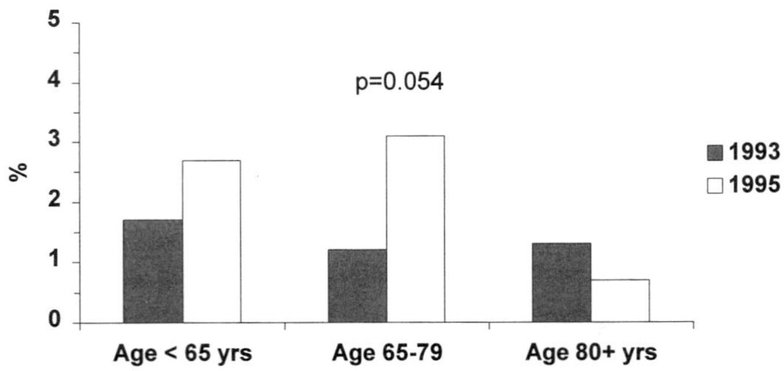

Figure 6. Comparison between readmission rates according to age segments during the 1993 and 1995 GIFA surveys.[6]

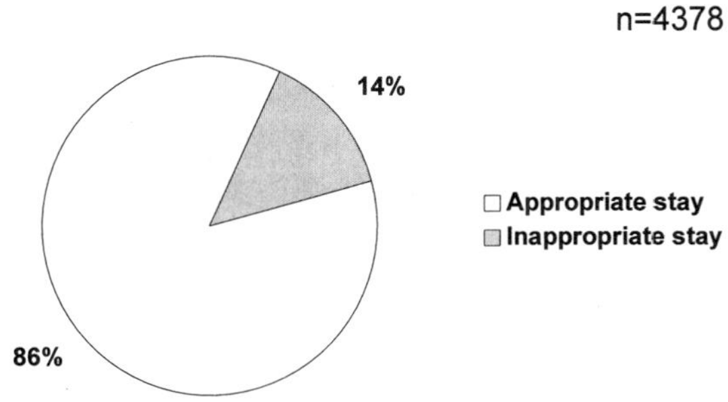

Figure 7. Rate of unnecessary hospital stays during the 1995 GIFA survey.

the issue of elderly care services may only derive from a strict cooperation of all members of the health system (including managers and operators) in transferring the resources from one compartment to another, according to validated criteria of efficacy and efficiency.

The validity of such a strategy, and the need for a political resolution, are supported by two interesting trials—implemented by our Geriatric Society—which evaluated new assistance models. Both these trials—coordinated by Professor Abate and Professor Bernabei, respectively—concerned the application of a multidimensional evaluation tool and the involvement of nonmedical health operators (such as nurses and social workers) as "case managers". Both trials proved that the simple application of this new assistance model improves some indices of quality of life, such as disability and mood, and significantly reduces hospitalization and institutionalization rates. This was obtained without additional costs, simply by education and optimal utilization of the existing personnel. One of these trials allowed an annual saving of over 3 million I£ per treated elderly (Table 4). The recent agreement with the Italian Society of General Medicine (SIMG) will allow to extend such trials to the whole national territory. Any attempt to implement continuous health care systems for older persons will depend upon full cooperation between GPs and geriatricians. The agreement protocol between SIMG and the Italian Geriatric Society represents a cornerstone for the forthcoming teamwork of General Medicine and Geriatrics. We can assume that the full realization of a model of integrated continuous care for the whole territory is at present more concrete. The adoption of the same multidimensional evaluation tool, which is another target of this agreement protocol, will allow comparison of the results from different regions, based on homogeneous data.

Another important issue in this protocol is the consensus on the definition of guidelines for care of older persons. Thus, GPs and geriatricians may implement a teamwork which will be essential to both home care and sheltered hospital discharge.

Table 4. One-year total expenditure (I£)

	Groups		
	Treatment (n=99)	Controls (n=100)	Difference
Hospital	447,000,000	688,000,000	–241,000,000
Nursing home	163,050,000	318,150,000	–155,100,000
Home care	166,600,000	215,096,000	–48,496,000
Home nursing	21,344,000	19,760,000	+1,584,000
Case manager	100,000,000	—	100,000,000
Total	897,994,000	1,241,006,000	–343,012,000

In a more general view, Italian geriatric and gerontological research has reached excellent results. A recent analysis by De Ferrari and Mela on Italian biomedical research has shown that, in an European context, Italian research in geriatrics is among the leading medical specialties.[7] A personal analysis of Italian geriatric schools has evidenced a satisfying mean impact factor (Figure 8), with many publications in prominent journals such as the New England Journal of Medicine, Lancet, JAMA, British Medical Journal, Archives of Internal Medicine, Journal of American Geriatric Society, etc.

However, our present situation is not a bed of roses. Our Geriatric Society has commanded a prominent role on the international scene; noticeably, a fellow of ours, Dr. Pahor, is currently Editor for the International Affairs of the Journal of American Geriatric Society. Nevertheless, the entry of geriatrics among medical specialties of the National Health Service is far from being accomplished. The sound work of Abate and coworkers in the context of the Progetto Finalizzato Invecchiamento shows that the recommendations of the Progetto Obiettivo Salute dell'Anziano (POSA) have not yet been fulfilled.[8] In many Italian regions the Geriatric Evaluation Units have not yet been implemented, and those which have been realized differ substantially in their composition from one region to another, and even between different AUSLs. A geriatrician is present in only 50% of cases, and different multidimensional evaluation tools are used, hindering any comparisons of the results achieved.

The transformation of the Health System into a firm is among the main obstacles to the reorganization of geriatric services. This can be deduced from the example of Great Britain, where Tatcher's reform was applied many years before the Italian one. The integrated geriatric service system was implemented in Great Britain about fifty years ago; the geriatrician who was a hospital consultant, and he operated in a teamwork with GPs and non-medical workers. Tatcher's reform has disjoined such a teamwork: the geriatrician currently operates in the hospital only, and GPs have to "buy" his services for patients. However, the target of reducing the institutionalization rates by increasing the levels of home care has been missed, since there has only been a transfer from public to private services, yet the number of institutional beds was unchanged.[9] Furthermore, the phenomenon of so-called "bed-blockers" was increased, as well as the legal actions by patients' relatives for forced hospital discharges.[10]

These obstacles, however, must not discourage us. The way is certainly long and hard to walk, but we have a firm starting point: the international research—and now Italian research, too—have definitely proved that multidimensional evaluation with team

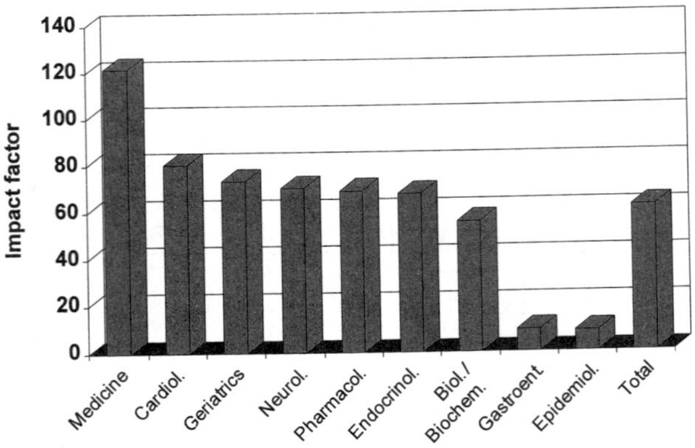

Figure 8. Mean impact factor of the main Italian specialties.

treatment represent the only way to improve the quality of continuous geriatric care and to optimize efficacy and efficiency rates. We must strongly believe in our pioneeristic task to build new medical strategies, and must keep on providing scientifically sound evidences that our proposed strategy is the only way to solve the complex care issues which derive from the aging of the population. This is the only process which may overcome the cultural and ethical gaps still underlying the lack of interest toward the instances of older subjects both at governmental and social levels. However, this situation is evolving.

More recently, the editorial production on aging has been enriched by many sound contributes. Among these, Spagnoli's book on Joung and Freud,[11] Scalfari's skilful interview to Gassman and Mastroianni in "La Repubblica",[12] and the enjoyable Sordi's lesson on gerontology held at the Catholic University[13] deserve mention. Yet, Bobbio's recent book,[14] and the related Riotta's comment in the "Corriere della Sera"[15] are the most impressive contributes. Bobbio declares he has nothing new to say, so that he prefers to keep silent: "I belong to the former Republic; thus, I will say nothing, as I belong to the past". Indeed, according to Riotta's interpretation, such an attitude does not represent a retirement into himself; rather, it is provocative: "this is the artistry of first detecting the novel paradigm, the boldness of leaving the old to bet on the new, this is the challenge of Bobbio's silence". According to the thought of philosopher of science Thomas Kuhn: "Science does not progress by steps. Einstein did not update Newton, after Newton updated Aristotle. Aristotle's physics is not a simpler Newton's physics, it is just another world". Thus, the new paradigm implies a cultural leap which is hardly accepted; therefore, the challenge of silence is sometimes necessary.

However, the "new" paradigm of geriatrics is not really so new; indeed, geriatrics has prompted a requirement of the holistic principles of medicine, not just on speculative bases, but rather proving the feasibility of clinical application of such principles on clinical bases, using multidimensional evaluation.[16] First, among medical specialties, geriatrics converted its final target from disease to functional ability.[16] Such a switch is hard to understand for those physicians who have so far privileged the advances in technology and experimental research.

The paradigm of geriatrics is the same of Virchow,[17] even though adjusted for the changes which have occurred in our society. Last century, Virchow said: "Medicine is a social science, and politics is nothing more than medicine in a larger extent". This is the same principle which underlies geriatric multidimensional evaluation. Geriatricians are on the right track; clinical medicine will have to recognize the validity of this view. Let me report the conclusions of a Task Force of the Rockefeller Foundation which were published in JAMA, 1989: "The educational response to the demographic realities of aging and long-term illness also is unbalanced. As mentioned previously herein, clinical education for the past half-century has focused on the care of patients in the acute-care hospital, the clinical paradigm being the search for cure to achieve full return of function. This model is appropriate for 35-year-old patients with acute pneumococcal pneumonia or acute appendicitis, but less so for 80-years-olds with chronic dementia or end-stage organ failure. By continuing to structure clinical education along the acute-care model, while neglecting the more difficult problems of how to preserve or improve function in the disabled, medical education has failed to respond to a societal need".[18]

I would like to conclude making a reference to the ethical principle of human value, which is unchanging from birth to death. This principle represents to the geriatrician the moral basis and stimulus to overcome all the restraints to his profession.

Also, I would like to remind our thought-master, Professor Antonini. He enclosed in his enjoyable book entitled "The age of masterpieces"[19] a fascinating self-portrait made by

Goya during the last stage of his life. Goya's crude representation of the devastating impact of time and diseases on his own body was inclement. Yet, the attention is attracted by the vivid glance of that bent, unsteady old man staying up by two sticks. The flash in his eyes and the inscription on the top of the portrait "aun aprendo" ("I'm still learning") testify the freeing of his mind and spirit from the restraints of his body. There is always something relevant left to say, so that life is worth being lived even in old age. In those days, a few months before dying, Goya depicted the milkwoman from Bordeaux who is a hymn to youth, "to colors and beauty: the light droops on her hair and shoulders, breaking the tones and reverberating an harmony of blue and green colors; Renoir was not born yet, but the impressionism has already a Master".[19]

These are our patients. Even a little gain for them will represent a great conquest to us. Firm in this belief, geriatricians will never be arrested in their task.

REFERENCES

1. Lori A, Golini A, Cantalini B. Atlante dell'invecchiamento della popolazione. CNR, Progetto Finalizzato Invecchiamento, Roma, 1995.
2. UNICEF: Crisis of mortality, health and nutrition. 1995.
3. Worrall A, Rea JN, Ben-Shlomo Y. Counting the cost of social disadvantage in primary care: retrospective analysis of patient data. Br Med J 314: 38, 1997.
4. Maggi S, Minicucci N, Grigoletto F, Amaducci L. I livelli di disabilità e relativi indicatori dei costi. CNR, Progetto Finalizzato Invecchiamento: I costi sociali dell'invecchiamento della popolazione italiana, Roma, 191, 1995.
5. The Merck Manual of Geriatrics, 2nd Edition, 265, 1995.
6. GIFA: Caratteristiche dell'ospedalizzazione dei pazienti anziani prima e dopo l'avvio del pagamento a prestazione (sistema DRG-ROD). Ann Ital Med Int 11: 220, 1996.
7. De Ferrari G, Mela GS. La ricerca biomedica nello scenario europeo. Università e Ricerca 7: 13, 1996.
8. Abate G, Bavazzano A, Di Iorio A. Assistenza Domiciliare Integrata. Indagine conoscitiva sulla situazione nazionale. CNR, Progetto Finalizzato Invecchiamento Roma, 1995.
9. Impallomeni M, Starr J. The changing face of community and institutional care for the elderly. J Publ Health 17: 171, 1995.
10. BGS News Letter, July 1996.
11. Spagnoli A. E divento sempre più vecchio: Jung, Freud, la psicologia del profondo e l'invecchiamento. Bollati Boringhieri 1995.
12. Scalfari E. D'amori e teatro per non parlar di vecchiaia. La Repubblica, 8 luglio 1996.
13. Sordi A. Gerontologo con qualche scongiuro. La Repubblica, Spettacoli, Roma 5 maggio 1996.
14. Bobbio N. De senectute. Einaudi, 1996.
15. Riotta G. Il Corriere della Sera, 20 ottobre 1996.
16. Feinstein AR. Clinical judgment revisited: the distraction of quantitative models. Ann Int Med 120: 799, 1994.
17. Virchow R. Die mediszinische Reform. Eine Wochenschrift. Berlin, Duch und verlag von G. Reiner, 1848.
18. Schroeder SA, Zones JS, Showstack JA. Il ruolo della medicina universitaria oggi. JAMA 2: 23, 1990.
19. Antonini F, magnolfi S. L'età dei capolavori. FIDIA ed, 217: 88, 1991.

2

BODY COMPOSITION IN THE ELDERLY

Giuliano Enzi, Mauro Bussolotto, Anna Ceccon, Paolo Beninca̓,
Alessandra Coin, and Giuseppe Sergi

Department of Internal Medicine
University of Padova

1. INTRODUCTION

Accurate evaluation of body composition is of primary importance in studying the nutritional condition of elderly people where the perturbation of body compartments is closely related to morbidity and mortality.

Aging is associated with changes in body composition. The decrease of fat free mass (1,2) related to the reduction of cell mass and the changes in extracellular to intracellular water ratio (3–7) are associated to the decline of cell function and to the perturbation of energy balance. The reduction of bone mineral content is also associated to high risk of fractures.

The nutritional assessment is traditionally based upon the antropometrical parameters (weight, weight variability, body mass index, body circunferences). In elderly, the problematical record and interpretation of several antropometrical data have led to application of new techniques in body composition analysis.

The availability of accurate methods for quantification of body compartments—as well as the dual energy X-ray absorptiometry (DEXA) and bioelectrical analysis (BIA)—permit to introduce the body composition parameters (fat-free mass, fat mass and total body water) in the nutritional assessment.

2. ANTHROPOMETRY

The collection of anthropometric measurements in the elderly presents special problems, because many elderly persons frequently have difficulty standing or maintaining an erect posture; in many elderly individuals the stature cannot be measured accurately because of the increased prevalence of spinal curvature, which is reported to be as high as 30%.

The measurement of body weight is generally possible, but it may require special equipment such as portable bed or wheelchair scales (8).

The body mass index (BMI) is a common index of body composition that is highly correlated with levels of fatness, and with morbidity and mortality (9). However, BMI

Recent Advances in Geriatrics, edited by Barbagallo, Licata, and Sowers.
Plenum Press, New York, 1998.

may not be as informative in the elderly as it is at younger ages. First of all, there is little information about the relationship between BMI and body composition parameters in elderly, especially at very old ages. Moreover, with age occur significant loss of stature and changes of body composition (decrease of fat-free mass and increase of fat mass with troncular redistribution) that led to only slightly variation of body mass index.

The epidemiological observation about the surviving in elderly indicate that the prognostic significance of BMI is quite different from adult, since the overweight did not reduce life expectancy and the modest higher weight seemed to be protective against death (10).

Among the anthropometric parameters, involuntary weight loss is the single best predictor for risk of malnutrition and death; a weight loss greater than 10% over a time interval of less than six months is considered clinically significant.

In the elderly the collection of skinfold thickness and their clinical applications present special problems because of the change in body composition distribution. The changes in the elasticity, hydration and compressibility of subcutaneous adipose tissue can alter the relationship between the skinfold thickness and body fatness. With age, adipose tissue thicknesses decrease on the arm and the leg, but the thicknesses of subcutaneous and internal adipose tissue are reported to increase on the trunk. Therefore, skinfold thicknesses and circumference measurements from the limbs decrease, but abdominal circumference increases (8).

In elderly subjects, however, other body measurements such as circumferences of the trunk may provide more important information regarding stores of body fat than the skinfolds, since the correlations of skinfold thicknesses with total body fat and percent body fat are reported to be less in older than in younger adults (11).

The midarm circumference (MAC) measured at midpoint of the right upper arm combined with the triceps skinfold permits to estimate the midarm muscle area (MAMA) that is the most commonly clinical indicator of lean tissue or muscle in the body.

The most important anthropometric measures for the nutritional status are available in NHANES III for United States population and Euronut Seneca studies (12). Anthropometric values less than the 5th percentile or less than twice standard deviation from the mean are suggestive of a seriously impaired nutritional state.

3. BODY COMPOSITION

3.1. Principles of the Body Composition

The entire body may be distinguished into separate homogeneous fractions based upon different chemical and/or physical characteristics, and depending on the method used for body composition study. Therefore, it is possible to consider the whole body according to four different levels: atomic, molecular, cellular and tissue-system (13) (Figure 1).

The methods for body composition analysis can be ordered in a hierarchical scale according to the degree of invasiveness and accuracy as shown in Figure 2 (14). The highest level of accuracy and invasiveness is represented by the physico-chemical analysis of body tissues obtained from cadaver dissection. From these studies are derived weights, proportions, densities and chemistry of elemental body constituents.

At level 2 there are the techniques of *in vivo* quantification of specific chemical or anatomical structures, as well as neutron activation analysis (NAA), magnetic resonance imaging (MRI) and dual X ray absorptiometry (DEXA). These techniques are relatively new and require expensive and sophisticated instrumentation, and the results obtained

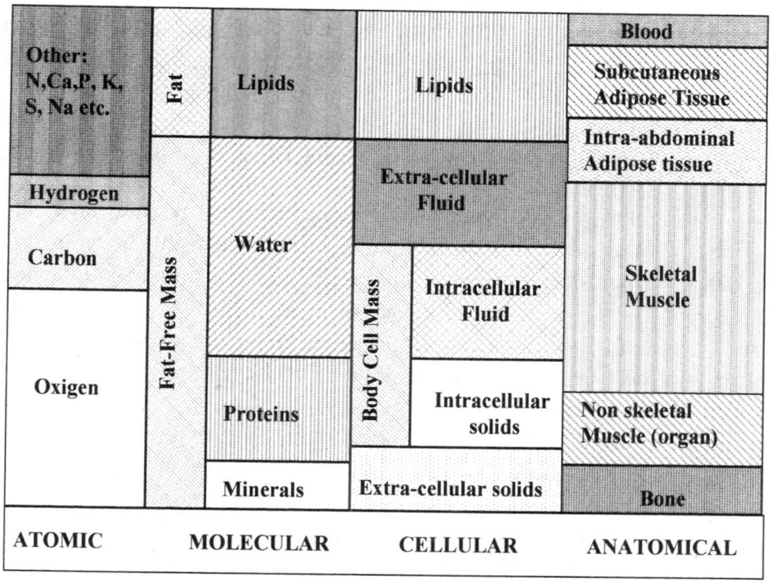

Figure 1. Body composition models.

must be validated against data from level 1. The methods at level 3 estimate two or more components of body composition using models that require assumptions regarding densities, proportions, or ratios of the various measured constituents. Most methods for body composition analysis are based upon the model in which the body consists of two chemically distinct compartments, fat mass (FM) and fat-free mass (FFM). This model requires the assumption of certain constants in FFM composition. For example, the hydrodensitometric method assumes that FFM density is a constant of 1.10 gr/cc; the total body water method assumes a constant level of FFM hydration (73.2%); the K method assumes a potassium content in FFM of 2.5 gr/Kg in men and 2.3 gr/Kg in women. Level 4 includes methods (Bioelectrical Impedance Analysis, Anthropometry) that measure somatic or

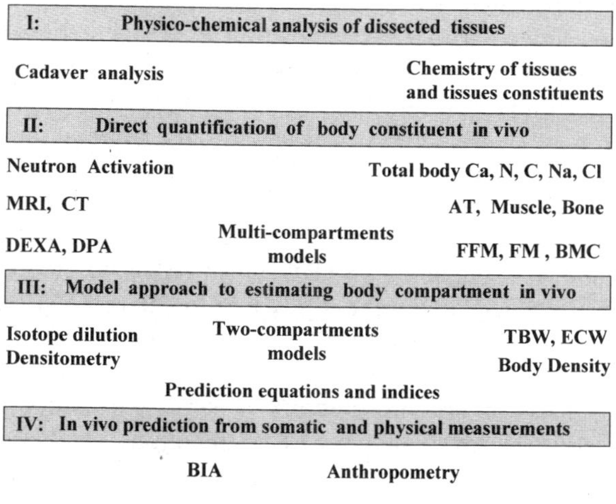

Figure 2. Methods of body composition.

physical properties of the body that are correlated to its principal components (total body water, FFM) and can be used to predict these compartments using equations validated in specific populations.

3.2. Body Composition Assessment in the Elderly

With advancing age the fat-free mass decreases (15,16) and the fat mass generally increases (17,18), with a redistribution of the adipose tissue from the limbs to the trunk. Also, the amount of minerals in the FFM changes (19), as does the ratio of extracellular to intracellular water (20–24). With age a decrease in total body water has been observed mainly due to decrease of intracellular water. Furthermore, the variability of the FFM hydration is larger in elderly with respect to adults an it may interfere with a two compartment model in body composition study.

Several methods are available for the assessment of body composition but it can be questioned whether some methods can be used in an older population. In clinical practice the methods that may be proposed for body assessment in elderly are the dual X-ray absorptiometry (DEXA) and the bioelectrical impedance analysis (BIA).

Dual-Energy X-ray Absorptiometry (DEXA) represents an important technological development for estimation of body composition. DEXA is based on a three-compartment model. By attenuation measurements at two discrete energy radiations (40 and 70 keV) of different tissues, it is possible to quantitate bone mineral content (BMC), and soft tissue mass (STM) which is composed of FM and lean soft tissue mass (LTM); FFM from DEXA is calculated as the sum of BMC and LTM. The advantages of DEXA include the low radiation dose (1.5 mR), rapidity of performance (6 minutes for scanning of total body) and the possibility of segmental measurements of body composition.

DEXA directly measures the three principal components of the body with an in vivo precision error (CV%) for fat-tissue mass, lean-tissue mass and total-body bone mineral of 6.6%, 2–3% and 1.5%, respectively (25,26). Furthermore, recent studies have demonstrated that DEXA is able to detect small individual changes in total mass and soft-tissue mass and it is also useful for detection of group changes in lean-tissue mass (27). The main problem with DEXA is the standardization of phantom for calibration; moreover, the accuracy of FFM detection either when FFM hydration is altered or in obesity has not yet been adequately verified.

Bioelectrical Impedance Analysis (BIA) is a non-invasive, rapid and repeatable method recently introduced in body composition assessment (28–30). This method is based on the behaviour of biological structures when they are subjected to a constant low-level alternating current (31,32). The body fluids behave as electrical conductors offering a resistance which is inversely correlated to the volume of water compartment. Because FFM contains virtually all the water and the conducting electrolytes in the body, conductivity is far greater in FFM than in FM; therefore, total body resistance is dependent on the proportion of FFM and FM. Using current flow at 50 kHz and 800 μA, several authors demonstrated that the best predictor of TBW and FFM were Height^2/Resistance. When TBW is obtained from BIA-equation, it is possible to derive FFM assuming FFM hydration relatively constant (FFM = TBW/0.732); then FM is calculated as the difference between total body weight and FFM (33).

Nevertheless, FFM hydration presents a large variability in healthy subjects (69–82%) (34) which increases with age (63.6–80.4%) (35), in obese subjects (36) and in patients with several water and metabolic disorders. Therefore, BIA is an accurate method in TBW estimation with a standard error of 1–4%, but it can underestimate or overestimate the FFM in fluids dehydration and retention states, respectively.

Furthermore, the introduction of the multi-frequency bioelectrical instruments permit the estimation of body fluid compartments and their changes frequently observed in clinical management of elderly patients. This application is based upon the principle that using low and high frequencies is possible to estimate extracellular (ECW) and total body water (TBW), respectively (37–39).

The BIA method has been used successfully in adults (40–42), however the validity of this method in body composition study in elderly population is not sufficiently investigated. In particular the prediction equations proposed for the adults can not be applied in elderly without introduction of a significant error. Our unpublished data demonstrate for the principal BIA equations a wide variability in accuracy of fat free mass estimation.

In conclusion, in elderly, the anthropometry cannot adequately estimate the nutritional status and the measure of fat mass and fat-free mass are recommended. Among the different methods, DEXA is the best method to evaluate FFM and FM, independently of FFM hydration; BIA estimates with accuracy body fluids (total body water and extracellular water); however, its accuracy to evaluate the fat free mass is dependent on hydration status.

REFERENCES

1. Forbes GB: The adult decline in lean body mass. Hum Biol 1976; 48:161–73.
2. Novice LP: Aging, total body potassium, fat free mass and cell mass in males and females between ages 18 and 85 years. J Gerontol 1972; 27:438–43.
3. Forbes GB: Human body composition. New York: Springer Verlag, 1988.
4. Friis-Hansen B: Hydrometry of growth and aging; in Brozek J (ed): Human body composition. Pergamon Press, Oxford 1965; pp 191–209.
5. Borkan GA, Norris AH: Fat redistribution and the changing body dimensions of the adult male. Hum Biol 1977; 49:495–514.
6. Steen B, Isaksson B, Svanborg A: Body composition at 70 and 75 years of age; a longitudinal population study. J Clin Exp Gerontol 1979; 1:185–200.
7. Steen B: Body composition and aging. Nutr Rev 1988; 46:40–46.
8. Chumlea WM, Guo SS, Vellas B, Guigoz Y: Techniques of assessing muscle mass and function (Sarcopenia) for epidemiological studies of the elderly. J Gerontol Series A 1995, 50 A (Special Issues): 45–51.
9. Van Itallie T. Health implications of overweight and obesity in the United States. Ann Intern Med 1985; 103:983–988.
10. Mattila K, Haavisto M, Rajala S: Body mass index and mortality in the elderly. Brit Med J 1988; 292:867–868.
11. Chumlea WM, Roche AF, Mukherjee D: Some anthropometrics indices of body composition for elderly adults. J Gerontol 1986; 41:36–39.
12. De Groot CPGM, Sette S, Zajkàs G, Carbajal A, Amorim Cruz JA: Euronut-Seneca study; Nutritional status: anthropometry. Eur J Clin Nutr 1991; 45(suppl 3): 31–42.
13. Wang ZM, Pierson RN Jr, Heymsfield SB: The five level model: a new approach to organizing body-composition research. Am J Clin Nutr 1992; 56: 19–28.
14. Heymsfield SB, Wang J, Lichtman S, Kamen Y, Kehayas J, Pierson RN: Body composition in elderly subjects: a critical appraisal of clinical methodology. Am J Clin Nutr 1989; 5:1167–1175.
15. Forbes GB: The adult decline in lean body mass. Hum Biol 1976; 48:161–73.
16. Novak LP: Aging, total body potassium, fat free mass and cell mass in males and females between ages 18 and 85 years. J Gerontol 1972;27:438–43.
17. Noppa H, Andersson M, Bengtsson C, Bruce A, Isaksson B: Body composition in middle-aged women with special reference to the correlation between body fat mass and anthropometric data. Am J Clin Nutr 1979; 32:1388–95.
18. Durnin JVGA, Womersley J: Body fat assessed from total body density and its estimation from skinfold thickness: measurements on 481 men and women aged from 16 to 72 years. Br J Nutr 1974; 32:77–97.
19. Mazess RB: On aging bone loss. Clin Orthop Res 1982; 165:239–52.
20. Forbes GB: Human body composition. New York: Springer Verlag, 1988.
21. Friis-Hansen B: Hydrometry of growth and aging; in Brozek J (ed): Human body composition. Pergamon Press, Oxford 1965; pp 191–209.

22. Borkan GA, Norris AH: Fat redistribution and the changing body dimensions of the adult male. Hum Biol 1977; 49:495–514.
23. Steen B, Isaksson B, Svanborg A: Body composition at 70 and 75 years of age; a longitudinal population study. J Clin Exp Gerontol 1979; 1:185–200.
24. Steen B: Body composition and aging. Nutr Rev 1988; 46:40–46.
25. Mazess RB, Barden HS, Bidek JP, Hanson J: Dual energy x-ray absorptiometry for total-body and regional bone-mineral and soft-tissue composition. Am J Clin Nutr 1990; 51:1106–1112.
26. Haarbo J, Gotfredsen A, Hassager C, Christiansen C: Validation of body composition measurement by dual energy x-ray absorptiomety (DEXA). Clin Physiol 1991; 11: 331–341.
27. Going SB, Massett MP, Hall CM, Bare LA, Root PA, Williams DP, Lohman TG: Detection of small changes in body composition by dual-energy x-ray absorptiometry. Am J Clin Nutr 1993, 57:845–850.
28. Lukaski HC, Jhonson PE, Bolonchuk WW: Assessment of fat free mass using bioelectrical impedance measurements of the human body. Am J Clin Nutr1985; 41: 810–817.
29. Kushner RF, Schoeller MD: Estimation of total body water by bioelectrical impedance analysis. Am J Clin Nutr 1986; 44: 417–424.
30. Segal KR, Van Load M, Fitzgerald P: Lean body mass estimation by bioelectrical impedance analysis: a four site cross validation study. Am J Clin Nutr 1988; 47:7–14.
31. Thomasett A: Bio-electrical properties of tissue impedance measurements. Lyon Med 1962; 207: 107–118.
32. Thomassett A: Bio-electrical properties of tissues. Lyon Med. 1963; 209:1325–1352.
33. Kushner RF, Schoeller, DA, Fjeld CR: Is the impedance index (Ht/R) significant in predicting total body water? Am J Clin Nutr 1992; 56: 835–839.
34. Sheng HP, Huggins RA: A review of body composition studies with emphasis on total body water and fat. Am J Clin Nutr 1979; 32:630–647.
35. Sergi G, Perini P, Bussolotto M, Zurlo F, Malvasi L, Carraro R, Del Prato S, Giantin V, Enzi G: Body composition study in the elderly: comparison between tritium diluition method and dual photon absorptiometry. J Gerontol 1993; 48:M244–248.
36. Deuremberg P, Leenen R, Van der Kooy K, Hautvast JGAJ: In obese subjects the body fat percentage calculated with Siri's formula is an overestimation. Eur J Clin Nutr 1989; 43:569–575.
37. Deurenberg P, Schouten FJM: Loss of total body water and extracellular water assessed by multifrequency impedance. Eur J Clin Nutr 1992; 46:247–255.
38. Van Loan MD, Mayclin PL: Use of multi-frequency bioelectrical impedance analysis for the estimation of extracellular fluid. Eur J Clin Nutr 1992; 46: 117–124.
39. Segal KR, Burastero S, Chun A, Coronel P, Pierson RN,Wang J: Estimation of extracellular and total body water by multiple-frequency bioelectrical impedance measurements. Am J Clin Nutr 1991; 54: 26–29.
40. Lukasky HC, Bolonchuk WW, Hall CB, Siders WA: Validation of tetrapolar bio-electrical impedance method to assess human body composition. J Appl Physiol 1986; 60:1327–1332.
41. Segal KR, Gutin B, Presta E, Wang J, van Itallie TB: Estimation of human body composition by electrical impedance methods: a comparative study. J Appl Physiol 1985; 58:1565–71.
42. Segal KR, van Loan M, Fitzgerald PI, Hodgdon JA, van Itallie TB: Lean body mass estimation by bioelectrical impedance analysis: a four-side cross-validation study. Am J Clin Nutr 1985; 42:889–90 (editorial).

3

NEUROENDOCRINE SYSTEM AND AGING PROCESSES

G. Valenti

Department of Geriatrics
University of Parma
Italy

SUMMARY

Aging phenomena must be seen as a function more of the breakdown of the integrative mechanisms (endocrine and immune systems) than of the impairment in the individual cells. Focusing on endocrine age-related modifications, some of them appear to be adaptive mechanisms which should be preserved more than antagonized. Typical examples are represented by the decline of hypothalamus pituitary thyroid axis seen as an intelligent response to the new metabolic requests of the whole body, by the decrease of estrogens and testosterone as a prevention mechanism against endometrium and prostate cancers and finally by the downward adjustment of GH secretion as a protection against diabetes, osteoarthritis and hypertension.

Conversely most age-related endocrine changes seem to play an important role in the pathogenesis of aging phenomena. Muscle and bone tissue catabolism, psychosexual function decline, cognitive and mood performance deterioration are the most significant consequences of the estrogens and androgen deprivation in both sexes. As for the adrenal hormone secretion, DHEAS age-related decrease might accelerate atherosclerotic processes, decrease immunocompetence and exert catabolic effects at muscle and skeleton levels. The catabolic age-related processes seem to be connected also with the decreased GH pituitary secretion.

So far too many unanswered questions on this topic still remain opposing the proposal of hormone replacement strategy in order to antagonize aging processes.

INTRODUCTION

In contrast with unicellular organisms, animals and humans possess different levels of organization. Obviously one level is intracellular and is under the genomic control of each cell. A second level is represented by intercellular connections which can be realized on the one hand through cell to cell communications mechanisms at tissue level and on the

Recent Advances in Geriatrics, edited by Barbagallo, Licata, and Sowers.
Plenum Press, New York, 1998.

other through the activation of the integrative systemic mechanisms like endocrine and immune systems with the mediation of extracellular milieu (1).

Previous views tended to reduce the aging problem to only one level of organization namely the cell,ignoring the other levels,namely the homeostatic and integrative mechanisms of the body. In each cell the genome contains a program for aging as it has been demonstrated by the elegant in vitro experiments on human fibroblasts (2). Environmental agents, both external and internal, can interact directly with cellular genetic apparatus during the whole life period, being nutrition disorders, stress, temperature abnormalities, ionizing radiation, toxins, oxidative agents the most frequent components involved (3). More recently increasing attention has been devoted to the hypothesis which sees aging more a function of the breakdown of integrative mechanisms (endocrine and immune systems) than of the impairment in the individual cells (4) (Fig. 1).

In my opinion both these approaches are important and possibly may coexist in an unified view. The age-related modifications of the integrative mechanisms (second level) in fact can be seen as expression of a primary impairment (first level) of the critical "command" cells of the neuroendocrine and immune systems. Focusing the attention on the neuroendocrine system, the neurons of the cerebral cortex and of the hypothalamus seem to be the "command" cells primarily involved. On this line aging processes can be seen at least partly as expression of the breakdown of the homeostatic functions exerted by neuroendocrine system. A separate parallel issue must be considered that of immune system but here we cannot forget the tigth correlations between the two components. The neuroendocrine system has a powerful influence on immune functions. There is compelling evidence that thymus involution shortly after puberty is triggered by hormone secretions; adrenal and go-

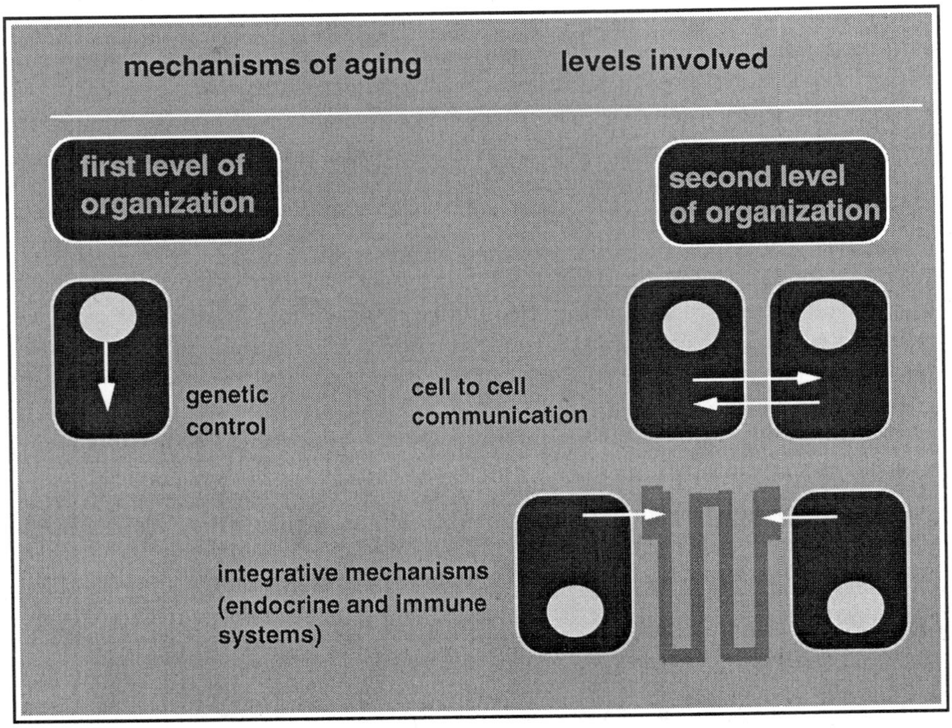

Figure 1. Schematic representation of the two different levels of organization: intracellular (genomic control) and intercellular (integrative systemic mechanisms) levels.

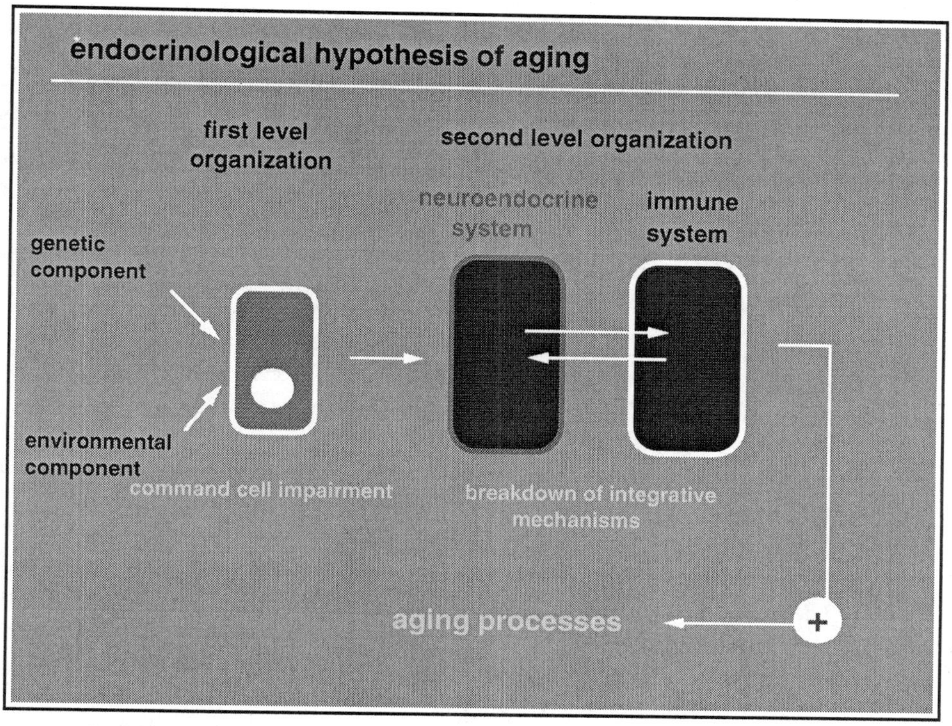

Figure 2. The scheme tries to represent in unified view the contemporary involvement of the two levels of organization in the activation of aging phenomena.

nadal steroids have a marked inhibitory effect on this gland (5). Furthermore in animals a significant correlation between the age dependent decline of endocrine secretions and thymus function has been demonstrated; consequently treatment of old mice with T4, hypothalamic extract or bovine GH seems to be able to restore the depressed circulating levels of thymic peptides (6,7). Reciprocally thymus produces general immunoregulatory substances active on endocrine circuits. TF5 (Thymosin fraction 5) and HTH (Homeostatic thymus hormone) are able to modulate TSH,GH and corticosterone secretion in animals: the response in old animals is much weaker suggesting that aging brings about a progressive desensitization of the neuroendocrine system to thymic signals (8–10) (Fig. 2).

RESULTS

In the present report the age-related modifications of neuroendocrine system have been extensively analysed with the purpose to focus their specific role in the development of aging phenomena. The age-related modifications of the neuroendocrine system develop in two different directions.

1. Some of them appear to be an intelligent response to the new metabolic requests of the whole body and therefore as adaptive mechanisms should be preserved more than antagonized.

   a. This is the case of hypothalamic-pituitary-thyroid axis which undergoes the following abnormalities:

i. reduction of TSH secretion that might be the consequence of a "supersensitivity" of the thyrotrophs to the negative feedback exerted by T4, even if other explanations such as reduced hypothalamic TRH secretion cannot be excluded;
ii. reduction of the secretion rate of T4 from the gland and of the degradation of T4 to T3 which shows in its plasma concentration a clear age dependent decline;
iii. increase in TBG concentration associated with a decrease of free fraction of thyroid hormones, even with conflicting results in experimental literature.

At the moment it is still an open question if these hormone changes are related to "normal" aging per se or to the coexistence of age-associated non thyroidal illnesses. Studies on healthy elderly subjects, selected by strict criteria, suggest that most thyroid function changes are tightly age-related and therefore might be seen as an adaptive mechanism to the new metabolic condition (11).

b. As for the well known drop in estrogen secretion at menopausal time we might suppose that also this endocrine change can be seen adaptive in some way as a sort of prevention mechanism against endometrial cancer. At the basis of this assumption we underline the results of a study performed with meta-analytic statistical methods concerning 35 epidemiologic studies which demonstrate the evidence that the long term supplementation of estrogen therapy increases risk for endometrial cancer. The same assumption cannot be repeated for breast cancer; in fact several meta-analyses concerning up to 39 epidemiological studies suggest that overall there is no increased risk of breast cancer in women who are taking estrogens (12).
c. Likewise the decline in testosterone secretion in men might be seen adaptive as prevention mechanism against atherosclerosis and prostatic cancer in elderly people. The negative effect of testosterone on lipoprotein metabolism has been suggested even if many observation studies concerning the effect of this steroid on HDL and LDL metabolism are controversial. Only some intervention studies are impressive showing that testosterone treatment is able to decrease HDL and apoproteins A-I and A-II concentrations and to increase LDL levels; opposite effect seems to be realized by chemical castration (13,14). Furthermore we cannot forget that many years ago the testosterone dependency of prostate cancer and the amelioration of prostate cancer by lowering the testosterone concentration by castration were demonstrated. Consequently the decline in testosterone secretion might be protective against the development of prostate cancer (15). Nevertheless there are no data able to show whether androgen can enhance the progression of preclinical to clinical cancer, while it is known that androgens will stimulate the growth of clinically diagnosed prostate cancers. As for benign prostate hypertrophy (BPH) recent studies have shown that decreasing the production of testosterone and of dehydrotestosterone in men with BPH, decreases prostate size and improves urine flow (16). Consequently the age-related decrease in testosterone production might be protective; nevertheless despite the theoretical considerations there is no evidence that the replacement of androgens in hypogonadal men will lead to the development of BPH or to aggravate the clinical status of BPH (17).

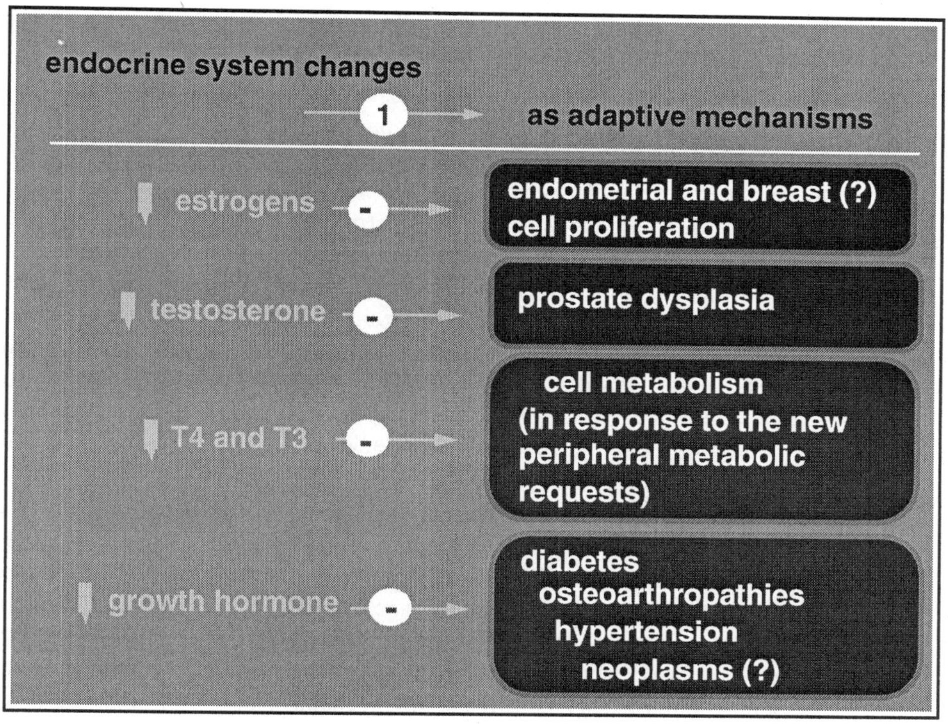

Figure 3. Summary of the age-related endocrine changes able to activate the protection mechanisms against the development of aging phenomena.

d. Finally we cannot leave out to theorize about the possible beneficial effects of the well documented downward adjustment of GH secretion in elderly. Chronic excess of GH in adult tends to cause diabetes, osteoarthritis, hypertension and possibly neoplasms. Therefore the diminishing activity of the somatotropic axis might reduce the risk of these medical hazards of old age (18) (Fig. 3).

2. Most age-related endocrine changes on the contrary seem to play an important role in the development of aging phenomena.

a. The declined secretion of estrogens means deprivation of all their antiaging properties. The first of them is represented by the antiatherogenic effect realized both through the positive interference on lipoprotein metabolism and through the direct effect on the vessel wall where specific estrogen receptors are diffusely present. At this level they suppress intimal proliferation,inhibit platelet aggregation,enhance endotelial degradation of LDL cholesterol and induce a vasodilating effect (19–21). Another antiaging property is represented by the anabolic effect on the skeleton realized through the activation of calcitonin secretion,the inhibition of osteoclasts and of local factors (interleukins 1 and 2, TNF and Prostaglandins) (22,23). Finally a significant interference on the central nervous system signified by positive interference on mood and cognitive performances has been extensively demonstrated. The effect might be realized both through a non genomic activational mechanism (modulation of noradrenergic,cholinergic and GABAergic systems) and through the activation of genetic apparatus and consequently of biosynthetic processes of the neuronal cells (24–27).

b. Also in men the gradual decline of testosterone secretion might signify a progressive deprivation of its antiaging properties. The first of them can be identified in its anabolic effect on muscle and skeleton systems. The effect seems to be realized through the activation of protein synthesis directly at cellular level or through the mediation of GH-IGF1 system (28,29). A second antiaging property consists in the capacity to positively affect psychosexual function and cognitive performances. The effect of testosterone on central nervous system seems to be realized through its previous aromatization to estrogens and consequently through the modulation of multiple neurotransmitter systems (30). Finally another antiaging property of testosterone might be identified in its capability to activate erythropoietic processes through a direct effect on bone marrow stem cells or through the activation of erythropoietin production by the kidney (13).
c. Another important age-related endocrine finding is represented by a primary derangement of steroidogenesis at adrenal level. The consequent decline in DHEAS synthesis,evident in males but even more in females, has led to investigation of the intriguing possibility that DHEAS feature might be related to the development of age associated diseases and consequently to the hypothesis of its antiaging properties. A first antiaging property might consist in its alleged antiatherogenic effect. The mechanism of action might be that of positively interfering on lipoprotein metabolism (decrease of LDL plasma concentration) (31–34), but more recently several experimental findings support the hypothesis that the effect might be realized through different mechanisms: DHEAS in fact has been proved to inhibit myocyte proliferation, platelet and macrophages adherence, free radical generation and to enhance fibrinolytic and lipolytic processes. There are also several findings corroborating the hypothesis for DHEAS to be protective against age-related impairment of central nervous system. The mechanism of action at this level might be that of a neuromodulation pointed mainly on GABAergic and serotoninergic systems; the activation of local IGF1 production able to promote a trophic and modulator neuronal effect cannot be ruled out (35,36). Another antiaging effect seems to be represented by the capability to antagonize the age-related decline of immune system through the activation of both humoral and cell mediated immunocompetence (37,38). Finally DHEAS has been demonstrated able to antagonize the age-related catabolic processes. The alleged anabolic effect might be realized directly on specific peripheral receptors or through the previous biotransformation of DHEAS to estrogens (in men and in postmenopausal women) and to androgen (in premenopausal women); the activation of the potent metabolic growth factor IGF1 cannot be excluded (32,39). The parallel age-related increase of cortisol secretion might make the metabolic condition worse.
d. GH and IGF1 is another hormonal secretion which declines with aging; many clinical phenomena globally called with the term of somatopause are at least partly related to such hormonal deficit. In fact, a first antiaging effect of GH-IGF1 system is that of protecting from the deterioration of body composition equilibrium: the increase in lean body mass and of the bone mineral density and the decrease of fat mass appear to be the most impressive biological ef-

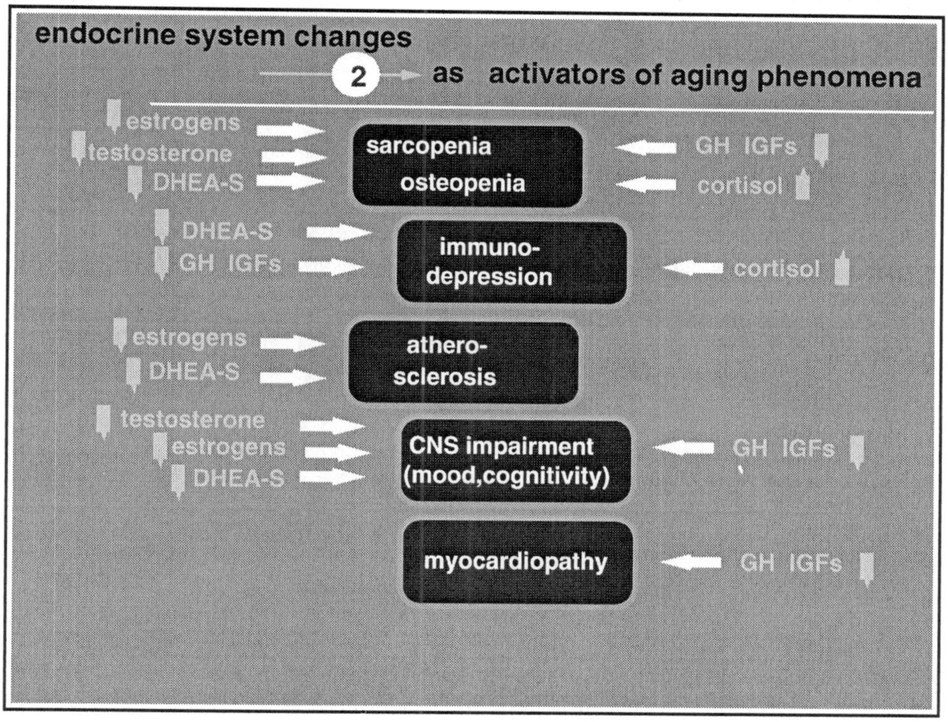

Figure 4. Summary of age-related endocrine changes able to promote the activation of aging processes at multiple levels.

fect of GH (40–42). A second antiaging effect of GH-IGF1 comes out from the capacity to positively affect brain function namely REM sleep, sense of well being, mental alertness and endurance (43–45). Lastly an important antiaging effect might be identified in the prevention of cardiovascular diseases both modulating lipoprotein profile and antagonizing heart failure in dilated cardiomyopathy (46,47) (Fig. 4).

These age-related changes of endocrine secretions totally taken can signify a decline of all their antiaging properties and consequently an acceleration of aging phenomena. From these premises the hypothesis of an hormone replacement strategy in order to antagonize aging processes comes out as an obvious consequence. Yet so far too many unanswered questions still remain. Which elderly people should be classified as being hormone deficient? What is the risk/benefit ratio for each hormone treatment, considering that the declining endocrine secretion is sometimes adaptive? These are some of the most impressive questions that the investigators interested in this area will try to answer in the very next future. This knowledge appears to be an indispensable premise for each kind of hypothetical hormonal supplementation strategy.

REFERENCES

1. Meites J, Goya R, Takahashi S: Why the neuroendocrine system is important in aging processes. Experimental Gerontology, 22, 1, 1987
2. Hayflick L: Theories of biological aging.Experimental Gerontology, 20, 145, 1985
3. Meites J: Neuroendocrine biomarkers of aging in the rat. Experimental Gerontology, 23, 349, 1988

4. Goya RG: The immune neuroendocrine homeostatic network and aging. Gerontology, 37, 208, 1991
5. Comsa J, Leonhardt H, Wekerle H: Hormonal coordination of the immune response. Rev Physiol Biochem Pharmacol 92; 115, 1982
6. Fabris N, Mocchegiani E: Endocrine control of thymic serum factor production in young adult and old mice. Cell Immunol 91; 325, 1985
7. Folch H, Eller G, Mena M: Neuroendocrine regulation of thymus hormones: hypothalamic dependence of facteur thymique serique level. Cell Immunol 102; 211, 1986
8. Hall Nr, McGillis PJP, Spangelo BL,: Evidence that thymosins and other biological response modifiers can function as neuroactive neurotrasmitters. J Immunol 135, 806s, 1985
9. Deschaux P, Binimbi M, Fontanges FR: Endocrine interaction of the thymus with the hypophysis, adrenals and testes: effects for two thymic extracts. Thymus 1, 95, 1979
10. Goya RG, Sosa YE, Quigley KL,: Homeostatic thymus hormone stimulates corticosterone secretion in a dose and age dependent manner in rats. Neuroendocrinology 51, 59, 1990
11. Mariotti S, Franceschi C, Cossarizza A, Pinchera A: The aging thyroid. E ndocrine Reviews; 16, 686, 1995
12. Grady D, Rubin SM, Petitti DB, Fox CS, Black D, Ettinger B, Ernster VL and Cummings SR: Hormone therapy to prevent disease and prolong life in postmenopausal women. Ann Intern Med 117, 1016, 1992
13. Swerdloff RS and Wang C: Androgens and aging in men. Exp Gerontol 28, 435, 1993
14. Denti L, Pasolini G, Cortellini P, Ferretti S, Sanfelici L, Ablondi F and Valenti G: Effects of androgen suppression by gonadotropin-realising hormone agonist and flutamide on lipid metabolism in men with prostate cancer: focus on lipoprotein (a). Clinical Chemistry 42,8,1176,1996
15. Schroder FH: Androgens and carcinoma of the prostate. In: Testosterone: action, deficiency, substitution. Nieschlang E and Behre HM (Editors) Springer Verlag, Berlin, Germany, 245, 1990
16. Mc Connell JD: Androgen ablation and blockade in the treatment of begnin prostatic hyperplasia. Urol Clin North Am 17, 661, 1990
17. Bardin CW, Swerdloff RS and Santen RJ: Androgens: risks and benefits. J Clin Endocrinol Metab 73, 4, 1991
18. Rudman D, Shetty KR: Unanswered questions conerning the treatment of hyposomatotropism and hypogonadism in elderly men. JAGS 42, 522, 1994
19. Fahraeus L, Wallentin L: High density lipoprotein subfractions during oral and cutaneous administrations of 17 beta-estradiol to menopausal women. Am J Obstet Gynecol 56, 797, 1983
20. Tikkanen MJ, Kuusi T, Kikkila EA, Stenman UH: Variation of postheparin plasma hepatic lipase by menstrual cycle. Metabolism 35, 99, 1986
21. Harder DR and Coulsom PB: Estrogen receptors and effect of estrogen on membrane electrical properties of coronary vascular smooth muscle. J Cell Physiol 100, 375, 1979
22. Soules MR and Bremner WJ: The menopause and climateric: endocrinologic basis and associated symptomatology. Jags 30, 547, 1992
23. Lowik CWGM, Va der Ppluijm G, Bloys H, Hoekman K, Bijvoet OLM, Aarden LA: Parathyroid hormone (PTH) and PTH-like protein (PLPL) stimulate interleukin-6 production by osteogenic cells: a possible role of interleukin-6 in osteoclastogenesis. Biochem Biophys Res Comm 162, 1546, 1989
24. Klaiber EL, Broverman DM, Vogel W: Estrogen replacement therapy for severe persistent depression in women. Arch Gen Psychitry 36, 550, 1979
25. Luine VN, Khylchevskaya RI and Mc Ewen BS: Effect of gonadal steroids on activities of monoamine oxidase and choline acetylase in rat brain. Brain Res 86, 293, 1975
26. Majewska MD, Harrison NL, Schwartz RD, Barker JL, Paul SM: Steroid hormone metabolites are barbiturate-like modulators of the GABA receptor. Science 232,1004, 1986
27. Frolkis VV, Tanin SA, Marcinko VI and Muradian KK: Effects of hormones on the fast axoplasmic transport of substances in central horns of the spinal cord in rats of different ages. Arch Geront Geriat 11, 33, 1990
28. Griggs RC, Kingston W, Jozefowicz RF, Herr BE, Forbes and Halliday DC: Effect of testosterone on muscle mass and muscle protein synthesis. J Appl Physiol 66, 498, 1989
29. Liu L, Merrian GR and Sherins RJ: Chronic sex steroid exposure increases mean plasma growth hormone concentration and pulse amplitude in men with isolated hypogonadotropic hypogonadism. J Clin Endocrinol Metab 64, 651, 1987
30. Swerdloff RS, Wang C, Hines M and Gorski R: Effect of androgens on the brain and other organs during development and aging. Psychoneuroendocrinology 17, 375, 1992
31. Nestler JE, Barlascini CO, Clore NJ, Backard WG: Dehydroepiandrosterone reduces serum low density lipoprotein levels and body fat but does not alter insulin sensitivity in normal men. J Clin Endocrinol Metab 66,57,1988
32. Morales AJ, Nolan JJ, Nelson JC: Effects of replacement dose of dehydroepiandrosterone in men and women in advancing age. J Clin Endocrinol Metab 78: 1360, 1994

33. Gordon GB, Bush DE and FW Weisman: Reduction of atherosclerosis by administration of dehydroepiandrosterone J Clin Inv 82, 712, 1988
34. Nestler JE, Beer NA, Jakubowicz DJ, Matt DW and Beer RM: Oral dehydroepiandrosterone (DHEA) administration enhances fibrinolysis in men. The Endocine Society - 77th Annual Meeting Proceedings p.60, 1995
35. Robel P, Baulieu EE: Neurosteroids: byosynthesis and function. Trend Endocrinol Metab 5,1,1994
36. Majewska MD: Neurochemical, physiological and behaviorel actions of neurosteroids: role in personality, learning, aging and disease. ISPNE 26th Congress Proceedings p.51,1995
37. Khorram O, Vu L and Yen SSC: Activation of immune function by DHEA in age-advanced men. J Gerontol Med Sci 52: M1–7,1997
38. Rasmussen KR, Martin EG, Arrowood MJ, Healey MC: Effects of dexamethasone and dehydroepiandrosterone in immunosuppressed rats infected with Cryptosporidium parvum. J Protozool 38,157S,1991
39. Mortola J, Yen SSC: The effects of oral dehydroepiandrosterone on endocrine-metabolic parameters in postmenopausal women. J Clin Endocrinol Metab 71,696,1990
40. Rudman D: Growth hormone, body composition and aging. JAGS 33,800,1985
41. De Boer H, Blok GJ, Voerman HJ, De Vries PMJM and Van Der Veen EA: Body composition in adult growth hormone-deficient men, assessed by anthropometry and bioimpedence analysis. J Clin Endocrinol Metab 75,833,1992
42. Rudman D, Feller AG, Nagraj HS, Gergans GA, Lalitha PY, Goldberg AF, Schlenker RA, Cohn L, Rudman IW, Mattson DE: Effects of human growth hormone in men over 60 years old. N Engl J Med 323,1,1990
43. Mendelson WB, Slater S, Gold P, Gillin CJ: The effect of growth hormone administraton on human sleep: a dose-response study. Biol Psychiatry 15,613,1980
44. Almqvist O, Thoren M, Saaf M, Eriksson O: Effects of growth hormone substitution on mental performance in adults with growth hormone deficiency: a pilot study. Psychoneuroendocrinology 11,347,1986
45. Degerblad M, Almkvist O, Grunditz R, Hall K, Kaijser L, Knuttsson E, Ringert H, Thoren M: Physical and psychological capabilities during substitution therapy with recombinant growth hormone in adults with growth hormone deficiency. Acta Endocrinol 123,185,1990
46. Yang R, Bunting S, Gillet N, Clark R, Hongkui J: Growth hormone improves cardiac performance in experimental heart failure. Circulation 92,262,1995
47. Fazio S, Sabadini D, Capalbo B, Vigorito C, Giordano A, Giuda R, Pardo F, Biondi B and Saccà L: A preliminary study of growth hormone in the treatment of dilated cardiomyopathy. N Engl J Med 334,809,1996

4

THE IONIC HYPOTHESIS OF AGING

Role of Intracellular Ions in the Development of Hypertension and Insulin Resistance

Mario Barbagallo,[1] Ligia J. Dominguez,[2] Anna Licata,[2] Lilia Granvillano,[1] Maria Adele Alessi,[1] Giuseppe Licata,[2] and Lawrence M. Resnick[3]

[1]Department of Geriatrics
University of Palermo
Via del Vespro, 141, 90144 Palermo, Italy
[2]Institute of Internal Medicine
University of Palermo, Italy
[3]Division of Endocrinology
Wayne State University
Detroit

INTRODUCTION

The clinical association of essential hypertension with metabolic abnormalities, such as hyperinsulinemia, insulin resistance, obesity, altered glucose tolerance and/or frank non-insulin dependent diabetes mellitus (NIDDM) has long been appreciated(1). Each of the above clinical conditions is extremely frequent in the elderly. The association of these different clinical states, that is also common at younger ages, has been termed "Syndrome X" and more recently "Generalized Cardiovascular-Metabolic Disease."(2,3) Although several hypothesis have been proposed, including a primary role of hyperinsulinemia and insulin resistance, the mechanism(s) of this linkage has not been established. This syndrome complex is frequently associated with target organ involvement, such as left ventricular hypertrophy (LVH) and atherosclerosis of the coronary and peripheral vascular beds.

The critical role of calcium and magnesium ions in cellular physiology is well known. Calcium ion is a universal cellular messenger for extracellular signals to regulate cell, tissue and organ function. The importance of calcium in cardiac and vascular smooth muscle contraction has been appreciated for over 100 years, since Ringer(4) first described the heart's requirement for extracellular calcium. Most contractile stimuli induce arterial smooth muscle contraction by increasing myoplasmic free calcium concentrations (Ca_i).(5) Calcium ion is unique among all the mineral ion species, due to the large intra- extracellular gradient (1:10.000), that is necessary to maintain the cellular responsiveness to a vari-

Recent Advances in Geriatrics, edited by Barbagallo, Licata, and Sowers.
Plenum Press, New York, 1998.

Table 1. Role of calcium in the regulation of vascular tone, blood pressure, and insulin sensitivity

- Calcium mediates stimulus-contraction coupling in cardiac, skeletal, and vascular smooth muscle
- Alterations in the ability of cells to accumulate and/or sequester Ca_i will affect the force of contraction, and the peripheral vascular tone.
- Calcium ions also regulate stimulus-secretion coupling in endocrine, neural, and renal tissues.
- Ca_i regulates insulin secretion and insulin action.
- Steady state Ca_i may determine cell responsiveness to insulin (ionic insulin resistance).

ety of extracellular stimuli, and the homeostasis of the cells. The cytosolic free calcium (Ca_i) concentrations in resting cells is ~100 nM. This concentration is constantly maintained in a very narrow range, and is regulated by a series of channels, pumps, and other transport mechanisms that controls the movements of calcium into and out of the cells and between the cytosol and the intracellular stores[(6–9)]. It is now understood that intracellular free calcium concentrations are not only involved in regulating cardiac and smooth muscle cardiac function, but acts as a final common factor in mediating cellular responses to a wide variety of stimuli, including stimulus-secretion coupling in endocrine cells, glycogen metabolism, cell division[(10)] (Table 1).

The role of magnesium ions in the physiologic regulation of cardiac and vascular smooth muscle activity is also established. Magnesium modulates the activity of many plasma membrane and intracellular ion transport pump mechanisms which maintain critical levels of cytosolic free calcium and sodium (Table 2). The role of calcium itself in stimulus-contraction coupling and relaxation is itself dependent on intracellular steady-state activities of magnesium. In particular, it is now clear that magnesium ion, although not directly involved in the biochemical process of contraction, modulates vascular smooth muscle tone and contractility by affecting calcium ion concentrations and its availability at critical sites. Magnesium ions actively promote relaxation, offset calcium-related excitation-contraction coupling, and decrease cellular responsiveness to depolarizing stimuli, by stimulating Ca^{++}-dependent K^+ channels, which offset the potential depolarizing influence of cellular calcium accumulation, by activating the membrane Na–K–ATPase pump, which is critical for the maintenance of the resting cellular membrane potential, by competitively inhibiting Ca binding to calmodulin, by stimulating both plasma membrane and sarcoplasmic reticulum Ca ATPases[(11–14)]. Consistent with the above, not only calcium-induced contraction in VSM is sensitive to changes in magnesium concentration[(11–13)], but direct reduction of extracellular magnesium raises smooth muscle Ca^{++} content, while conversely, elevations in Mg^{++} concentrations reciprocally lower calcium content in smooth muscle[(15)]. Moreover, magnesium directly affect uptake, distribution and content of calcium in vascular smooth muscle cells, and can itself function as a weak calcium channel blocker, modulating calcium-channel activity in heart cells[(16)], and causing vasodilatation comparable to pharmacologic calcium channel blockade[(17)]. Magnesium ions have shown

Table 2. Role of magnesium in the regulation of vascular tone, blood pressure, and insulin sensitivity

- Magnesium modulates the activity of many plasma membrane and intracellular ion transport pump mechanism, which maintain critical levels of sodium and calcium.
- By affecting calcium ion concentrations and its availability at critical sites, magnesium modulates vascular smooth muscle tone and contraction.
- Magnesium is also a necessary co-factor in all ATP-transfer reactions, thus regulating the tyrosyne-kinase insulin receptor activity and the rate limiting enzymes of glycolysis.

to directly alter baseline tension or tone of blood vessels[18–19]. Indeed, depletion of magnesium both in vitro and in vivo induce vascular hyperreactivity and frank hypertension[11–13]. Intracellular free magnesium (Mg_i) is not only involved in regulating cardiac and smooth muscle contractile function, but, as well as calcium, is critical to cellular responses to a wide variety of external stimuli, including stimulus-secretion coupling in endocrine cells, neurotransmitter release from nerve terminals both centrally and peripherally, and renal excretory function[10]. Similarly, magnesium is a necessary cofactor in all ATP-transfer reactions, and thus is critical in glucose metabolism for the action of tyrosine kinase activity and for the rate limiting enzymes of glycolysis, and depletion of magnesium. This has been demonstrated in patients with diabetes, insulin resistance, and hypertension[20].

WHAT DO INTRACELLULAR IONS HAVE TO DO WITH CLINICAL HYPERTENSION AND INSULIN RESISTANCE?

In the steady state, alterations of both calcium and magnesium levels are present in essential hypertension and in NIDDM. Erne et al., have first demonstrated a direct significant relationship between intracellular free calcium in platelets and blood pressure in essential hypertensive subjects[21]. Resnick et al. showed that subjects with essential hypertension, and/or with type II diabetes mellitus, compared with normotensive, nondiabetic subjects, display similar alterations of intracellular ions, characterized, at least in part, by increased cytosolic free calcium and/or reciprocally suppressed cytosolic free magnesium[22]. Resnick et al. also showed that blood pressure levels are not only directly related to cytosolic free calcium levels but also inversely linked to levels of intracellular free magnesium[23]. A connection is also present between intracellular ions and indices of glycemic metabolic control. In particular fasting blood sugar levels are directly related to Ca_i[24] and inversely related to Mg_i[22], and to the hyperinsulinemic response to oral glucose loading[25]. It appears that the greater is the intracellular ionic perturbation (the higher the free calcium and/or the lower the intracellular free magnesium), the worst is the metabolic compensation and the higher the blood pressure, and the peripheral insulin resistance[25]. The opposite relation of free calcium and free magnesium concentrations to these hemodynamic and metabolic events is explained because cytosolic free calcium and magnesium are themselves inversely related, that is the lower the free magnesium, the higher the free calcium[2,3].

The importance of calcium and magnesium in the regulation of cardiac and smooth muscle contraction as well as glucose utilization is itself a strong physiologic support to the hypothesis that an altered intracellular ionic profile, characterized by increased free calcium and suppressed free magnesium levels, might be the cellular basis of the peripheral insulin resistance of NIDDM, and essential hypertension. Thus, decreased availability of magnesium or excess cellular calcium accumulation would thus be expected to enhance vasoconstriction, and/or blunt cardiac and smooth muscle relaxation, and to decrease cellular glucose utilization, contributing to peripheral insulin resistance as a post-receptor defect[2,3,20].

WHAT DOES REGULATE INTRACELLULAR IONS?

To better understand the mechanism of these multiple, coordinate alterations of intracellular ion levels in hypertension and NIDDM we have assessed intracellular ionic levels dynamically, under a series of different clinical and physiological conditions, both in vivo and in vitro, including dietary salt loading, oral glucose tolerance testing, direct addition to cells systems in vitro of glucose, insulin and hormones, such as estrogen and dehydroepiandrosterone sulfate (DHEAS) that have been shown to have a vascular protective effect.

Salt

The ability of dietary salt loading to elevate blood pressure in some hypertensive subjects appears to be dependent on its ability to induce elevations in Ca_i and to reciprocally suppress Mg_i levels. These changes are proportionate to the pressor effects of salt, i.e., the greater the salt-induced rise in Ca_i and the greater the fall in Mg_i, the more the pressure rises. Consistent with the critical role of these ionic changes were the observation that the efficacy of calcium channel blockade to reverse salt-induced hypertension was closely related to its ability to reverse these ionic effects of salt-loading, nifedipine reducing Ca_i and elevating Mg_i levels[26].

Sugar

Not only salt, but elevations of blood sugar may also contribute to these ionic abnormalities, and thus to the hypertension and vascular disease of diabetes. First, research from our group indicated that the transient hyperglycemia of oral glucose loading reproduces the same altered ionic profile of increased Ca_i and depleted Mg_i levels that occur chronically in diabetic subjects[27]. Second, hyperglycemia in vitro, independently of insulin or other in vivo responses to oral glucose ingestion, directly induces these same cellular ionic changes in human erythrocytes[28]. Glucose in a concentration- and time-dependent manner, at levels achieved clinically, and independent of insulin, elevates intracellular free calcium content also in primary cultures of vascular smooth muscle cells[29], suggesting that these ionic effects of glucose might be relevant to the increased vasoconstriction present in chronic diabetic states. The mechanism(s) by which glucose modulates intracellular ion content remains unclear. Osmotic or other nonspecific effects seem ruled out by the failure of equiosmolar amounts of L-glucose or mannitol to reproduce the D-glucose effect. Davis et al., demonstrated a direct inhibitory effect of hyperglycemia on plasma membrane Ca–ATPase[30], possibly mediated by enzymatic glycosilation[31], which could promote calcium accumulation from the extracellular space. A second potential mechanism for the observed effect of glucose on intracellular free calcium involves glucose induced stimulation of protein kinase C[32], potentially recruiting calcium from intracellular storage sites via IP_3 formation. A third mechanism involves the activation of glycolysis by increased cellular glucose uptake, which would increase organic acid formation and thus lower intracellular pH. Regardless of the mechanism involved, however, this glucose-induced stimulation of Ca_i is clinically significant occurring at glucose concentrations (10 mM) observed in vitro in subjects with impaired glucose tolerance as well as frank diabetes mellitus, and consistent with the increased incidence of hypertension in diabetes. Hence, circulating glucose concentrations, even within the "normal" range, may be one physiologic determinant of basal cytosolic free calcium levels. As a support of the clinical significance of these glucose-induced changes, HbA1c levels, reflective of average glycemic levels over time, in diabetic subjects, are closely related to fasting basal cytosolic free calcium levels[24]. Thus, circulating glucose concentrations, even within the "normal" range, may be one physiologic determinant of basal cytosolic free calcium levels.

These glucose-related ionic alterations might also help to explain concomitant alterations of cardiac structure often present in NIDDM. We have analyzed divalent cellular ion concentrations in diabetic and matched control subjects, and compared them both with glucose and insulin levels before and after oral glucose loading, and with cardiac structural indices determined by prior echocardiographic examinations[24]. We found i) that even in the absence of overt hypertensive disease, NIDDM was associated with early changes of cardiac structure, while hypertensive NIDDM was associated with significantly increased cardiac mass; ii) that blood pressure and cardiac mass were significantly related to levels of glycemia, both fasting and post-glucose loading, but not to levels of circulating insulin; and iii) independently of diagnostic assignment, for all subjects, that glycemia as well as blood pressure and cardiac structural indices, were each directly related to basal, steady-state fasting cytosolic free calcium levels, while being inversely related to extracellular serum ionized calcium levels; iv) lastly, this glucose-calcium-cardiac link was further supported by multivariate regression analysis, in which glucose and Ca_i remained a determinant of LVMI, independently of BMI, age, insulin, and blood pressure. The above data, and the known direct cellular effects of glucose on intracellular divalent cations, elevating steady-state cytosolic free calcium and reciprocally suppressing magnesium levels, support the hypothesis that hyperglycemia may contribute to both the elevated blood pressure and cardiac hypertrophy of NIDDM[24].

Insulin

A variety of clinical studies have emphasized the association of hyperinsulinemia per se with blood pressure. In theSan Antonio heart study, hyperinsulinemia was correlated directly with systolic and diastolic blood pressure in men[33]. Lucas reported fasting serum insulin levels to be positively associated with systolic and diastolic blood pressure in obese women, independently of age, weight, and blood glucose values[34]. On the basis of epidemiological and clinical evidences, it has been suggested that insulin resistance represent the basic defect that may underlie the clinical association of hypertension, abnormal glucose tolerance and diabetes mellitus, all conditions that share hyperinsulinemia, peripheral insulin resistance and intracellular ion abnormalities[35,36]. On the other hand insulin itself is a vasodilator and may even induce frank hypotension in absence of an adequate, compensatory rise in cathecolamine activity[37]. Insulin have direct ionic actions, elevating Ca_i in erythrocytes[38], adipocytes[39], and VSMC. The mechanism by which insulin increase Ca_i is still in question. Insulin might induce alterations in ion fluxes particularly stimulating the Na/H^+ antiporter either directly or via diacylglycerol-protein-kinase C[40], or inhibiting Ca–ATPase activity. Insulin also significantly increases Mg_i[38,41,42]. However, the relationship between insulin and intracellular ion concentrations is not a simple one. Thus, insulin affects intracellular ion concentrations, but there are also evidence that both Ca_i and Mg_i mediate insulin action[39,42]. Basal ion levels are critical in determining insulin responsiveness[42]. Suppressed Mg_i levels, as found in hypertension and NIDDM may result in a defective tyrosine-kinase, and altered function of the insulin receptor level. This may lead to an impairment of insulin action and insulin resistance. As a result of these evidences the question arises to what extent alterations of intracellular ions contribute to or are just an indirect reflection of the insulin resistance of hypertension and NIDDM. To help to answer this question and to investigate the ionic actions of insulin we measured Ca_i and Mg_i in cells from normal and hypertensive patients, before and 30, 60, 120, and 180 min after the addition of insulin. In cells from hypertensive subjects the ionic action of insulin on both calcium and magnesium were blunted. Continuous relationship were observed between basal ionic values and insulin responses: the greater the intracellular calcium, the less the calcium rose (r: 0.574, p: 0.013); and the lower the intracellular magnesium, the less the magnesium rose in response to insulin (r: 0.524, p: 0.025)[42]. Furthermore, we have used cells from normal volunteers with physiologic ionic responses to insulin and depleted them of magnesium by treatment with either A23187, in a calcium free medium, or with high glucose concentrations (15 mM). A depletion of Mg_i induced a suppression of the magnesium responses to insulin, thus reproducing the behavior of hypertensive and NIDDM cells[42]. Altogether these data demonstrate ionic aspect of insulin resistance and suggest that Ca_i and Mg_i levels may regulate cellular responsiveness to insulin. To confirm the importance of the ionic environment in insulin resistance, drugs that are routinely used in the treatment of NIDDM and insulin resistance have also ionic actions. Dominguez and Sowers have shown that metformin is able to reduce calcium responses to thrombin[43], and more recently the same group have demonstrated that both pioglitazone and trioglitazone have a calcium antagonist action, significantly inhibiting the L-channel in vascular smooth muscle cells[44,45].

Calcium Regulating Hormones

Several of the hormones responsible for maintaining overall, total body calcium homeostasis are also vasoactive hormones, modulating cellular calcium metabolism and force generating capacity in cardiovascular tissues. As such, they may participate in the long-term regulation of vascular tone. Peptide hormones such as parathyroid hormone (PTH), calcitonin, 1,25$(OH)_2$ D_3, the calcitonin gene-related peptide (CGRP), all vary with age and by affecting the intra- and extracellular distribution of calcium, may all influence the modifications of vascular resistance and insulin sensibility with age[3]. In addition to the classical calcium regulating hormones, we have recently investigated the role of sex steroids and dehydroepiandrosterone sulfate in the regulation of vascular tone and calcium metabolism[3].

Sex Steroid Hormones

The involvement of sex steroid hormones in the regulation of cardiovascular function and vascular tone has been a topic of increasing interest. Despite an increasing number of studies describing the effects of sex steroids on the cardiovascular system, underlying mechanisms remain unclear. We have recently investigated the effect of estrogen and progesterone on blood pressure in the whole animal, on rat tail artery tension in vitro, and on intracellular free calcium concentrations and Ca^{++} channel current activity in cultured VSMC[46,47]. Administrations of estrogens did not affect basal blood pressure but inhibited pressor response to norepinephrine (NE). In isolated rat tail artery helical strips, estrogen inhibited contractile responses to KCl, AVP and NE. These effects of estrogen on vascular tissue may, at least in part, be explained by its effect on intracellular calcium metabolism, since estrogen significantly decreased L-type calcium channel current and concurrently blunted the rise in Ca_i induced by depolarizing stimuli in cultured VSMC[46]. Using the same experimental protocols, we recently found similar effects of progesterone on intracellular calcium metabolism in VSMC, progesterone blunting the calcium increment induced by KCl and decreasing L-type calcium currents in VSMC[47]. Since activation of L-type calcium channel activity and/or cellular calcium accumulation links electrical excitation to subsequent vascular contraction, the inhibition of these calcium-related events by sex steroids may underlie estrogen and progesterone-induced vasodilatation, and may also have protective effect on insulin resistance.

DHEAS

Dehydroepiandrosterone (DHEA) is the most abundantly produced adrenal steroid, and serum concentrations of its sulfate ester, DHEAS, are approximately 20-fold higher than those of any other circulating steroid hormone. Nevertheless, the physiologic function of this endogenous steroid remain undefined. DHEAS circulating levels progressively decrease with age, peak levels occurring between the third and fourth decade of life, and decreasing progressively thereafter by 90–95% after the age of 85[48–49]. The remarkable age-related decline in circulating DHEAS levels has been linked to the increased incidence of atherosclerotic and cardiovascular disease with age[50], while high plasma level in DHEAS levels have been associated with a reduction of mortality and cardiovascular diseases[51]. These observations, and several animal studies have added to the presumption that DHEAS may participate in the pathophysiology of vascular diseases associated with atherosclerosis and aging. A reduction in aortic atherosclerosis in rabbits fed a high cholesterol diet has been obtained after dietary supplementation with DHEA[52]. While its mechanism of action is unknown, direct vascular effects of DHEAS have also been suggested. We have recently confirmed that DHEAS, in doses reflecting circulating levels of the hormone in vivo exerts direct calcium-related effects on the vasculature at both tissue and cellular levels[53]. At the tissue level, DHEAS modulates the vasoconstrictor response to depolarizing stimuli and to specific endogenous agonists. In a parallel fashion, at the cellular level, DHEAS blunts depolarization-induced cellular calcium accumulation in VSMC. We hypothesize that DHEAS may function endogenously, to physiologically buffer vascular calcium-dependent responses to various electrophysiologic and hormonal stimuli. This may be one mechanism by which the well known, progressive decline of DHEAS with age contributes to atherosclerotic and cardiovascular diseases in the elderly.

INTRACELLULAR IONS AND AGING

In industrialized countries, aging is epidemiologically associated with an increase in blood pressure. Systolic blood pressure (SBP) rises throughout the life span. Diastolic blood pressure (DBP), in contrast rises much more modestly with age, increasing until the age of 55–60, and after the age of seventy starts to decline[54]. In the Framingham Heart Study, SBP increased about 25 mmHg in men and 35 mmHg in women between the fourth and the eight decades[55]. Arterial hypertension and "normal" aging, in absence of hypertension, have many similar effects on the cardiovascular system. An increased arterial stiffness, an increased systemic vascular resistance, an increased left ventricular mass, are common both between hypertensive patients and healthy normotensive old subjects.

A decrease of glucose tolerance with advancing age has also been longly recognized[56]. However, the mechanisms by which glucose metabolism is progressively impaired with increasing age are not completely understood. The association of age with impaired glucose handling has been first investigated in depth by De Fronzo[57], who focused on the role of tissue unresponsiveness to insulin (peripheral insulin resistance) as "primum movens", although other mechanism(s) may be involved. As discussed above a dysregulation of intracellular ions can itself increase vascular tone and impair insulin sensitivity[2,3].

Similar alterations of intracellular ion homeostasis, that we have previously shown in hypertension and NIDDM are also present in "normal" aging. We have recently shown that also in healthy "normal" subjects aging is associated with an increase of cytosolic free calcium[58,59]. It is well known that in blood vessels the calcium content rises linearly with advancing age[60]. Elkeles have proposed a "calcium shift theory" in old age, in which the progressive loss of calcium from bone and the correspondent accumulation of the ion in the cell and in the blood vessels, may lead to an increased incidence of osteoporosis and atherosclerosis with aging[61]. According to the hypothesis of Elkeles, the calcium deficiency state of aging, and a subsequent secondary hyperparathyroidism might be the primary mechanism of the shift of calcium from the extracellular to the intracellular compartment.

At the cellular level, in normal elderly subjects we observed an age-dependent cytosolic free calcium accumulation and a reciprocal depletion of cytosolic free magnesium[58,59]. These alterations are indistinguishable from those present in essential hypertension or type II, non insulin dependent diabetes mellitus, independently of age[3,58,59]. Since both the intracellular calcium accumulation and the magnesium depletion increase vascular contractility and vascular resistance, leading to a decreased blood flow, and increased systemic blood pressure, this ionic alteration occurring with age may be potentially important in the pathogenesis of the hypertension in the elderly. In the same fashion, we have proposed that the ionic alterations (suppression of intracellular free magnesium and increased cellular free calcium) leading to a reduced TK activity and ionic cellular resistance[3] may also be responsible of the increased peripheral insulin resistance and alterations of glucose metabolism associated with age. The derangement in intracellular ions may be important in the pathogenesis of abnormalities of insulin secretion and action and in the pathogenesis of macrovascular complication. As such, may also represent a common link among diabetes, hypertension, atherosclerosis and accelerated aging.

Fleckenstein empirically suggested an upper limit for the physiologic range of intracellular calcium (being in the different cells and tissues between 100–200 nM), above this physiologic range calcium concentrations being "cytotoxic". He hypothesized that these "cytotoxic" cellular calcium concentrations might be reached in old age, leading to cells and tissues dysfunction. Hypertension, and NIDDM accelerate and anticipate the reach of this "cytotoxic" range of cellular calcium, thus also providing a model of accelerated aging[62]. Our and other evidences suggest that depletion of cellular magnesium may also have a role in this process[3,58,59,63].

IONIC HYPOTHESIS OF AGING AND CARDIOVASCULAR-METABOLIC DISEASES

Although the cause of the intracellular free calcium accumulation with age have not been clarified yet, the possible mechanisms involved includes: i) Alterations of the permeability, fluidity and/or structure of the membrane; ii) alterations of calcium channels; iii) alterations of the mechanism of extrusion of calcium (reduced Na^{+}–Ca^{++} exchange and/or reduced ATPases Ca^{++}–Mg^{++} dependent); iv) alterations of the intracellular mechanisms of sequestration. We also cannot demonstrate here if these alterations of ionic environment occurring with age are genetically determined, or if life-long exposition to environmental inputs (some of them discussed above) and integrating hormonal signals have a major role in their determination (Figure 1).

The pivotal role of calcium in so many cellular processes imposes the need for a very fine regulation of its intracellular level. It is clear that to maintain constant the concentrations of intracellular free calcium, in the cytosol, is of extreme importance to preserve the cell function and the cell responsiveness. A dysregulation in the intracellular

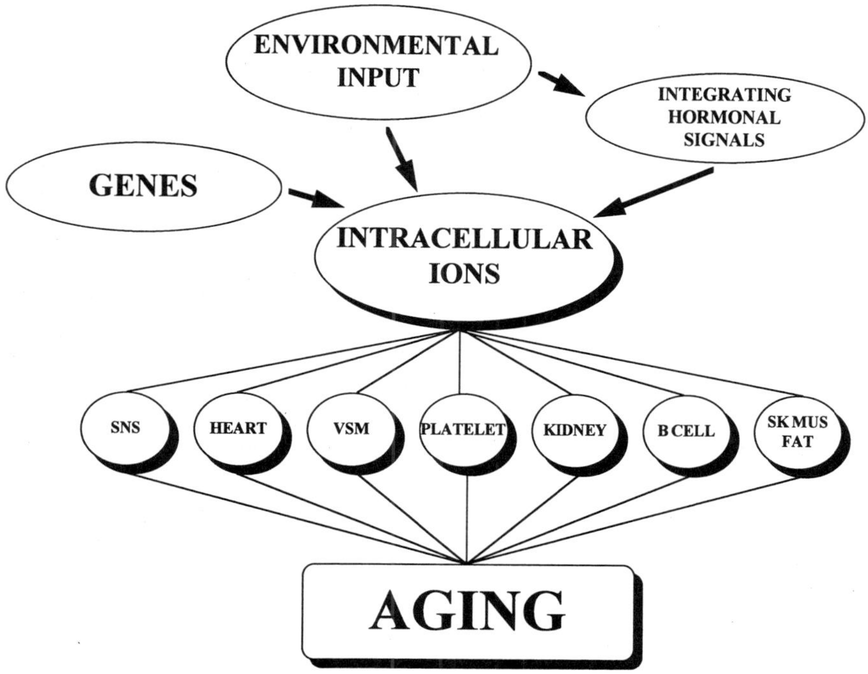

Figure 1. Ionic hypothesis of aging, in which cellular ionic alterations, independently of any initiating contribution of genetic, environmental or hormonal factors, promote a spectrum of altered tissue responses, resulting in clinical disease states, and/or in an accelerated aging process.

concentrations may lead to dramatic changes in the cell function. An excess of calcium in the cytoplasm is a major threat to the viability of cells. Moreover, an accumulation of intracellular free calcium is also the final pathway leading to cell degeneration and death in response to a wide variety of environmental and toxic noxious stimuli[64,65]. In the heart, it is well known the risk of reperfusion, after a prolonged ischemic period, due to the overload of calcium in the cells, leaking from the plasma membrane altered by the ischemia. An excessive rise in calcium threatens cells in several ways. Adverse effects of a massive rise in intracellular calcium involve altered protein phosphorylation, proteolysis, lipolysis. A rise in calcium also activates enzymes that lead to production of free radicals[64,65]. There is a complex interaction between the amount and the duration of this perturbation of the intracellular calcium homeostasis. Kachaturian have proposed that a small change in intracellular free calcium concentrations sustained for a long period of time (years) may cause the same toxic effect induced by high calcium concentrations for a short time (minutes, seconds)[66].

$$\Delta \, Ca_i \times \Delta \, T = K$$ [66]

Thus the calcium hypothesis of aging and metabolic and cardiovascular diseases hypothesize that a dysregulation of Ca_i and of the calcium mediated signaling system that are part of the final common pathways leading to cell dysfunction and death, might also play a critical role in the development of hypertension and metabolic diseases with age (Figure 1).

CONCLUSIONS

We propose that the cellular ionic dysfunction found in healthy, elderly subjects, similar to that present in young hypertensives and NIDDM subjects, may be the missing link responsible for the frequent coexistence of cardiovascular and metabolic diseases with aging , and may accelerate the aging process itself (Figure 1). The ionic hypothesis of aging postulates that with "normal" aging, cells become more vulnerable to calcium dysregulation, leading to possible elevation of intracellular free calcium and to concurrent magnesium depletion. Specifically, these cellular ionic defects, present in multiple different organ systems, would be expected to produce a spectrum of altered tissue responses, resulting in either the above mentioned clinical disease states and/or what we currently term the normal aging process, including universal cellular hypofunction and hyporesponsiveness to stimuli associated with aging. We propose that an alteration in the cellular mechanisms for maintaining the homeostasis of cytosolic calcium concentrations play a key role in aging. According to the ionic hypothesis, a sustained accumulation of cellular calcium and/or the depletion of cellular magnesium could provide the final common pathway for many aging-associated diseases, including hypertension and NIDDM.

REFERENCES

1. Jarret RJ, Keen H, McCartney M, Fuller JH, Hamilton PJS, Reid D, Rose G.: Glucose tolerance and blood pressure in two population samples. Their relationship to diabetes mellitus and hypertension. Am.J.Epidemiol., 1978, 7: 15–24.
2. Resnick LM.: Ionic basis of hypertension, insulin resistance, vascular disease and related disorders. The mechanism of "Syndrome X". Am.J.Hypertens., 1993, 6: 123S-134S.
3. Barbagallo M., Resnick LM, Calcium and Magnesium in the regulation of smooth muscle function and blood pressure. in: Endocrinology of the Vasculature, JR Sowers editor, Humana Press Inc. NJ, USA, pp. 283–300.
4. Ringer S.: A third contribution regarding the infusion of the inorganic constituents of the blood on the ventricular contraction. J.Physiol., 1883, 222–5.
5. Kuriyama H., Uishi I., Suaky H., Kitamura K., Itoh T.: Factors modifying contraction-relaxation in vascular smooth muscle. Am.J.Physiol., 1982, 243: H641-H662.
6. Borle AB: Control, modulation and regulation of cell calcium. Rev. Physiol. Biochem. Pharmacol., 1981, 90: 13–153.
7. Rasmussen H.: Calcium messenger system. N.Engl.J.Med., 1986, 314:1094–1107, 1164–1170.
8. Eggermont J.A., Vrolix M., Raeymaekers L., Wuytack F., Casteels R.: Ca^{++} transport ATPases of vascular smooth muscle. Circ.Res., 1988, 62: 266–278.
9. Nabel E.G., Berk B.C., Brock T.A., Smith T.W: Na^{+}- Ca^{++} exchange in cultured vascular smooth muscle cells. Circ.Res., 1988, 62: 486–489.
10. Rubin RP: The role of calcium in the release of neurotransmitter substances and hormones. Pharmacol. Rev. 1970; 22: 389–427.
11. Altura BM, Altura BT: Magnesium ions and contractions on vascular smooth muscles: relationship to some vascular diseases. Fed Proc. 1981; 40: 2672–79.
12. Altura BM, Altura BT, Carella A, Turlapaty PDMV: Ca^{++} coupling in vascular smooth muscle: Mg^{++} and buffer effects on contractility and membrane Ca^{++} movements. Can.J.Physiol. 1982; 60: 459–482.
13. Altura BM, Altura BT: Magnesium and contractions of arterial smooth muscle. Microvasc Res.1974; 7: 145–155.
14. Woods WT, Katholi RE, Urthaler F, James TN: Electrophysiological effects of magnesium on cells in the canine sinus node and false tendon. Circ. Res. 1979; 44: 182–188.
15. Turlapaty PDMV, Altura BM: Extracellular magnesium ions control calcium exchange and content of vascular smooth muscle. Eur J Pharmacol. 1978; 52: 421- 23.
16. Agus ZA, Kalipourie E, Dukes I, Morad M.: Cytosolic magnesium modulates calcium channel activity in mammalian ventricular cells. Am.J.Physiol. 1989; 256: C452–455.

17. Ji BH, Erne P, Kiosky W, Buhler FR, Bolli P.: Magnesium-induced vasodilatation is comparable to that induced by calcium channel blockade. J.Hypertension 1983; 1(suppl.2): 368–71.
18. Altura BM, Altura BT.: Role of magnesium ions in contractility of blood vessels and skeletal muscle. Magnesium Bull. 1981; 3: 102–114.
19. Altura BM, Altura BT, Gebrewold A, Ising H, Guntter T: Magnesium deficiency and hypertension: correlation between magnesium deficient diets and microcircolatory changes in situ. Science 1984; 223: 1315–17.
20. Paolisso G, Barbagallo M., Hypertension, Diabetes Mellitus and Insulin Resistance. The role of intracellular magnesium. Am.J. Hypertens., 1997, 10, 346–355.
21. Erne P., Bolli P., Burgissen E., Buhler F.: Correlation of platelets calcium with blood pressure: Effects of antihypertensive therapy. N.Engl.J.Med., 1984, 319: 1084–8.
22. Resnick L.M., Gupta R.K., Bhargava K.K., Gruenspan H., Alderman M.H., Laragh J.H.: Cellular ions in hypertension, diabetes, and obesity: A nuclear magnetic resonance spectroscopic study. Hypertension, 1991, 17: 951–957.
23. Resnick LM, Gupta RK Sosa RE Corbett ML, Laragh JH. Intracellular free magnesium in erythrocyte of essential hypertension. Proc.Nat.Acad.Sci. USA, 1987, 84: 7663–7667.
24. Barbagallo M., Gupta RK, Resnick LM. Cellular ions in NIDDM: Relation of calcium to hyperglycemia and cardiac mass. Diabetes Care, 1996, 19, 1393–1398.
25. Resnick L.M., Gupta R.K., Gruenspan H., Alderman M.H., Laragh J.H.: Hypertension and peripheral insulin resistance: mediating role of intracellular free magnesium. Am.J.Hypertens., 1990, 3: 373–379.
26. Resnick LM, Gupta RK, Di Fabio B, Barbagallo M, Marion R, Laragh JH: Intracellular ionic consequences of dietary salt loading in essential hypertension. J Clin Invest, 1994;94:1269–76.
27. Resnick LM, Gupta RK, Gruenspan H., Laragh JH: Intracellular ion response to glucose tolerance: Relation of hypertension, obesity and insulin resistance. Circulation, 1988, 78(suppl.II): II-570.
28. Resnick L.M., Barbagallo M., Gupta R.K., Laragh J.H.: Ionic basis of hypertension in diabetes mellitus: role of hyperglycemia. Am.J.Hypertens., 1993, 6: 413–417.
29. Barbagallo M., Shan J., Pang PKT, Resnick LM: Glucose-induced alterations of cytosolic free calcium in cultured rat tail artery vascular smooth muscle cells. J.Clin.Invest., 1995, 95: 763–767.
30. Davis FB, Davis PJ, Gerard N, Blas S, MacGillivray S, Gutman S, Feldman J.: The effect of in vivo glucose administration on human Ca-ATPase activity and on enzyme responsiveness in vitro to thyroid hormone and calmodulin. Diabetes, 1985, 34: 639–646.
31. Deziel MR, Safeer RS, Blas S, Davis FB, Davis PJ: Hexose-specific inhibition in vitro of human red cell Ca^{++}-ATPase- ATP-ase activity. Biochem.Biophys.Acta, 1992, 1110: 119–122.
32. Draznin B., Leitner W., Sussman KE, Sherman N.: Insulin and glucose modulate protein kinase C in rat adipocytes. Biochem.Biophys.Res.Commun., 1988, 156: 570–575.
33. Haffner SM, Fong D, Hazude HP, Pugh J.A, Patterson J.K: Hyperinsulinemia, upper body adiposity and cardiovascular risk factors in non diabetics. Metabolism, 1988, 37, 338–345.
34. Lucas C.P., Estigarribie J.A., Darza L.L., Reaven G.M.: Insulin and blood pressure in obesity and hypertension. Hypertension, 1985, 7, 702–706.
35. Reaven G.M., Hoffman B.B.: A role for insulin in the aetiology and course of hypertension. Lancet, 1987, 2, 435–437.
36. Ferrannini E., Buzzigoli G., Bonadonna R., Giorico M.A., Oleggini M., Graziadei L., Pedrinelli R., Brandi L., Bevilacqua S.: Insulin resistance in essential hypertension. N.Engl.J.Med., 1987, 317, 350–357.
37. Mathias C.J., daCosta D.F., Fosbraey P., Christensen N.J., Bannister R.: Hypotensive and sedative effect of insulin in autonomic nervous failure. Br..Med.J., 1987, 295, 161–163.
38. Barbagallo M., Gupta R.K., Resnick LM:: Cellular ionic effects of insulin in normal human red cells: a nuclear magnetic resonance study. Diabetologia, 1993, 36: 146–149.
39. Draznin B., Sussman K.E., Eckel R., Kao M., Yost T., Sherman N.A.: Possible role of cytosolic free calcium concentration in mediating insulin resistance of obesity and hyperinsulinemia. J.Clin.Invest., 1988, 82: 1848–1852
40. Hoffman J.M., Ishizuka T., Farese R.V.: Interrelated effects of insulin and glucose on diacylglycerol-protein kinase-C signaling in rat adipocytes and soley muscle in vitro and in vivo in diabetic rats. Endocrinology, 128, 2937–2948, 1991.
41. Paolisso G., Sgambato S., Passariello N., Giugliano D., Scheen AJ., D'Onofrio F., Lefebvre PJ.: Insulin induces opposite changes in plasma and erythrocyte magnesium concentration in normal man. Diabetologia 1986; 29: 644–647.
42. Barbagallo M., Gupta RK, Bardicef M, Bardicef O., Resnick LM: Altered ionic effect of insulin in hypertension: Role of basal ion levels in determining insulin responsiveness. J.Clin.Endocrinol.Metab., 1997, 82, 1761–1765.

43. Dominguez LJ, Davidoff AJ, Srinivas PR, Standley PR, Walsh MF, Sowers JR: Effects of metformin on tyrosine-kinase activity, glucose transport and intracellular calcium in rat vascular smooth muscle. Endocrinology, 1996, 137, 113–121.
44. Zhang F., Sowers JR, Ram JL, Standley PR, Peuler JD.: Effect of pioglitazone on L-type calcium channel in vascular smooth muscle. Hypertension, 1994, 24, 170–175.
45. Song J., Walsh MF, Igwe R, Ram JL, Barazi M, Dominguez LJ, Sowers JR: Trioglitazone reduces contraction by inhibition of vascular smooth muscle cell Ca^{++} currents and not endothelial nitric oxide production. Diabetes, 1997, 46, 659–664.
46. Shan J., Resnick LM, Liu Q, Wu X, Barbagallo M, Pang PKT: Vascular effect of 17 estradiol in male SD rats. Am.J.Physiol, 1994;266:H967-H973.
47. Barbagallo M, Shan J, Pang PKT, Resnick LM: Vascular effects of progesterone : role intracellular calcium metabolism. Am J Hypertens, 1995;8(part2):66A.
48. Orentreich N, Brind JL, Rizer RL, Vogelamn JH: Age changes and sex differences in serum dehydroepiandrosterone sulfate concentrations throughout adulthood. J Clin Endocrinol Metab, 1984;59:551–555.
49. Yamaji T, Ibayashi H: Plasma dehydroepiandrosterone sulfate in normal and pathological conditions. J Clin Endocrinol Metab, 1969;29:273–78.
50. Marmoston J, Griffith GC, Geller PJ, Fishman EL, Welsch F, Weiner JM: Urinary steroids in the measurement of aging and atherosclerosis. J Am Geriat Soc, 1975;23:481–492.
51. Barret-Connor E, Khaw KT, Yen SSC: A prospective study of dehydroepiandrosterone sulfate, mortality and cardiovascular disease. N Engl J Med, 1986;315:1519–24.
52. Gordon GB, Bush DE, Weishman HF: Reduction of atherosclerosis by administration of dehydroepiandrosterone. J Clin Invest, 1988;82:712–720.
53. Barbagallo M, Shan J, Pang PKT, Resnick LM: DHEAS effects on VSMC cytosolic free calcium and vascular contractility. Hypertension, 1995; 26(part 2): 1065–69.
54. Gordon T.: Blood pressure of adults by age and sex, USA 1960–62. National Center for Health Statistics, 1964, PHS publication 1000, series 11, n.4.
55. Kannel W.B.: Blood pressure and the development of cardiovascular disease in the aged. In: Cardiology in Old Age. Caird FL, Dall JLC, Kennedy RD eds. New York, NY, Plenum Press publisher, 1976, 143–175.
56. Andres R.: Aging and diabetes. Med.Clin.North Am., 1971, 55: 835–45.
57. DeFronzo R.A.: Glucose intolerance and aging. Evidence for tissue insensitivity to insulin. Diabetes, 1979, 28: 1095–1101.
58. Barbagallo M., Gupta R.K., Resnick L.M. Effect of aging on cellular divalent cations: Relation to hypertension and diabetes. J.Invest. Medicine, 1995, 43, suppl.2: 300A.
59. Barbagallo M., Dominguez LJ, Putignano E., Barbagallo Sangiorgi G., Resnick LM: Effect of aging on intracellular divalent cation metabolism: a link to the increased incidence of hypertension and non-insulin dependent diabetes mellitus in the elderly? Arch. Gerontol. Geriatr. , 1996(suppl 5), pp. 233–238.
60. Lansing AI, Alex M, Rosenthal TB.: Calcium and elastin in human atherosclerosis. J.Geront., 1973, 5: 112–117.
61. Elkeles A: A comparative radiological study of calcified atheromas in males and females over 50 years of age. Lancet, 1957, ii: 714–715.
62. Fleckenstein A., Frey M., Zorn S., Fleckenstein-Grun G.: Experimental basis of long term therapy of arterial hypertension with calcium antagonists. Am.J.Cardiol., 1995, 56: 3H-14H.
63. Orimo H., Ouchi Y.: The role of calcium and magnesium in the development of atherosclerosis. Experimental and clinical evidence. Ann.NY.Acad.Sci., 1990, 598: 444–57.
64. Orrenius S, McConkey DJ, Bellomo G., Nicotera P.: Role of Ca^{++} in toxic cell killing. Trends Pharmacol. Sci., 1989, 10: 281–285.
65. Fujita T.: Aging and calcium. Mineral Electrolyte Metab., 1986, 12: 149–156.
66. Kachaturian ZS: Hypothesis on the regulation of cytosol calcium concentration and the aging brain. Neurobiol. Aging, 1987, 8, 345–346.

5

RECENT ASPECTS OF RENAL PATHOPHYSIOLOGY IN THE ELDERLY

A. Ungar,[1] C. Cantini,[1] A. Altobelli,[1] B. Vallotti,[1] C. Di Serio,[1] G. La Cava,[3] M. Pellegri,[3] S. Castellani,[2] and G. Masotti[1]

[1]Istituto di Gerontologia e Geriatria
[2]Istituto di Clinica Medica Generale e Cardiologia
[3]Unità Operativa di Medicina Nucleare
Dipartimento di Fisiopatologia Clinica
Università di Firenze

1. INTRODUCTION

The aging kidney is characterized by both anatomical and functional changes. However, renal modifications that are currently observed in the elderly are often due not only to the physiological renal senescence but also to the overlapping of various pathological conditions that may be subclinical or unrecognized. Therefore the present chapter will deal with the consequences of physiological aging of the kidney and the reasons will be examined why these modifications in the elderly are capable of conditioning a different reaction in the presence of a stressful or pathological situation in respect to the young.

1.1. Anatomic Changes of the Aging Kidney

Aging is associated with a gradual reduction in renal mass, affecting preferentially the cortex, so that renal weight decreases from 250–270 g to 180–200 g between the ages of 30 to 90 years (1,2). Glomerulosclerosis is the main factor related to these changes and the number of sclerotic glomeruli increases from 1% in the young adult to 20–30% at age 80 (3). The functional glomeruli show a mesangial expansion and thickness in the glomerular basal membrane (4). Also the vascular component with age undergoes typical changes. In the cortex, afferent arterioles undergo complete atrophy. In the juxtamedullary area a different pattern of change in arteriolar-glomerular units occurs: afferent and efferent arterioles become continuous so forming a shunt. The result is that while in the cortex blood flow is reduced, it is maintained in the medulla (5). This relative increase in medullary blood flow may interfere with the capacity of the countercurrent system and may compromise the urinary concentrating mechanism in the elderly subjects (6).

In the tubules, the aging process leads to a decrease in number and length of proximal tubules and distal tubules develop more diverticula (5,7).

Recent Advances in Geriatrics, edited by Barbagallo, Licata, and Sowers.
Plenum Press, New York, 1998.

1.2. Functional Changes

The anatomical alterations of the aged kidney are also associated with functional changes. Many cross sectional studies have found a fall in renal blood flow (RBF) after the age of fourty of about 10% per decade so that RBF decreases from 600 ml/min/1.73 m^2 in the adult to 300 in the elderly aged 80 years (Fig. 1) (8,9). The decrease in RBF is associated with a significant increase in afferent and efferent arteriolar resistance (8).

Hollenberg et al. (10) using the xenon washout technique in 311 healthy potential kidney donors, showed a progressive decrease in RBF per unit of renal mass with aging, suggesting that the decrease in RBF is not secondary to the reduction of mass but is primarily involved in causing the parenchymal loss. Cross-sectional studies, using a variety of methodologies, have shown that GFR progressively decreases with aging, falling after 30 years at the rate of 8 ml/min/1.73 m^2 per decade (11). These results were confirmed in the Baltimore Longitudinal Study of Aging in which a large number of normal volunteers were followed for at least 23 years. The mean decrease in creatinine clearance was 0.75 ml/min per year and there was a normal distribution around the mean. Of particular interest however, was a 36% of subjects that had no absolute decrease in creatinine clearance (12). These data suggest that the age-related loss of glomerular function is not a phenomenon necessarily connected with aging but dietary, metabolic, hormonal or hemodynamic factors may play a role. The GFR decreased less than the RBF so that filtration fraction is increased (11,12). The mechanism is probably due to a vasoconstriction of efferent arteriole greater than in afferent arteriole, with a consequent increase in intraglomerular pressure. This hyperfiltrating condition of the aging kidney represents the adaptation to a reduced number of functioning glomeruli, but this rise in intraglomerular pressure may lead in time to glomerulosclerosis (13,14). The fall in creatinine clearance with age is not accompanied by a rise in serum creatinine that remains substantially unchanged due to the parallel reduction of daily production of creatinine secondary to decreasing muscle mass. Thus, the serum creatinine concentration usually underestimates the decline in GFR in the elderly (12).

Also the renal tubular function is impaired with aging and in particular there is an age-related decrease in the capacity to concentrate urine. The reason for this change is a reduced responsiveness of collecting duct cells to ADH and a decreased capacity of the kidney to elaborate maximally concentrated urine. In fact in the aging kidney, as mentioned above, the countercurrent system has a reduced capacity in generating medullary hypertonicity (15,16). In consequence, elderly patients need a larger urine volume to excrete the obligatory daily solute load of 600 mOsm. The ability to dilute urine and to excrete a water load has not been extensively evaluated but seems to decrease with age

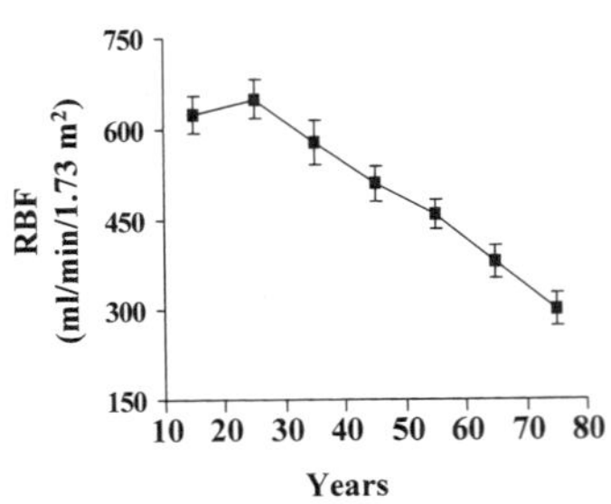

Figure 1. Age-related decline of renal blood flow (RBF). From (9) modified.

consequently to the fall in GFR (17). Acid excretion, glucose and aminoacid transport are narrowed in the aging kidney (18,19). The aging kidney is also unable to achieve sodium balance and it reacts to salt deprivation with an impaired sodium conservation. It may be due to defects in the renin-aldosterone axis that have been repeatedly demonstrated in the elderly (17). Tsunoda et al. (20) found that, although the total renin is normal in the aged, there is an age-dependent decline in active renin and in aldosterone concentration. Elderly people have a defect in urinary acidification that may be unapparent under baseline conditions when the acid-base parameters, such as serum bicarbonate and pH, may be normal. Frequently, however, the serum bicarbonate level is low, normal or slightly depressed due to an age-related reduction in the capacity of excreting an acid load (21).

2. RENAL RESPONSE TO ADRENERGIC STIMULATION

In normal conditions the aging kidney carries out its function until very advanced age. However, the various age-related alterations and in particular the condition of increased glomerular pressure leads to a reduction in renal physiologic reserve. This concept may explain the well-known clinical observation that the aging kidney is particularly vulnerable to chronic diseases such as diabetes or high blood pressure (14,22). But this frailty also reveals itself under non pathological conditions, in particular when involving vasoconstrictive stimuli, such as stress provoking situations (23,24), or administration of drugs usually well tolerated by the young (25).

However, the problem of selectively testing the way in which the aging kidney bears the impact of vasoconstrictive challenges has not yet been specifically addressed. Equally unexplored in these conditions is the participation of many vasoactive systems, such as renal eicosanoids, renin-angiotensin and various endothelium-derived substances. All these factors participate in the regulation of renal hemodynamics (26,27) but are altered during the aging process (28,29).

To have some understanding of the possible mechanisms of the shift from vasoconstriction to ischemic damage or renal failure, it is mandatory to explain the physiologic renal response to adrenergic stimulation in its integrated setting of hormonal reactions. These considerations prompted us systematically to investigate the differences between the young and elderly in their response to an acute adrenergic stimulation. In the first part of this section we present the hemodynamic and neurohumoral response induced in the young by applying a reproducible method of adrenergic stimulation. The second part deals with preliminary data concerning the changes, associated with aging, in the response to adrenergic stimulation.

2.1. Effects of Adrenergic Stimulation in the Young

Adrenergic stimulation was induced by a well-defined mental stress such as the Fair Culture Test, a multiple-choice image questionnaire. This test was preferred to other forms of psychological stimuli, given that it does not require any degree of cultural background, such as the solving of arithmetic problems or the reading of a text. Indeed, the Fair Culture Test can be administered at any age, without any regard to scholastic level (30,31). The test is made up of 50 questions, subdivided into four sets; each set is preceded by a full explanation and a preliminary test. To elicit a maximal anxiety reaction, the time given for answering all questions is carefully controlled. This is a fundamental feature of the stimulus, given that time dependence is known to elicit significant and increasing anxiety whenever an intellectual performance is urged. All aspects of the testing have to be completed within 30 minutes, according to the study protocol.

The study was performed after sodium and potassium balance had reached equilibration. To achieve a constant urinary flow, subjects were studied under moderate hydration. Experiments were performed with the subject in the supine position. A catheter was inserted into the urinary bladder to collect urinary samples and a catheter needle into the antecubital vein to collect blood samples. Renal clearances of iodine ^{131}I-labeled hyppurate and iodine ^{125}I-labeled iotalamate were used for measurement of renal plasma flow and glomerular filtration rate respectively. The study consisted of four successive 30-minute experimental periods: baseline determinations, mental stress and two recovery periods. Experiments were carried out in women, given that in males urinary prostaglandins may have an extrarenal origin.

In young volunteers mental stress induced sympathetic activation as evidenced by significant increase in blood pressure, heart rate (Fig. 2) and plasma norepinephrine that were limited to the period stimulus administration (30). Mental stress was also associated with significant changes in renal hemodynamics almost limited to the period of adrenergic activation. Renal plasma flow significantly decreased and renal vascular resistance increased during mental stress (Fig. 3). On the contrary, the GFR did not vary throughout the experiment and filtration fraction increased during mental stress and the first recovery period (Fig 3).

Together with the hemodynamic changes, MS induced complex neuroendocrine response in the kidney characterized by a significant increase in endothelin-1 and PGE_2 (Fig. 4). Urinary endothelin-1 increased during mental stress and the first recovery period when compared with baseline values. $UPGE_2$ increased with growing intensity up to the second recovery period, when it reached a peak value that was four times higher than the baseline (Fig. 4). Urinary 6-Keto-$PGF_1\alpha$ increased during mental stress and the two recovery periods (15.0 ± 6.0; 17.0 ± 8.0 and 15.0 ± 4.0 pg/ERPF respectively vs. a baseline value of 12.0 ± 0.1, $p < 0.001$). $UPGF_2\alpha$ and $UTXB_2$ did not significantly increase. Cyclic GMP rose only during the stimulus (71.8 ± 39.9 pmol/ERPF during mental stress vs. 40.4 ± 21.4 pmol/ERPF; $p < 0.05$) and subsequently dropped to baseline value during the first recovery period.

In conclusion, in the healthy young individual sympathetic stimulation induced by mental stress provokes a hemodynamic response which is characterized by a transient reduction in renal plasma flow, while glomerular filtration rate is maintained constant. This renal response is mediated by changes and interactions of several local neurohumoral systems. Sympathetic activation stimulates renal endothelin-1, whose long-lasting vasoconstrictive activity is modulated by renal vasodilating systems in two successive phases. In the first rapid phase the modulating activity of nitric oxide prevails. In the second phase the activity of ET-1 is mainly counteracted by renal PGE_2 during at least a 60-minute period.

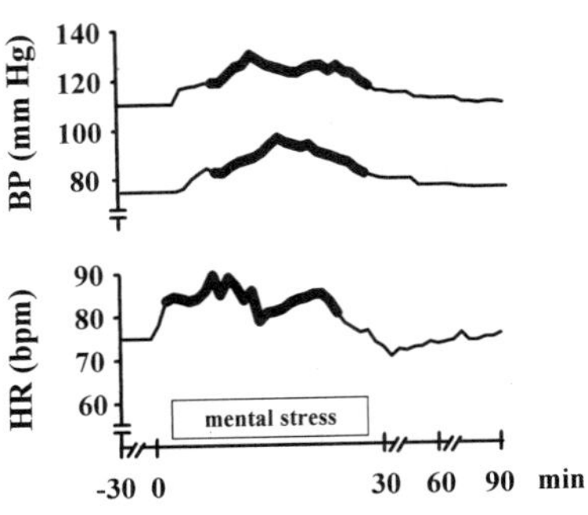

Figure 2. Effects of mental stress on blood pressure (BP) and heart rate (HR) in 8 healthy, young volunteers (age 31±6 years). The extra heavy line indicates values significantly different from baseline ($p < 0.001$ for each curve, LSD test, ANOVA). From (30) with permission.

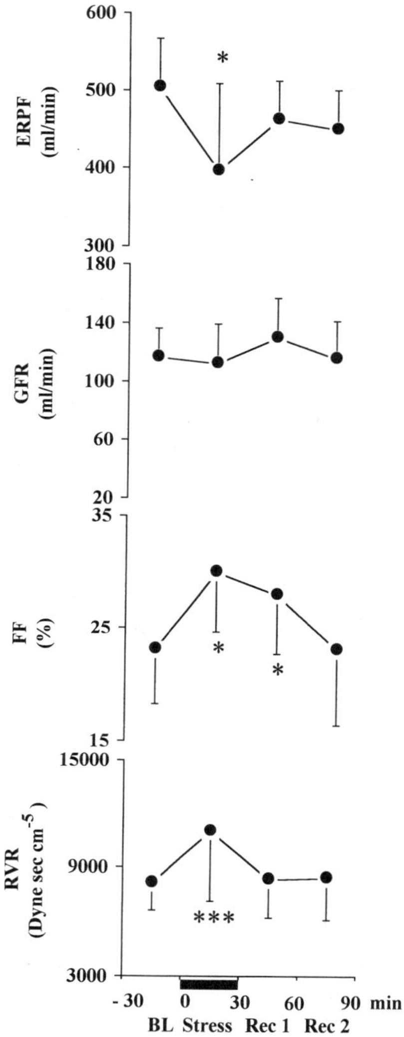

Figure 3. Effects of mental stress on renal hemodynamics in 8 healthy, young volunteers (age 31±6 years) (mean values ± SD). * $p < 0.05$ and *** $p < 0.001$ vs baseline, respectively (LSD test, ANOVA). Effective renal plasma flow (ERPF): $F = 3.60$, $p = 0.03$, ANOVA for the whole curve. Glomerular filtration rate (GFR): $F = 1.03$, p = ns, ANOVA for the whole curve. Filtration fraction (FF): $F = 3.53$, $p = 0.03$, ANOVA for the whole curve. Renal vascular resistance (RVR): $F = 8.50$, $p = 0.0001$, ANOVA for the whole curve.

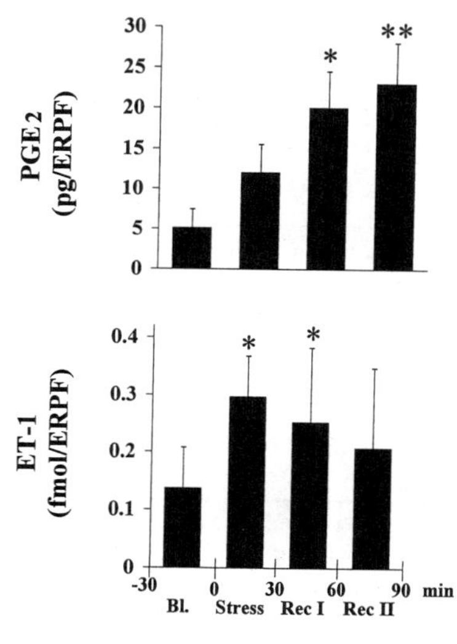

Figure 4. Effects of mental stress on urinary prostaglandin E2 (UPGE2) and endothelin 1 (UET-1) in 8 healthy, young volunteers (age 31 ± 6 years) (mean values ± SD). * $p < 0.05$ and ** $p < 0.01$ vs baseline, respectively (LSD test, ANOVA).

2.2. Effects of Adrenergic Stimulation in the Elderly

In the elderly, changes in systemic hemodynamics (blood pressure, heart rate and plasma catecholamines) induced during the application of mental stress were similar to the young. On the contrary, the effects on renal hemodynamics were significantly different. While in the young changes in renal blood flow were limited to the period of mental stress, in the elderly ERPF decreased progressively reaching the greatest fall 60 minutes after mental stress. Renal vascular resistance began to rise during MS and peaked during the second recovery period (Tab. 1).

Therefore in the elderly, MS causes a renal vasoconstriction which was both greater in magnitude and longer lasting than in the younger subjects. But in spite of the pronounced and prolonged reductions in renal blood flow, the aging kidney was still capable of maintaining a constant glomerular filtration rate during the whole experiment. This was achieved at the expense of a further and marked increase in intraglomerular pressure, as indicated by the increase in filtration fraction which was prolonged throughout the second recovery period (Tab. 1).

These data are still preliminary because limited to the hemodynamic compartment. The study is still in progress and is going to be completed with the definition of the renal neurohormonal profile, which will allow a better understanding of renal changes with aging. However, hemodynamic changes themselves already seem to outline the reason for the greater vulnerability of the aging kidney in certain conditions. The hemodynamic pattern of the aging kidney is characterized by a vasoconstrictive response to a stressful event, albeit with a preserved capability to maintain a constant glomerular filtration rate. It is not surprising that when the stressful event superimposes itself not on a normal physiological pattern but on a condition of increased activity of either renin-angiotensin or adrenergic systems, renal failure may be initiated. Conditions of increased activation of the renin-angiotensin system may be primed by the occurrence of hypovolemia and/or hypotension (23,24). A strong adrenergic stimulation, on the other hand, is a constant feature of acute myocardial infarction or heart failure. However, an increased risk for the aging kidney may also be represented by the use of nonsteroidal anti-inflammatory drugs leading to inhibition of vasodilating renal prostaglandins (32). And finally chronic conditions such as

Table 1. Effects of mental stress on renal hemodynamics in 6 healthy elderly (72.3 ± 5.0 years) and in 8 healthy, young volunteers (age 31 ± 6 years) (mean values ± SD)

	Age	Baseline (30 min)	Mental stress (30 min)	Recovery 1 (30 min)	Recovery 2 (30 min)	ANOVA for the whole curve F	p
ERPF (ml/min)	E	391.8 ± 84.5	307.2 ± 95.6*	299.0 ± 74.4*	253.0 ± 50.8**	3.58	0.04
	Y	503.7 ± 63.3	395.8 ± 113.0***	462.4 ± 50.2	450.1 ± 50.9	5.92	0.01
GFR (ml/min)	E	99.6 ± 13.1	90.3 ± 17.9	91.5 ± 19.5	86.5 ± 13.7	1.04	ns
	Y	116.4 ± 19.9	112.2 ± 27.0	129.9 ± 27.3	116.0 ± 25.7	0.69	ns
FF (%)	E	25.9 ± 4.7	30.6 ± 5.4	31.5 ± 5.3*	35.2 ± 6.5**	3.32	0.05
	Y	23.0 ± 4.0	30.3 ± 6.0*	28.0 ± 7.0*	23.0 ± 5.0	5.18	0.01
RVR (Dyne sec cm^{-5})	E	10500 ± 3200	14620 ± 3040*	15040 ± 6020*	16600 ± 5550**	3.50	0.04
	Y	8100 ± 1500	11000 ± 3900***	8300 ± 2100	8400 ± 2300	10.2	0.0006

E = elderly (n=6); Y = young (n=8). ERPF, effective renal plasma flow, F=32.8, p<0.0001 (MANOVA between the two curves); GFR, glomerular filtration rate, F=21.0, p<0.0001 (MANOVA between the two curves); FF, filtration fraction, F=7.7, p<0.01 (MANOVA between the two curves); RVR, Renal vascular resistance, F=24.3, p<0.0001 (MANOVA between the two curves). * = p < 0.05, ** = p<0.01; *** = p<0.001 vs. baseline (LSD test, ANOVA), ns, not significant.

high blood pressure or diabetes (14,22,33) may interfere with the normal aging process of the renal vasculature therefore enhancing the vasoconstrictive response of the aging kidney to stressful situations, ultimately leading to renal failure.

REFERENCES

1. McLachlan M: Anatomic structural and vascular changes in the aging kidney, in Nunez JFM, Cameron JS (eds): *Renal Function and Disease in the Elderly*. London, Butterworths, 1987, pp 3–26.
2. Anderson S, Brenner BM: Effects of aging on the renal glomerulus. *Am J Med* 80:435–442, 1986
3. Brown WW, Davis BB, Spry LA, Wongsurawat N, Malone JD, Domoto DT: Aging and the kidney. *Arch Intern Med* 146:1790–1796, 1986
4. Kappel B, Olsen S: Cortical interstitial tissue and sclerosed glomeruli in the normal human kidney, related to age and sex. *Virchows Arch A Path Anat and Histol* 387:271–277, 1980
5. Fliser D, Ritz E, Franek E: Renal reserve in the elderly. *Seminars in Nephrology* 15, 463–467, 1995
6. Goyal VK: Changes with age in the human kidney. *Exp Gerontol.* 17: 321–331, 1982
7. Takazakura E, Sawabu N, Handa A, Takada A, Shinoda A, Takeuchi J: Intrarenal vascular changes with age and disease. *Kidney Int* 2: 224–230, 1972
8. Darmady EM: The parameters of the aging kidney. *J Pathol* 109: 195–201, 1977
9. Davies DF, Shock NW: Age changes in glomerular filtration rate, effective renal plasma flow, and tubular excretory capacity in adult males. *J Clin Invest* 29: 496–507, 1950
10. Hollenberg NK, Adams DF, Solomon HS, Rashid A, Abram LA, Merril JP: Senescence and the renal vasculature in normal man. *Circ Res* 34, 309- 316, 1974
11. Meyer BR: Renal function in aging. *J Am Geriatr Soc* 37: 791–860, 1989
12. Rowe JW, Andres RA, Tobin JD, Norris AH, Shock NW: The effect of age on creatinine clearance in man: a cross sectional and longitudinal study. *J Gerontol.* 31: 155–163, 1976
13. Brenner BM, Meyer TW, Hostetter TH: Dietary protein intake and progressive nature of kidney disease: the role of hemodinamically mediated glomerular injury in the pathogenesis of progressive glomerular sclerosis in aging, renal ablation and intrinsic renal disease. *N Engl J Med* 307: 652–659, 1982
14. Guasch A, Hashimoto H, Sibley RK: Glomerular disfunction in nephrotic humans with minimal changes or focal glomerulosclerosis. *Am J Physiol* 260: F728, 1991
15. Rowe JW, Shock NW, DeFronzo RA: The influence of age on the renal response to water deprivation in man. *Nephron* 17:270–278, 1976
16. Epstein M, Hollenberg NK: Age as a determinant of renal sodium conservation in normal man. *J Lab Clin Med* 7: 411–417, 1979
17. Belmin J, Lewy BI, Michel JB: Changes in the renin-angiotensin-aldosterone axis in later life. *Drugs Aging* 5: 391–400, 1994
18. De Santo NG, Anastasio P, Coppola S, Barba G, Jadanza A, Capasso G: Age-related changes in renal reserve and renal tubular function in healthy humans. *Child Nephrol.Urol.* 11, 33–40, 1991
19. Crowe MJ: Alterated water excretion in healthy elderly men. *Age Ageing* 16: 285–290, 1987
20. Tsunoda K, Abe K, Goto T, Yasujima M, Sato M, Omata K, Seino M, Yoshinaga K: Effect of age on the renin-angiotensin-aldosterone system in normal subjects: simultaneous measurement of active and inactive renin, renin substrate and aldosterone in plasma. *J Clin Endocrinol Metab* 62:384–389, 1986
21. Adler S, Lindeman RD Yengst MJ: Effects of acute acid loading on urinary acid excretion by the aging human kidney. *J Lab Clin Med* 72: 278–289, 1968
22. Klag MJ, Whelton PK, Randall BL, Neaton JD, Brancati FL, Ford C, Shulman NB, Stamler J: Blood pressure and end stage renal disease in men. *N Engl J Med* 334: 13–18, 1996
23. Kenney WL, Zappe DH: Effect of age on renal blood flow during exercise. *Aging Clin Exp Res* 6: 293–302, 1994
24. Tinetti ME: Effects of stress on renal function in the elderly. *J Am Geriatr Soc* 31:174–181, 1983
25. Taha A, Lenton RJ, Murdoch PS, Peden NR: Non-oliguric renal failure during treatment with mefenamic acid in elderly patients: a continuing problem. *Br Med J* 291:661–662, 1985
26. Schnermann J, Briggs JP, Weber PC: Tubuloglomerular feedback, prostaglandins and angiotensin in the autoregulation of glomerular filtration rate. *Kidney Int* 25: 53–64, 1984
27. Rabelink TJ, Kaasjager KHA, Boer P, Stroes EG, Braam B, Koomans HA: Effects of endothelin-1 on renal function in humans: implications for physiology and pathophysiology. *Kidney Int* 46: 376–381, 1994.

28. Luft FC, Fineberg NS, Weinberger MH: The influence of age on renal function and renin and aldosterone responses to sodium-volume expansion and contraction in normotensive and mildly hypertensive humans. *Am J Hypertens* 5:520–528, 1992
29. Rathaus M, Greenfeld Z, Podjarny E, Brezis M, Green J, Bernheim J: Altered prostaglandin synthesis and impaired sodium conservation in the kidneys of old rats. *Clinical Science* 83: 301–306, 1992
30. Castellani S, Ungar A, La Cava G, Cantini C, Stefanile C, Camaiti A, Messeri G, Coppo M, Vallotti B, Di Serio C, Brocchi A, Masotti G: Renal adaptation to stress: a possible role of endothelin release and prostaglandins modulation in the human. *J Lab Clin Med* 129: 462–469, 1997.
31. Cattel RB, Feingold SN, Sarason SB: A culture free intelligence test. II. Evaluation of cultural influences on test performance. *J Educ Psychol* 32:81–100, 1941
32. Stillman MT, Schlesinger PA: Nonsteroidal anti-inflammatory drug nephrotoxicity. *Arch Intern Med* 150: 268–270, 1990.
33. Anderson S, Brenner BM: Effects of aging on the renal glomerulus. *Am J Med* 80: 435–442, 1986

6

AGING AND ENDOTHELIAL FUNCTION

Stefano Taddei, Agostino Virdis, Lorenzo Ghiadoni, and Antonio Salvetti*

Cattedra di Medicina Interna
Dipartimento di Medicina Interna
University of Pisa, Italy

INTRODUCTION

Endothelial cells play an important local regulatory role by secreting substances that control both vascular tone and structure[1]. The best characterized endothelium-derived relaxing factor (EDRF) is nitric oxide (NO)[2,3], which is derived from the metabolism of L-Arginine[4], by NO synthase (NOS)[5], a constitutive enzyme present in endothelial cells.

NO is produced and released both tonically and under the influence of endothelial agonists, such as acetylcholine, bradykinin, substance P, serotonin and others acting on specific receptors[1], and by mechanical forces, such as shear stress[6].

In several pathological conditions such as hypertension, diabetes mellitus, atherosclerosis, vasospasm and reperfusion injury, activation of endothelial cells can lead to the production and release of contracting factors. Such substances are mainly cyclooxygenase-derived endothelium-dependent contracting factors (EDCFs), at this time partially identified with prostanoids (TXA2 and PGH2)[7,8] and superoxide anions[9], which counteract the relaxing activity of NO.

However it is worth noting that superoxide anions can also impair endothelial function by causing NO breakdown[10].

As shown in Fig. 1, NO and EDCFs not only exert an opposite effect on vascular tone but also respectively inhibit and activate those mechanisms such as platelet aggregation[11,12], vascular smooth cell proliferation[13] and migration[14], monocyte adhesion[15] and adhesion molecule expression[16] that exert an important role in the genesis of thrombosis and atherosclerotic plaque. Thus endothelial dysfunction, caused by an impairment of the L-Arginine-NO pathway[17] and production of EDCFs[18], can be considered a relevant mechanism causing atherosclerosis and thrombosis.

This hypothesis is in agreement with the finding that endothelial dysfunction is detectable in presence of various cardiovascular risk factors, such as hypertension[17–20], hypercholesterolemia[21,22], diabetes mellitus[23,24] and smoking[25,26], and that the association of several risk factors further impairs endothelial function[26]. In the present paper we will

* Address for correspondence: Antonio Salvetti, Cattedra di Medicina Italiana, Clinica Medica I, Via Roma 67, 56100 Pisa, Italy. Fax: +39-50-553407

Recent Advances in Geriatrics, edited by Barbagallo, Licata, and Sowers.
Plenum Press, New York, 1998.

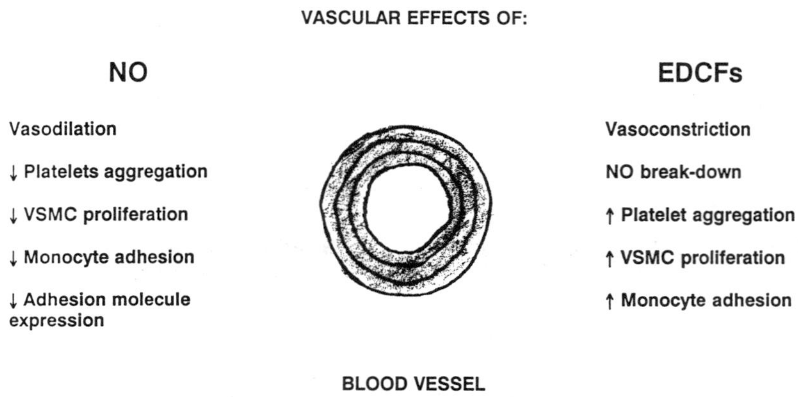

Figure 1. Functional and structural effects of endothelium-derived nitric oxide (NO) and contracting factors (EDCFs) on blood vessel wall.

examine the influence of aging on endothelial function both in normotensive subjects and in hypertensive patients, the mechanism(s) through which aging can modify endothelial function and finally the relationship between aging, gender and endothelial function.

AGING AND ENDOTHELIAL FUNCTION

Experimental data indicate that aging alters endothelium-dependent relaxation in rat large and small resistance arteries[27–31]. These findings have been documented in both epicardial coronary arteries and coronary microcirculation in humans[32–35].

However human coronary arteries can be affected by early atherosclerosis not detectable by angiography, a process known to impair endothelial function[33]. To avoid the presence of this confounding factor, we performed a study on normocholesterolemic normotensive subjects to examine whether aging can alter endothelial function in the forearm, which is a district not usually affected by atherosclerosis[36]. Data obtained so far indicate that the maximum forearm vasodilating response to acetylcholine, as well as the slope of the forearm blood flow response to acetylcholine, showed a significant inverse correlation with increasing age (maximum FBF response: $r = -0.86$, $p < 0.001$; slope of the FBF response: $r = -0.83$, $p < 0.001$) (Fig. 2). On the other hand, vasodilation to sodium nitroprusside, an endothelium-independent vasodilator, was minimally affected by aging (maximum FBF response: $r = -0.37$, $p < 0.01$; slope of the FBF response: $r = -0.37$, $p < 0.01$). These data, which were thereafter confirmed by others, clearly indicate that aging per se impairs endothelium-dependent vasodilation in healthy subjects with no cardiovascular risk factors, such as diabetes, hypercholesterolemia and hypertension[36].

Similar findings have been obtained in patients with essential hypertension[36]. As compared to normotensive subjects, hypertensive patients showed an impaired endothelial-dependent vasodilation. However, in these patients we found also an inverse relationship between increasing age and the maximum forearm blood flow response to acetylcholine ($r = -0.85$; $p < 0.001$) as well as to the slope of the forearm blood response to acetylcholine ($r = -0.83$; $p < 0.001$) (Fig. 2). In contrast, forearm vasodilation to sodium nitroprusside was showed a poor inverse correlation with patient age (maximum FBF response : $r = -0.36$, $p < 0.01$; slope of the FBF response : $r = -0.30$, $p < 0.05$). Thus, aging impairs endothelium-dependent vasodilation not only in normotensive subjects but also in essential hypertensive

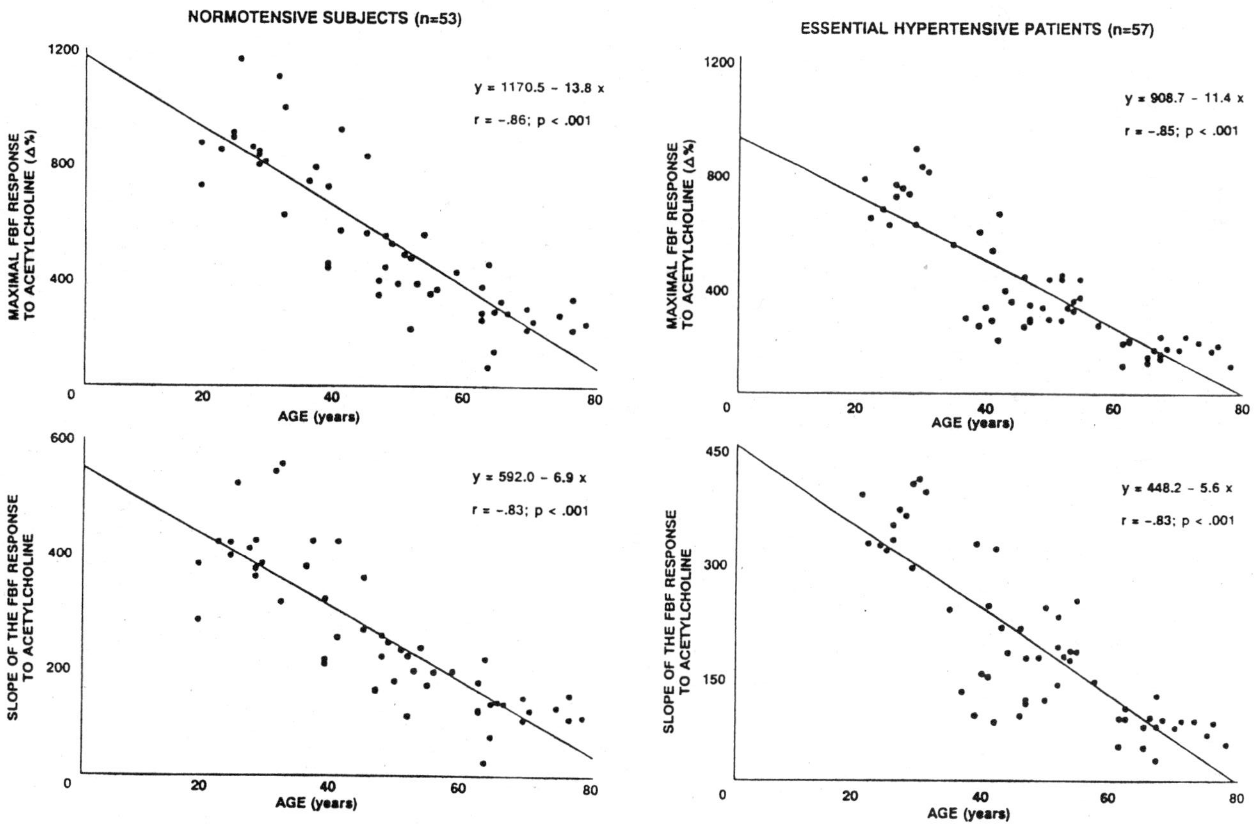

Figure 2. Scatterplot of relation between age (x axis) and maximum (top) or slope (bottom) of the forearm blood flow (FBF) to acetylcholine (y axis) in normotensive control subjects (left) and essential hypertensive patients (right). The maximum effect is calculated as percent increase above basal level, and the slope (percent increase in blood flow/log[dose]) is determined using a linear regression analysis. Adapted from ref 36, with permission.

patients. This latter finding is of particular interest since it indicates that advancing age is such a powerful inductor of endothelial dysfunction that it is possible to detect its negative effect even in the presence of hypertension, which itself is a clinical condition able to cause impaired endothelium-dependent vasodilation.

MECHANISMS OF AGE-INDUCED ENDOTHELIAL DYSFUNCTION

The mechanisms through which aging impairs endothelium-dependent vasodilation may involve various different alterations. In a study evaluating endothelial function in normotensive subjects and essential hypertensive patients at different ages (from 18 to 70 years)[37], the integrity of the L-arginine NO-pathway was tested by evaluating the effect of L-arginine, the substrate for NO-synthase, on vasodilation to acetylcholine, while the production of cyclooxygenase dependent EDCF was evaluated by testing the effect of indomethacin. In normotensive subjects younger than 30 years neither L-arginine nor indomethacin affected the vasodilation induced by acetylcholine, indicating that at this age endothelial function is preserved (Fig. 3). In normotensive subjects aged between 31 and 60 years, while indomethacin was still devoid of any effect on acetylcholine-induced vasodilation, L-arginine restored endothelial function as compared to the youngest subgroup (Fig. 3). Finally, in normotensive individuals older than 60 years, both L-arginine and indomethacin were able to increase the vascular response to acetylcholine (Fig. 3). These results seem to indicate that in normotensive subjects endothelial dysfunction starts after 30 years, and up to 60 years is mainly caused by an alteration in the L-arginine-NO pathway. Only after 60 years does EDCF production participate in causing dysfunction of endothelium-dependent vasodilation. The same mechanisms operate in essential hypertensive patients, the only difference being time of appearance. Thus in young (< 30 years) essential hypertensive patients the blunted response to acetylcholine was restored by intrabrachial administration of L-arginine while indomethacin was ineffective (Fig. 3). In older hypertensives, on the other hand (between 31 and 45 years) L-arginine still augmented the vasodilation to acetylcholine and indomethacin also increased the response to the highest concentration of the muscarinic agonist (Fig. 3). In two further groups of older essential hypertensive patients (46–60 and > 60 years, respectively) L-arginine no longer improved the vasodilation to acetylcholine, which, in contrast, was potentiated by indomethacin (Fig. 3). Thus the relationship between aging and endothelial dysfunction seems to be mediated by different mechanisms according to which age range is considered. In essential hypertensive patients younger than 30 years, endothelial dysfunction seems to be selectively caused by a defect in the L-arginine-NO pathway. In patients older than 30 years the alteration in the L-arginine-NO pathway is still present and reversible when production of cyclooxygenase-dependent EDCF starts to be detectable, although when endothelial cells are stimulated by high concentrations of the agonist. After the age of 45, the defective NO production and/or release is no longer reversible by administration of L-arginine and, in addition, EDCF production is augmented. Given this finding that the mechanisms responsible for aging and hypertension related endothelial dysfunction are the same, and that the only difference consists in time of appearance, it is conceivable that impaired endothelium-dependent vasodilation in essential hypertension could be a mere acceleration of changes seen in advancing age.

What is the nature of EDCF, whose production, as described above, seems to be associated with increasing age? First, the possibility that these substances could curtail endothelium-dependent vasodilation not only by inducing vasoconstriction, but also by

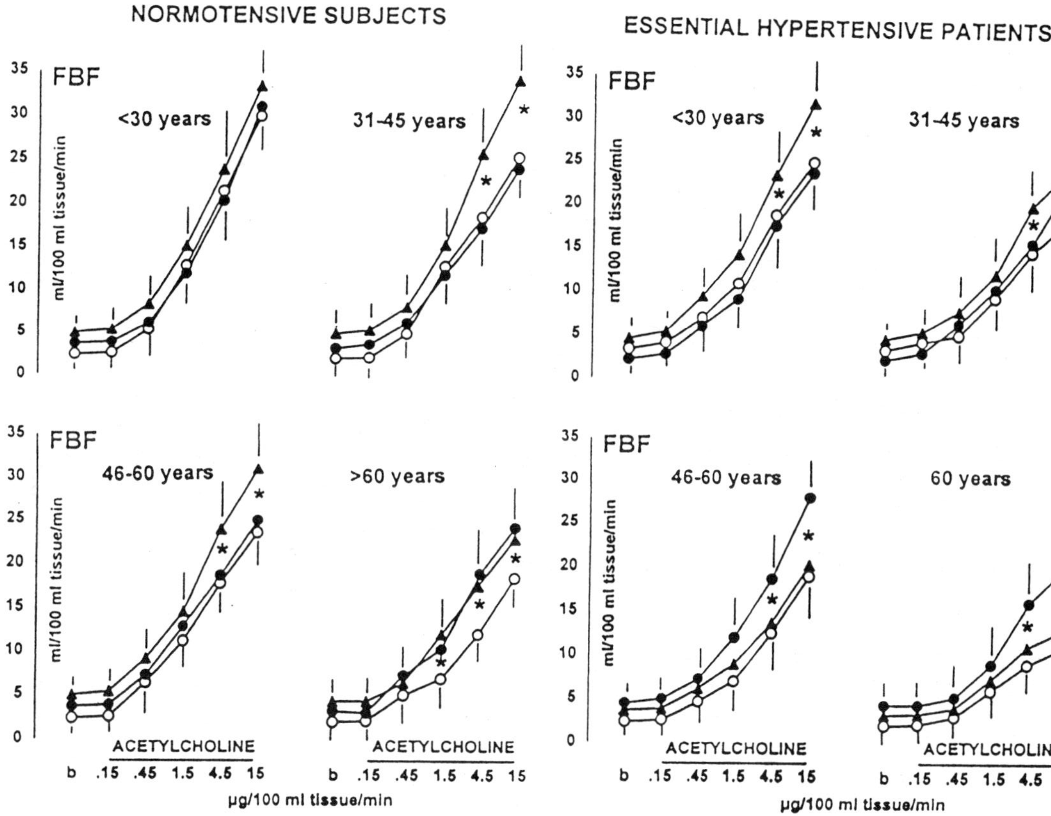

Figure 3. Line graphs show forearm blood flow increase above basal (b) induced by intra-arterial acetylcholine under control conditions (○; saline infusion) and in presence of intra-arterial L-arginine (▲; 1 μmol/100 ml forearm tissue/min) or indomethacin (●; 50 μg/100 ml forearm tissue/min) in four groups of normotensive subjects (left) and essential hypertensive patients (right) characterized by a different age profile (<30 years, n=10 normotensive, n=10 hypertensive; 31–45 years, n=12 normotensive, n=14 hypertensive; 46–60 years, n=11 normotensive, n=12 hypertensive; >60 years, n=10 normotensive, n=11 hypertensive). Data shown as means ± SEM and expressed as absolute values. *Significant difference between saline and L-arginine or indomethacin ($p < 0.05$ or less). Adapted from ref 37, with permission.

impairing the L-arginine-NO pathway was tested. It was shown that in essential hypertensive patients (aged around 50 years) cyclooxygenase blockade by indomethacin restores the facilitating and inhibiting effect of L-arginine and L-NMMA on vasodilation to acetylcholine respectively, indicating that cyclooxygenase-derived EDCFs can at least partially impair the NO-system[38]. On the basis of the experimental literature, the most likely candidates as the cause of NO breakdown are superoxide anions[10]. In line with this possibility, preliminary observations[39] showed that intrabrachial administration of vitamin C, a superoxide anion scavenger, increases the vasodilating response to acetylcholine in the forearm vasculature of essential hypertensive patients, but not of normotensive controls. Since vitamin C does not alter vasodilation to sodium nitroprusside, these findings support the hypothesis that production of superoxide anions could be one of the mechanisms responsible for endothelial dysfunction in essential hypertension. Whether and to what degree cyclooxygenase-dependent prostanoids also take part in this vascular abnormality is still to be established, since at the present time selective antagonists for the thromboxane A_2/prostaglandin H_2 receptor or inhibitors of thromboxane synthase are not available for intraarterial human utilization.

In conclusion, this line of evidence makes it possible to assume that aging-related endothelial dysfunction starts as an alteration in the NO pathway and only in old age does EDCF production start to be detectable. In essential hypertensive patients the onset of L-arginine-NO pathway dysfunction is anticipated as compared to normotensive subjects, although the dysfunction is still reversible by L-arginine administration. At around 45 years, EDCF production starts to be detectable and L-arginine can no longer correct blunted endothelium-dependent vasodilation. Thus it is tempting to speculate that at this age, cyclooxygenase-dependent superoxide anion production causes a further impairment in the L-arginine-NO pathway by NO breakdown and, as a consequence, the NO-pathway alteration is no longer reversible by increasing substrate availability.

AGING, GENDER, AND ENDOTHELIAL FUNCTION

It is well documented that menopause and consequent estrogen deprivation increase the risk of cardiovascular disease in women[40,41]. However the mechanisms responsible for the cardioprotective effect of estrogen in women are not clear. Although the estrogen-mediated favourable affect on lipid profile can explain around 50% of the beneficial effect of the hormone on cardiovascular risk[42–44], increasing evidence supports the possibility that estrogens can act directly on the arterial wall by improving endothelial function[45–47]. Therefore the possibility exists that the augmented prevalence of cardiovascular disease in post-menopausal women could be related to endothelial dysfunction caused by endogenous estrogen deficiency.

To address this issue we examined whether the onset of menopause is associated with detectable impairment of endothelium-dependent vasodilation either in healthy women or female patients with essential hypertension[48]. To distinguish the possible role of menopause from the age-related decline in endothelial function, we compared endothelium-dependent vasodilation in matched women and men, to ascertain whether females are characterized by an attenuation of age-dependent endothelial dysfunction when still menstruating and by a sharp worsening after menopause compared to males.

In our study population we confirmed the presence of endothelial dysfunction in essential hypertension. In addition, in both normotensive and hypertensive subjects a highly significant inverse correlation was confirmed between increasing age and response to acetylcholine (normotensive subjects: $r = -0.88$, $p < 0.001$; hypertensive patients: $r = -0.87$, $p < 0.001$) while only a weaker negative correlation was observed between the vasodilating effect of sodium nitroprusside and aging (normotensive subjects: $r = -46$, $p < 0.01$; hypertensive patients: $r = -48$, $p < 0.01$). Taken together this evidence reinforces the possibility that aging is associated with endothelial dysfunction[36,37].

However the main finding of our study was that menopause affects endothelium-dependent, but not endothelium-independent, vasodilation both in normotensive subjects and essential hypertensive patients. Thus in normotensive males endothelial responses started to decline after age 30 years and the derangement was gradual and progressive until old age (Fig. 4). In contrast, in premenopausal normotensive women, advancing age only slightly affected endothelium-dependent vasodilation while after menopause endothelium-dependent vasodilation showed a steeper decline as compared to men (Fig. 4). It is important to observe that the gender-related difference in endothelium-dependent vasodilation was no longer evident after 60 years. In male essential hypertensive patients advancing age was associated with a decrease in endothelium-dependent vasodilation to acetylcholine, which was more evident up to 40 years, after which the rate of decline started to slow (Fig. 4). The more rapid decline in endothelium-dependent vasodilation in younger hypertensive men as compared to those aged over 40 years reinforces the possibility, previously discussed, that

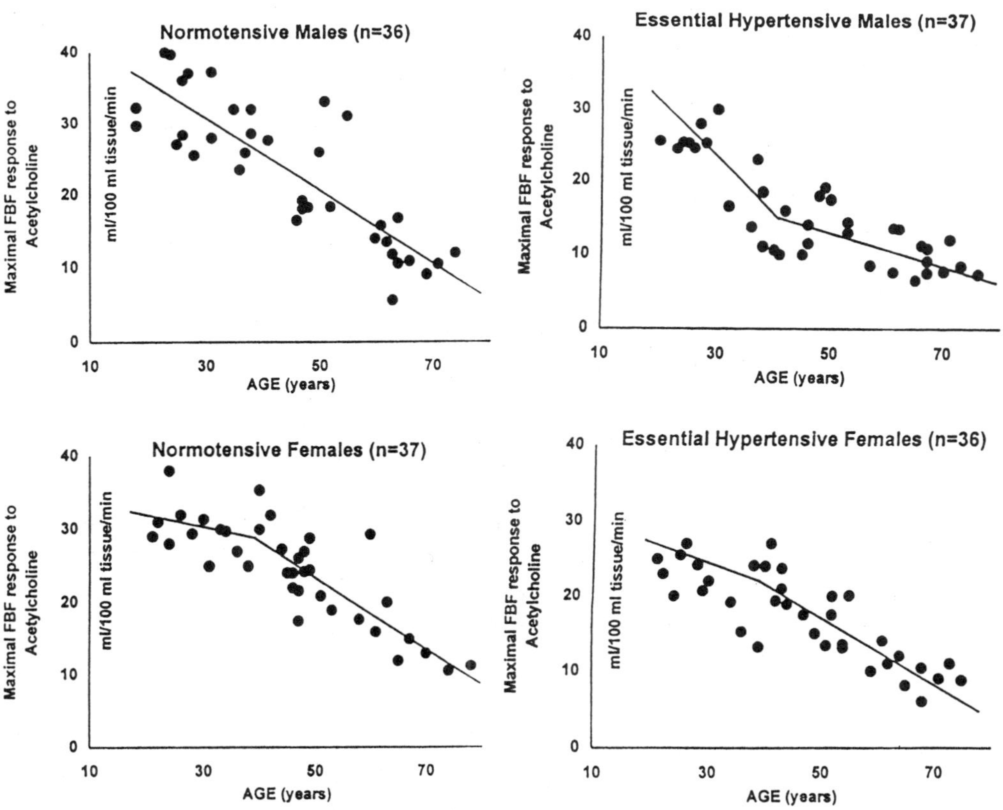

Figure 4. Relation between age (x axis) and maximum of the forearm blood flow (FBF) to acetylcholine (15 μg/100 ml forearm tissue/min) (y axis) in male (top) and female (bottom) normotensive subjects (left) and essential hypertensive patients (right). The broken line describes the change point of the age-related decline in endothelium dependent vasodilation. Data are expressed as absolute values. Adapted from ref 48, with permission.

hypertension anticipates age-related endothelial dysfunction. Moreover, the fact that after a certain age (around 40 years) the decline seems to slow is probably because the response to acetylcholine cannot be depressed above a certain degree. At variance with results observed in hypertensive males, the pattern of endothelial dysfunction seems to be the opposite in hypertensive women. Thus the rate of age-related dysfunction in vasodilation induced by acetylcholine was evident but slower up to 44 years, while a steeper decline commenced at around the age of menopause (Fig. 4). In older groups (> 60 years), no difference was observed in the age-related decrease in endothelial function in men compared to women. In both normotensive subjects and essential hypertensive patients we observed no gender difference in the response to sodium nitroprusside.

Taken together, these results seem to indicate that while in normotensive males endothelial dysfunction associated with increasing age is a constant and homogenous event, in normotensive females menopause is a crucial moment characterized by a remarkable deterioration of endothelial function. Worth of noting that in both male and female essential hypertensive patients an impairment in endothelium-dependent vasodilation is already detectable in early age. However in early maturity age-related endothelial dysfunction is more accentuated in male than in female hypertensive patients, while after age 60 the extent of impairment of endothelium-dependent vasodilation is lower in men than in postmenopausal women. These findings indicate that endogenous estrogen can protect endothelial function against the negative influence of aging both in normotensive and hypertensive women.

In conclusion, the present study indicates that both in normotensive and essential hypertensive females menopause is associated with onset or worsening of aging-associated endothelial dysfunction respectively, a finding which suggests that loss of endogenous estrogen could be a possible mechanism responsible for the acceleration of cardiovascular risk in postmenopausal women.

CONCLUSIONS

Aging is associated with the development of cardiovascular structural and functional alterations, which can explain the age-related increase in cardiovascular risk[49]. Available data indicate that aging causes endothelial dysfunction both in normotensive subjects and in essential hypertensive patients. This alteration is caused by impairment of the L-arginine-NO pathway and production of cyclooxygenase-dependent EDCFs, including possibly superoxide anions which in turn can cause a further impairment in the L-arginine-NO pathway by NO breakdown. Essential hypertension seems to anticipate the mechanisms and therefore to amplify the negative influence of aging on endothelial function, while endogenous estrogen seems to protect premenopausal women by the negative effect of aging. Thus age-related endothelial dysfunction could be one rational explanation for age-related cardiovascular risk.

This hypothesis is reinforced by our recent results showing that in a population of never treated essential hypertensive patients with recent onset of hypertension and a low cardiovascular risk profile, intima-medial thickness of carotid arteries, an early marker of atherosclerosis, was positively related with age and inversely related with endothelium-dependent vasodilation[50]. This evidence of a possible relationship between aging, impaired endothelium-dependent vasodilation and early atherosclerosis further supports the possibility that endothelial dysfunction is one of the main mechanisms through which advancing age leads to the development of atherosclerotic lesions and therefore of cardiovascular events. If this hypothesis is correct, the correction of endothelial dysfunction could be a rational therapeutic target. It is tempting to speculate that any therapeutical intervention which prevents or reverses endothelial dysfunction associated with advancing age could reduce age-related vascular alterations and the therefore age-related increase in cardiovascular risk.

REFERENCES

1. Luscher TF, Vanhoutte PM: The endothelium: modulator of cardiovascular function. Boca Raton, Fla, CRC Press, 1990.
2. Furchgott RF, Zawadzky JV: The obligatory role of endothelial cells in the relaxation of arterial smooth muscle by acetylcholine. Nature 1980;288:373–376.
3. Palmer RMJ, Ferrige AG, Moncada S: Nitric oxide release accounts for the biological activity of endothelium-derived relaxing factor. Nature 1987;327:524–6.
4. Palmer RMJ, Ashton DS, Moncada S: Vascular endothelial cells synthesize nitric oxide from L-arginine. Nature 1988;333:664–6.
5. Bredt DS, Hwang PM, Glatt CE, Lowenstein C, Reed RR, Snyder SH: Cloned and expressed nitric oxide synthase structurally resembles cytochrome P-450 reductase. Nature 1991;351:714
6. Rubanyi GM, Romero JC, Vanhoutte PM: Flow-induced release of endothelium-derived relaxing factor. Am J Physiol 1986; 250: H1145-H1149
7. Miller VM, Vanhoutte PM: Endothelium-dependent contractions to arachidonic acid are mediated by products of cyclooxygenase. Am J Physiol 1985; 248: H432-H437.
8. Altiere RJ, Kiritsy-Roy JA, Catravas JD: Acetylcholine-induced contractions in isolated rabbit pulmonary arteries: Role of thromboxane A_2. J Pharmacol Exp Ther 1986; 236: 535–541
9. Katusic ZS, Vanhoutte PM: Superoxide anion is an endothelium-derived contracting factor. Am J Physiol 1989; 257: H33-H37.
10. Gryglewski RJ, Palmer RMJ, Moncada S: Superoxide anion is involved in the breakdown of endothelium-derived vascular relaxing factor. Nature 1986; 320: 454–456.
11. Radomski MW, Palmer RMJ, Moncada S: The anti-aggregating properties of vascular endothelium: Interactions between prostacyclin and nitric oxide. Br J Pharmacol 1987;92:639–646. New York: Raven Press, 1989:1–13.
12. Radomski MW, Palmer RMJ, Moncada S: Endogenous nitric oxide inhibits human platelet adhesion to vascular endothelium. Lancet 1987;2:1057–68.
13. Garg UC, Hassid A: Nitric oxide-generating vasodilators and 8-bromo-cyclic guanosine monophosphate inhibit mitogenesis and proliferation of cultured rat vascular smooth muscle cells. J Clin Invest 1989;83:1774–7.
14. Dubey OB, Lüscher TF: Nitric oxide inhibits angiotensin II induced migration of vascular smooth muscle cells. Hypertension 1993;22:412.
15. Kubes P, Suzuki M, Granger DN: Nitric oxide: an endogenous modulator of leucocyte adhesion. Proc Natl Acad Sci USA, 1991;88;4651–4655.
16. De Caterina R, Libby P, Peng HB, Thannickal VJ, Rajavashisth TB, Gimbrone MA, Shin WS, Liao JK: Nitric oxide decreases cytokine-induced endothelial activation. J Clin Invest 1995; 96: 60–68.
17. Panza JA, Casino PR, Kilcoyne CM, Quyyumi AA: Role of endothelium-derived nitric oxide in the abnormal endothelium-dependent vascular relaxation of patients with essential hypertension. Circulation 1993;87:1468–74.
18. Taddei S, Virdis A, Mattei P, Salvetti A. Vasodilation to acetylcholine in primary and secondary forms of human hypertension. Hypertension 1993; 21: 929–33.
19. Linder L, Kiowski W, Buhler FR, Luscher TF: Indirect evidence for the release of endothelium-derived relaxing factor in the human forearm circulation in vivo: Blunted response in essential hypertension. Circulation 1990; 81: 1762–1767
20. Panza JA, Quyyumi AA, Brush JE Jr, Epstein SE: Abnormal endothelium dependent vascular relaxation in patients with essential hypertension. N Engl J Med 1990;323:22–7.
21. Creager MA, Cooke JP, Mendelsohn ME, Gallagher SJ, Coleman SM, Loscalzo J, Dzau VJ: Impaired vasodilation of forearm resistance vessels in hypercholesterolemic humans. J Clin Invest 1990; 86: 228–234.
22. Casino PR, Kilcoyne CM, Quyyumi AA, Hoeg JM, Panza JA. The role of nitric-oxide in endothelium-dependent vasodilation of hypercholesterolemic patients. Circulation 1993; 88: 2541–2547.
23. Williams SB, , Cusco JA, Roddy M-A, Johnstone MT, Creager MA. Impaired nitric oxide mediated vasodilation in patients with non insulin-dependent diabetes mellitus. J Am Coll Cardiol 1996; 27: 567–574.
24. Ting HH, Timini FK, Boles KS, Creager SJ, Ganz P, Creager MA: Vitamin C improves endothelium-dependent vasodilation in patients with non-insulin-dependent diabetes mellitus. J Clin Invest 1996; 97: 22–28.

25. Celermajer DS, Adams MR, Clarkson P, Robinson J, McCredie R, Donald A, Deanfield JE. Passive smoking and impaired endothelium-dependent arterial dilatation in healthy young adults. N Engl J Med 1996; 334: 150–154.
26. Heitzer T, Ylä-Herttauala S, Luoma J, Kurz S, Münzel T, Just H, Olschewski M, Drexeler H: Cigarette smoking potentiates endothelial dysfunction of forearm resistance vessels in patients with hypercholesterolemia. Role of oxidized LDL. Circulation 1996; 93:1346–1353.
27. Soltis EE: Effect of age on blood pressure and membrane-dependent vascular responses in the rat. Circ Res 1987; 61:889–897.
28. Moritoki H, Hosoki E, Ishida Y. Age-related decrease in endothelium-dependent dilator response to histamine in rat mesenteric artery. Eur J Pharmacol. 1986; 126: 61–67.
29. Hongo K, Nakagomi T, Kassel NF, Sasaki T, Lehmann M, Vollmer dg, Tsukahara T, Ogawa H, Torner J: Effects of aging and hypertension on endothelium-dependent vascular relaxation in rat carotid artery. Stroke 1988;19:892–897.
30. Mayhan WG, Faraci FM, Baumbach GL, Heistad DD : Effects of aging on responses of cerebral arterioles. Am J Physiol 1990; 258 (Heart Circ Physiol 27) :H1138-H1143.
31. Dohi Y, Thiel MA, Bühler FR, Lüscher TF: Activation of endothelial L-arginine pathway in pressurized mesenteric resistance arteries: effect of age and hypertension. Hypertension 1990;15:170–5.
32. Vita JA, Treasure CB, Nabel EG, Mclenacham JM, Fish RD, Yeung AC, Vekshtein VI, Selwyn AP, Ganz P : Coronary vasomotor response to acetylcholine relates to risk factors for coronary artery disease. Circulation 1990; 81:491–497.
33. Yasue H, Matsuyama K, Matsuyama K, Okumura K, Morikami Y, Ogawa H: Responses of angiographically normal human coronary arteries to intracoronary injection of acetylcholine by age and segment. Possible role of early coronary atherosclerosis. Circulation 1990;81:482–490.
34. Egashira K, Inou T, Hirooka Y, Kai H, Sugimachi M, Suzuki S, Kuga T, Urabe Y, Takeshita A: Effects of age on endothelium-dependent vasodilation of resistance coronary artery by acetylcholine in humans. Circulation 1993;88:77–81.
35. Zeiher AM, Drexter H, Saurbier B, Just H: Endothelium-mediated coronary blood flow modulation in humans. Effects of age, atherosclerosis, hypercholesterolemia, and hypertension. J Clin Invest 1993;92:652–62.
36. Taddei S, Virdis A, Mattei P, Ghiadoni L, Gennari A, Basile-Fasolo C, Sudano I, Salvetti A: Aging and endothelial function in normotensive subjects and essential hypertensive patients. Circulation, 1995;91:1981–1987.
37. Taddei S, Virdis A, Mattei P, Ghiadoni L, Basile-Fasolo C, Sudano I, Salvetti A: Hypertension causes premature aging of endothelial function in humans. Hypertension, 1997; 29 :736–743
38. Taddei S, Virdis A, Ghiadoni L, Magagna A, Salvetti A: Cyclooxygenase inhibition restores nitric oxide activity in essential hypertension. Hypertension, 1997; 29(part 2) :274–279.
39. Virdis A, Taddei S, Ghiadoni L, Salvetti A: Effect of vitamin C on vasodilation to acetylcholine in the forearm of essential hypertensive patients. Hypertension, 1996;28:695(abs).
40. Kannel WB, Hjortland MC, Mc Namara PM: Menopause and the risk of cardiovascular disease: The Framingham Study. Ann Intern Med 1976;8S:447–456.
41. Barrett-Connor E, Bush TL: Estrogen and coronary heart disease in women. JAMA 1991;265:1861–1867.
42. Lobo RA: Estrogen and cardiovascular disease. Ann NY Acad Sci 1990;592:286–294.
43. Wahl P, Walden C, Knopp R, Hoover J, Wallace R, Heiss G, Rifkind B: Effect of estrogen/progestin potency on lipid/lipoprotein cholesterol. N Engl J Med 1983;308:862–867.
44. Walsh BW, Schiff I, Rosner B, Greenberg L, Ravnikar V, Sacks FM: Effects of postmenopausal estrogen replacement therapy on the concentrations and metabolism of plasma lipoproteins. N Engl J Med 1991;325:1196–1204.
45. Collins P, Rosano GMC, Jiang C, Lindsay D, Sarrel PM, Poole-Wilson PA: Hypothesis: cardiovascular protection by oestrogen - a calcium antagonist effect? Lancet 1993;341:1264–1265.
46. Gisclard V, Miller VM, Vanhoutte PM: Effect of 17ß-estradiol on endothelium-dependent responses in the rabbit. J Pharmacol Exp Ther 1988;244:19–22.
47. Hayashi T, Fukuto JM, Ignarro LJ, Chaudhuri G: Basal release of nitric oxide from aortic rings is greater in female rabbits than in male rabbits: implications for atherosclerosis. Proc Natl Acad Sci USA 1992;89:11259–11263.
48. Taddei S, Virdis A, Ghiadoni L, Mattei P, Sudano I, Bernini GP, Pinto S, Salvetti A: Menopause is associated with endothelial dysfunction in women. Hypertension, 1996; 28: 576–582.
49. Salvetti A, Ghiadoni L, Gennari A, Taddei S : Age influence on some aspects of cardiovascular adaptation to hypertension. High Blood Press, 1995; 4: 87–96.
50. Ghiadoni L, Taddei S, Virdis A, Sudano I, Di Legge V, Meola M, Di Venanzio L, Salvetti A: Endothelial function and common carotid wall thickening in essential hypertensive patients. Submitted to publication.

7

VASCULAR CHANGES AND AGING

Salvatore Novo,[1*] Agostino Geraci,[2] and Claudio Pernice[2]

[1]Department of Clinical Pathophysiology
[2]Department of Internal Medicine II
Institute of Internal Medicine and Geriatrics
University of Palermo

1. INTRODUCTION

The progress of cardiovascular prevention and the large use of antibiotics have determined in the last fifty years a progressive increase of life duration, especially in the western countries, and so, a noticeable increase of elderly subjects in the population (1,2).

The morbidity and mortality of elderly people is mainly due to cardiovascular diseases (1). For this reason, in all countries there is a growing interest for the study and the detection of vascular damage in the elderly (1,2).

The physiological vascular aging is characterized by a progressive thickening of the arterial wall layers—the intima/media complex (3,4)—with reduction of elastic fibers and increase of collagen and calcium deposition into the media (5). This process determines an alteration of the collagen/elastin ratio and a progressive medial hypertrophy with increased distance between the elastic layers (5).

The consequence of the physiological vascular aging is a progressive loss of elasticity of the arterial wall (6), with diminution of the Windkessel function (3) and increase of the propagation speed of the sphygmic wave (3,7,8). The loss of elasticity of the arterial wall induces also a diminution of the arterial wall distensibility against the increase of cardiac output, determining a slight rise of the systolic blood pressure (SBP) and of the pulse pressure (PP) with a mild thickening of interventricular septum (IVS) and of the posterior wall (PW) of the heart (2,3,7–9).

This pathophysiological process normally is named "arteriosclerosis" (10). We demonstrated a progressive but mild increase of casual SBP at rest (2) (Table 1), at the maximal common work (Table 2) during ergometer test (2) and during ambulatory monitoring (9) (Table 3), parallel to aging, with a mild increase of the thickeness of the cardiac walls as evaluted by M-Mode and 2D by echocardiography (Table 4) and a slow decrease of

* Address for correspondence: Prof. Salvatore Novo, Chair of Clinical Pathophysiology, Institute of Internal Medicine and Geriatrics (Head: Prof. Serafino Mansueto), University of Palermo, Via del Vespro 141, 90127 Palermo, Italy. Tel: 0039-91-51.13.75/655.29.86. Fax: 0039-91-655.29.62

Recent Advances in Geriatrics, edited by Barbagallo, Licata, and Sowers.
Plenum Press, New York, 1998.

Table 1. Behaviour of SBP, DBP, and HR at rest in apparently healthy subjects of both genders, without risk factors, of three different age groups (2)

	Group 1 25M/18F 25–35 years	Group 2 26M/26F 45–55 years	Group 3 22M/16F 65–75 years
SBP (mmHg)			
Males	118.75 ± 11.43	119.23 ± 7.16	124.54 ± 10.11*
Females	114.44 ± 13.26	116.15 ± 14.30	128.43 ± 13.99*
DBP (mmHg)			
Males	78.75 ± 7.53	80.38 ± 7.99	80.00 ± 10.80
Females	76.22 ± 10.89	74.61 ± 10.09	78.31 ± 16.23
HR (bpm)			
Males	79.85 ± 18.39	74.07 ± 10.73	74.40 ± 12.63
Females	83.55 ± 14.55	81.00 ± 16.31	78.31 ± 16.25

SBP: Systolic blood pressure; DBP: Diastolic blood pressure; HR: Heart rate
*$p < 0.01$ Group 3 vs Groups 1 and 2.

heart rate as consequence of both the increase of SBP and of the resetting of baroceptorial reflex with aging (5).

Of course, the physiological aging of vascular system can be strongly influenced by the presence of risk factors such as arterial hypertension, diabetes mellitus, smoking, hypercholesterolemia and others (2).

The modifications of the arterial system with the aging complains: 1) changes of the large arteries compliance (proximal compliance); 2) structural changes of the small arteries (distal compliance); 3) endothelial dysfunction and 4) asymptomatic or symptomatic atherosclerotic lesions.

2. ALTERATIONS OF LARGE ARTERIES COMPLIANCE (PROXIMAL COMPLIANCE)

The age-related loss of elasticity is particularly evident in large arteries. Reneman (11) in 1985 firstly evaluated the absolute diameters, and the relative changes during the cardiac cycle, of the common carotid artery (CCA) and of the internal carotid artery (ICA)

Table 2. Behaviour of SBP, DBP, and HR, at the maximal common work during ergometer test, in apparently healthy subjects, without risk factors, of three different age groups (2)

	Group 1 25M/18F 25–35 years	Group 2 26M/26F 45–55 years	Group 3 22M/16F 65–75 years
SBP (mmHg)			
Males	143.41 ± 15.92	151.53 ± 13.83	162.50 ± 20.28*
Females	134.44 ± 14.23	148.65 ± 25.51	164.37 ± 19.05*
DBP (mmHg)			
Males	87.40 ± 12.50	91.92 ± 10.86	91.81 ± 8.66
Females	84.16 ± 10.74	87.46 ± 13.33	91.87 ± 10.46
HR (bpm)			
Males	107.48 ± 14.52	102.84 ± 11.62	101.81 ± 15.94
Females	123.61 ± 18.62	120.03 ± 24.16	112.31 ± 29.38

SBP: Systolic blood pressure; DBP: Diastolic blood pressure; HR: Heart rate
* $p < 0.05$ Group 3 vs Group 1.

Table 3. 24 hours mean values of SBP, DBP, and HR, during non-invasive, automatic, intermittent monitoring, in three groups of normotensive subjects, without risk factors, of three different age groups (9)

	Group 1 7M/7F 20–39 years	Group 2 7M/7F 40–59 years	Group 3 7M/7F > 60 years
SBP (mmHg)	116.40 ± 13.80	121.8 ± 9.1*	128.4 ± 10.1**
DBP (mmHg)	72.1 ± 7.2	75.9 ± 5.3*	76.4 ± 7.8*
HR (bpm)	80.2 ± 6.8	74.9 ± 9.4*	70.81 ± 8.4**

SBP: Systolic blood pressure; DBP: Diastolic blood pressure; HR: Heart rate
*$p < 0.005$ Group 3 vs Group 2 and Group 2 vs Group 1.
**$p < 0.0005$ Group 3 vs Group 2.

in young and oldest subjects. In oldest subjects the absolute diameters of CCA and ICA were greater, while the changes during the cardiac cycle were less.

A similar effect on carotid structure is exerted by arterial hypertension. In fact, comparing two groups of hypertensives with mild or severe hypertension, and different degree of left ventricular hypertrophy and monitored blood presssure, Licata and coworkers (12) showed a more evident intima-media thickening and a greater diameter of the popliteal artery in subjects with more severe hypertension.

We studied the behaviour of proximal arterial compliance, as related with aging, by using the Aortic Index (13), obtained by the pulse pressure/stroke volume ratio, this latter as calculated by echocardiography (14). Elderly normotensive subjects when compared with middle-aged normotensive subjects show an increase of pulse pressure and of aortic index, as expression of reduced arterial compliance (2,9,15) (Table 5). This finding was more and more evident in hypertensive subjects, both of middle-age and especially elderly (14,15). So, it appear that hypertension is a risk factor worsening the alterations of proximal compliance due to physiological aging (16) (Table 5).

Some drugs, such as calcium antagonists, can improve arterial compliance (17). In our experience, chronic treatment of elderly sybjects with isolated systolic hypertension, with slow release nifedipine, decreases BP and improves proximal compliance (18).

3. STRUCTURAL ALTERATIONS OF SMALL VESSELS (DISTAL COMPLIANCE)

In the small vessels, such as arterioles, the physiological aging induces structural changes with reduced lumen/wall ratio and with a loss of the maximal vasodilation capacity after appropriate stimuli (19). This aspect can be investigated by direct methods including

Table 4. Behaviour of interventricular septum (IVS) and posterior wall (PW) telediastolic thickening as evaluated by M-mode echocardiography, in three groups of normotensive subjects, apparently healthy, without risk factors, of three different age groups (2)

	Group 1 7M/7F 25–35 years	Group 2 7M/7F 45-55 years	Group 3 7M/7F 65-75 years
IVS (mm)	9.4 ± 1.0	9.5 ± 1.9*	10.7 ± 1.5*
PW (mm)	9.0 ± 0.9	9.2 ± 1.3*	10.4 ± 1.7*

*$p < 0.005$ Group 2 vs Group 1 and Group 3 vs Group 2.

Table 5. Behaviour of pulse pressure, aortic index and other haemodynamic parameters in normotensive and hypertensive subjects of middle-age and elderly (14,15)

	Middle-aged		Elderly	
	Normotensives 20 subjects 47.24 ± 11.7 yrs	Hypertensives 20 subjects 44.34 ± 9.14 yrs	Normotensives 10 subjects 68.4 ± 4.3 yrs	Hypertensives 10 subjects 73.7 ± 5.4 yrs
SBP (mmHg)	125.2 ± 5.1	160.94 ± 6.37**	142.0 ± 14.0	193.7 ± 20.0**
DBP (mmHg)	74.8 ± 4.1	104.25 ± 4.75**	79.7 ± 7.3	81.2 ± 14.0
PP (mmHg)	50.4 ± 2.59	56.09 ± 2.41**	63.0 ± 17.0	113.5 ± 15.0*
HR (bpm)	74.2 ± 7.98	77.10 ± 7.01	70.3 ± 5.9	59.0 ± 2.9**
SV (ml)	76.75 ± 8.53	77.25 ± 12.36	84.9 ± 6.0	108.0 ± 16.2*
SVR (dyne.sec.cm^{-5})	1378.2 ± 207.5	1602.7 ± 339.4**	1311.0 ± 334.1	1505.2 ± 430.4*
AI (%)	0.66 ± 0.05	0.73 ± 0.07**	0.74 ± 0.06	1.04 ± 0.1*

SBP: Systolic blood pressure; DBP: Diastolic blood pressure; HR: Heart rate; PP: Pulse pressure; SV: Stroke volume as obtained by 2D-Echo using the Sympson's formula; SVR: Systemic vascular resistances as calculated by the following formula: (mean blood pressure x 60x1332)/cardiac output; AI: Aortic index as obtained by PP/SV ratio.
*p < 0.01 Group 4 vs Group 3.
**p < 0.005 Group 2 vs Group 1 and Group 4 vs Group 3.

the evaluation of the maximal vasodilation capacity of biopsized vessels in vivo (20), or indirectly, using plethysmography and calculating the minimal vascular resistances (MVR), obtained after an ischemic stimulus alone (21) or associated with physical exercise.

We have performed this evaluation by using the strain-gauge plethysmography. Using a counterpressure of 50 mm Hg on the cuff above the strain-gauge we obtained the rest flow (RF); with a counterpressure of 250 mm Hg, for three minutes (21) or more (22), one may obtain the peak flow (PF) or post-ischemic flow. By the ratio between mean blood pressure and RF and PF respectively, it is possible to allow the basal (BVR) and minimal (MVR) vascular resistance (21).

In our experience, elderly normotensives, as compared to middle-aged normotensives, show only a slight increase of MVR, as expression of structural changes in the arteriolar bed (23,24). This phenomenon is present also in borderline hypertensives (25) and is especially evident in stable middle-aged and elderly hypertensives (23,24) (Table 6).

Chronic treatment with the ACE inhibitor captopril partially reversed these alterations (26) and a similar but less effect was exerted by the alpha- and beta-blocker labetalol (27). One possible explanation of this phenomemom is the following: both nor-epinephrine and angiotensin II have a stimulating action on the growth and proliferation of smooth muscle cells in the arteriolar wall. So, an antagonist of noradrenaline or of angiotensin II can reverse the alterations of the arterial wall, while a simple beta-blocker doesn't exert this action.

4. ENDOTHELIAL DYSFUNCTION

Physiological aging also causes a progressive endothelial dysfunction with changes in the balance of TXA2/PGI2 system, ET-1/NO system, and S1/S2 serotoninergic receptors, increases the oxidant free radicals, and hyperfunctioning of platelets with enhanced release of PF4 and beta-thromboglobukin, and depression of fibrinolysis with altered PAI/tPA ratio (28). All these alterations of the endothelial function and, in general, the process of vascular aging are certainly enhanced by the presence of risk factors, mainly hypertension, diabetes, smoking and hypercholesterolemia (30,31).

Table 6. Behaviour of blood flow and vascular resistance at the calf in normotensive and hypertensive subjects of middle-age and elderly (23,24)

	Middle-aged		Elderly	
	Normotensives 13M/7F 47.24 ± 11.7 yrs	Hypertensives 55M/30F 41.4 ± 10.4 yrs	Normotensives 12M/8F 69.2 ± 4.06 yrs	Hypertensives 10M/15F 68.5 ± 2.7 yrs
SBP (mmHg)	125.2 ± 5.1	175.21 ± 18.5*	137.25 ± 14.73	178.84 ± 15.29*
DBP (mmHg)	74.8 ± 4.1	104.53 ± 13.86*	85.75 ± 12.06	101.15 ± 15.29*
MBP (mmHg)	92.5 ± 3.4	128.01 ± 14.01*	102.81 ± 10.59	127.04 ± 15.84*
HR (bpm)	76.2 ± 7.98	73.33 ± 12.1	71.6 ± 11.3	71.33 ± 7.2
RF (ml/min/100 gr)	3.98 ± 0.88	3.93 ± 2.1	4.05 ± 2.47	3.09 ± 1.82***
PF (ml/min/100 gr)	25.11 ± 5.45	21.03 ± 7.7**	23.34 ± 6.48	15.11 ± 7.24*
BVR (AU)	25.24 ± 5.98	46.03 ± 7.7*	26.00 ± 14.98	57.91 ± 13.34*
MVR (AU)	3.68 ± 0.91	8.72 ± 6.8***	4.27 ± 1.08****	11.12 ± 6.5*

SBP: Systolic blood pressure; DBP: Diastolic blood pressure; MBP: Mean blood pressure; HR: Heart rate; RF: Rest flow as evaluated by strain-gauge plethysmography; PF: Peak flow (after ischemic stimulus); BVR: Basal vascular resistance; MVR: Minimal vascular resistance; AU: arbitrary units

*p < 0.0005 Group 2 vs Group 1 and Group 4 vs Group 3. **p < 0.025 Group 2 vs Group 1. ***p < 0.0025 Group 4 vs Group 3. ****p < 0.01 Group 3 vs Group 1.

Recently, Gerhard et al. (32) demonstrated that aging progressively impairs the endothelium-dependent vasodilation in forearm resistance vessels of humans, showing that age, total- and LDL-cholesterol were univariate predictors of endothelium vasodilation. In this study, age remained the most significant predictor of endothelium-dependent vasodilator response by stepwise regression analysis (32).

Similar results were obtained by Salvetti and co-workers (22). These authors demonstrated that ACh induces a dose-dependent vasodilation, significantly lower in essential hypertensives patients than in normotensive control subjects. Moreover, in this study a significant negative correlation between ACh-induced vasodilation and age was shown, both in normotensive ($r = 0.86$, $p < 0.01$) and in hypertensive patients ($r = 0.85$, $p < 0.001$). Therefore, these authors conclude that the impaired endothelium-dependent vasodilation in essential hypertension could be a mere acceleration of the changes seen in aging (33).

Ledda and co-workers were also able to demonstrate that the vasodilating response to ACh decreases with aging and hypertension showing that the main mechanism responsible for the effect of Ach in vessels of young animals consist of the activation of K+ channels (34).

5. ASYMPTOMATIC AND SYMPTOMATIC ATHEROSCLEROTIC LESIONS

The presence of hypertension and other risk factors is able not only to enhance the process of physiological aging "arteriosclerosis", but also to promote the atherosclerotic lesions of carotids (35), coronary arteries (36), iliac-femoral-popliteal arteries (37) or contemporaneously in several districts (35,38). These lesions can be symptomatic or asymptomatic (38,39); they can progressively or suddenly evolve determining target organs complications or show regression spontaneously or after pharmacologic treatment (40–42).

We evaluated the relationship between risk factors, aging and asymptomatic carotid lesions in the contest of the multicenter research project (1988–1994) on "Cardiovascular Aging", promoted in Italy by the Ministry of the University and the Scientific and Technological Research (MURST) in cooperation with GESCO (43).

Table 7. Frequency of IMT, ACP, and IMT plus ACP in subjects without RF or with a single RF (43)

	Normal findings (%)	IMT (%)	ACP (%)	IMT + ACP (%)
Subjects without RF	83.8	10.8	5.4	16.2
Subjects with RF	52.8	32.5*	14.7*	47.2*
Hypertension	34.5	44.8*	20.7*	65.5*
Diabetes	58.3	25.0	16.7*	41.7*
Hyper-C	73.4	13.3	13.3*	26.6**
CVD+ history	80.6	12.9	6.5	19.4
Smoking	66.7	33.3**	0	33.3*
Hyper-TG	75.0	25	0	25

IMP: Intima media thickening; ACP: Asymptomatic carotid plaque; RF: Risk factors
*p < 0.001, **p < 0.05

Table 8. Frequency of normal findings, IMT and ACP in subjects without RF according to the subdivision into three groups of age (43)

	Normal findings (%)	IMT (%)	ACP (%)	IMT + ACP (%)
<35 years	100	0	0	0
≥35 <65 years	91.7	5.5	2.8	8.3
≥65 years	58.6	27.6*	13.8*	41.4*

IMP: Intima media thickening; ACP: Asymptomatic carotid plaque; RF: Risk factors
* p < 0.01

We studied 755 subjects, asymptomatic for cerebrovascular disease, of both sex. The presence of asymptomatic atherosclerotic plaque was significantly higher in subjects with RF in comparison with those without RF, in males in comparison with females and in elderly people in comparison with young population (Table 7 and Table 8) (43).

6. CONCLUSIONS

The process of vascular aging named "arteriosclerosis" is a pathophysiological process that involves the old people, more or less, with the aging. Physiological vascular aging induces: 1) alterations of large arteries compliance (proximal compliance), with partial loss of the Windkessel function (43); 2) structural changes of small vessels (distal compliance), with increased vascular resistance (43); 3) impaired endothelial function with increased risk of atherosclerotic lesions. This process can be accelerated by some risk factors such as hypertension, diabetes, hypercholesterolemia, and smoking (44); it can be partially reversed by the correction of risk factors or by drugs administration (45). But risk factors are very important to begin and promote the process of atherogenesis, both asymptomatic, or symptomatic with manifestation of target organs complications.

Age is one of the most important risk factor for asymptomatic atherosclerosis, especially if associated with hypertension (22). Age, male gender, hypertension, hypercholesterolemia, diabetes and smoking are, in our experiencxe, the most important risk factors for the beginning of atherosclerotic lesions at the univariate analysis (43).

The modifications of life-style and the correction of risk factors by diet and/or pharmacologic treatment (45) can perhaps modify this dangerous evolution (41, 42).

REFERENCES

1. Safar M. Ageing and its effects on cardiovascular system. Drugs 1990; 39 (Suppl. I): 1–8
2. Strano A., Barbagallo Sangiorgi G., Novo S., Putignano E., Longo B., Liquori M., Failla G., Nardi E., Giovenco E., Calcara L., Corda M., Abrignani M.G.: Non invasive evaluation of cardiovascular alterations in the physiological aging. Cardiologia 1991; 36 (Suppl. 1 to n. 12): 237–246
3. O'Rourke M.F. Arterial function in health and disease. Churchill Livingstone, Edinburgh-London-Melbourne-New York, 1982: pp 53–66, 153–169, 196–252
4. Safar M.E., Simon A.Ch., Levenson J. A. Structural changes of large arteries in sustained essential hypertension. Hypertension 1984; 6 (Suppl. III): 117–121
5. Yin F.C.P. The aging vasculature and its effect on the heart. In: Weisfeldt M.L. (Ed.). The aging heart: its function and response to stress. Raven Press, New York, 1980: pp. 137–213
6. Safar M.E., London G.M. Blood pressure in relation to physical aging process in the arterial wall. Handbook of Hypertension 1989; 12: 70–84
7. Nichols W.W., O'Rourke M. F. Avolio A.P., Yaginuma T., Murgo J. P. Effects of age on ventricular-vascular coupling. Am J Cardiol 1985; 56: 1179–1184
8. Walsh R. A. Cardiovascular effect of the aging process. Am J Med 1987; 82 (Suppl. 1B): 34–40
9. Novo S., Alaimo G., Abrignani M.G., Corrao S., Longo B., Strano A. Blood pressure and heart rate variability in normotensives in relation to their age. J Ambulatory Monitoring 1989; 2: 143–151
10. Novo S., Failla G., Liquori M., Longo B., Gennaro C., Corda M., Barbagallo M., Abrignani M.G., Barbagallo Sangiorgi G., Strano A. Vascular alterations in arterial hypertension: non invasive evaluation. Cardiologia 1991; 36 (Suppl. 1 to n. 12): 323–337
11. Reneman R.S., van Merode P., Hick P., Hoeks A.P. Flow velocity patterns and distensibility of the carotid artery bulb in subjects of various ages. Circulation 1985; 71:500–509.
12. Pinto A., Scaglione R., Galati D., Paterna S., Parrinello G., Arnone S., Licata G. Evaluation of regional haemodynamics and alterations of vascular wall of the lower limbs in hypertensive subjects. Eur Heart J 1995; 16:1692–1697
13. Tarazi R.C., Magrini F., Dustan H.P. The role of aortic distensibility in hypertension. In: Miller P., Safar M.E., eds. International Symposium on hypertension.. Munchen 1975, Boehringer Ingelheim, pp 133–138.
14. Novo S., Scaglione R., Abrignani M.G., Liquori M., Sanguigni V., Licata G., Strano A. Arterial compliance and its relationship with the severity of the hypertensive state.In: Strano A., Novo S. (Eds.). Advances in Vascular Pathology 1989. Elsevier Excerpta Medica, Amsterdam, 1989: pp. 875–880
15. Novo S., Nardi E., Noto G., Zingone F., Abrignani M.G., Strano A. Arterial compliance in elderly patients with isolated systolic hypertension. In: Strano A., Novo S. (Eds.). Advances in Vascular Pathology 1989, Elsevier Excerpta Medica, Amsterdam, 1989: pp. 869–875
16. Novo S., Liquori M., Longo B., Licata G., Barbagallo Sangiorgi G., Strano A. Proximal and distal compliance in relation to ageing and arterial hypertension. Am J Hypertension 1994; 7 (Part. 2 - Abstract Issue):
17. Chalmers J.P., Smith S.A., Wing M.H.: Hypertension in the elderly. The role of calcium antagonists. J Cardiovasc Pharmacol 1989; 12 (Suppl. 8): S147-S155
18. Novo S., Nardi E., Noto G., Licata G., Strano A. Effects of Nifedipine on blood pressure, arterial compliance and left ventricular mass in elderly patients with isolated systolic hypertension. In: Omae T. and Zanchetti A. (Eds). How should elderly hypertensive patients be treated?. Springer-Verlag, Tokyo 1989: pp. 189–195
19. Folkow B., Karlstom G. Age- and pressure dependent changes of systemic resistance vessels concerning the relationship between geometric design, wall distensibility, vascular reactivity and smooth muscle sensitivity. Acta Physiol Scand 1984; 122: 17–33
20. Aalkjaer C., Eiskjaer H., Mulvany M.J.: Abnormal structure and function of isolated subcutaneous resistance vessels from essential hypertensive patients despite antihypertensive treatment. J Hypertension 1989; 7: 305–309
21. Novo S., Pinto A., Licata G., Davi' G., Avellone G., Galati D., Strano A. Arterial flow and vascular reactivity in the lower limbs in uncomplicated essential arterial hypertension. Giorn Ital Cardiol 1982; 12: 348–354
22. Aging and endothelial function in normotensive subjects and patients with essential hypertension. Circulation 1995; 91: 1981–1987
23. Novo S., Pinto A., Abrignani M.G., Galati D., Giordano U., Fasulo S., Alaimo G., Strano A. Calf blood flow and vascular resistance in middle-aged and elderly hypertensives. Int Angiol 1985: 4 (Suppl. 4): 133–136
24. Strano A., Novo S., Pinto A., Fasulo S., Alaimo G. Calf blood flow and vascular resistance in middle-aged and elderly hypertensives. J Hypertension 1985; 3 (Suppl. 3): S351-S353

25. Novo S., Pinto A., Alaimo G., Galati D., Strano A.: Calf blood flow and vascular resistance in borderline hypertensives in comparison with control subjects. J Cardiovasc Pharmacol 1986; 8 (Suppl. 5): S122-S124
26. Novo S., Abrignani M.G., Liquori M., Corda M., Pinto A., Cosentino F., Strano A. Regression of structural vascular changes after chronic treatment in hypertensives. J Hypertension 1991; 9 (Suppl. 6): S2O2-S2O3
27. Novo S., Abrignani M.G., Pinto A., Strano A. Regression of structural vascular changes in hypertensives after captopril treatment. Eur Heart J 1992; 13: 1135–1137
28. Novo S., Abrignani M.G., Liquori M., Strano A. Partial regression of vascular structural alterations in hypertensive patients treated with the alpha-betablocker labetalol. Int Angiol 1992; 11: 137–141
29. Vanhoutte P. M. Endothelium-derived vasoactive factors, platelets and coronary disease. In: Nakamura M. and Vanhoutte P. M. (Eds). Coronary circulation in physiological and pathological states. Spinger-Verlag, Tokyo, 1991: pp. 89–102
30. Vita J. A., Treasure C. B., Nabel E. G., McLenacham J. M., Fish R.D., Yeung A.C., Vekshtein V. I., Selwyn A. P., Ganz P. Coronary vasomotor response to acetylcholine relates to risk factors for coronary heart disease. Circulation 1990; 81: 491–497
31. Salvetti A., Ghiadoni L., Gennari A., Taddei S. Age influence on some aspects of cardiovascular adaptation to hypertension. High Bloob Press 1995; 4: 87–96
32. Gerhardt M., Roddy M. A., Creager S. J., Creager M. A. Aging progressively impairs endothelium-dependent vasodilation in forearm resistance vessels of humans. Hypertension 1996; 27: 849–853
33. Taddei S., Virdis A., Mattei P., Ghiadoni L., Gennari A., Fasolo CB., Sudano I., Salvetti A. High blood pressure ages vessels. Hypertension 1997; 29: 736–742
34. Mantelli L., Amerini S., Ledda F. Role of nitric oxide and endothelium-derived hyperpolarizing factor in vasorelaxant effect of acetylcholine as influenced by aging and hypertension. J Cardiovasc Pharmacol 1995; 25: 595–602
35. Pujia A., Rubba P., Spencer M.P. Prevalence of extracranial carotid disease detectable by echo-Doppler in an elderly population. Stroke 1990; 21: 1567–1572
36. Waller B.F., Morgani R. The very elderly heart. Cardiovasc Clin 1987; 18: 361–410
37. Novo S., Avellone G., Di Garbo V., Abrignani M.G., Liquori M., Panno A.V., Strano A. Prevalence of risk factors in patients with peripheral arterial disease: a clinical and epidemiological evaluation. Int Angiol 1992; 11: 218–229
38. Ciccone M., Di Noia D., Di Michele L., Corriero F., Di Biase M., Biasco M.G., Novo S., Strano A., Rizzon P. The incidence of asymptomatic extracoronary atherosclerosis in patients with coronary atherosclerosis. Int Angiol 1993; 12: 25–28
39. Novo S., Pernice C., Geraci A. M., Longo B., Barbagallo C.M., Caruso R., Liquori M., Putignano E., Barbagallo Sangiorgi G., Strano A. Risk factors, ageing and asymptomatic catotid plaque. Cardiologia 1995; 40 (Suppl. 1 to n. 12): 263–272
40. Norris J.W., Bernstein N.M. Progression and regression of carotid stenosis. Stroke 1986; 17: 755–757
41. Colins P., Fox K. The pathogenesis of atheroma and the rationale for its treatment. Eur Heart J 1992; 13: 560–565
42. Hughenoltz P.G., de Feyter P.J. Is regression of atherosclerosis possible? Cardiologia 1992; 37: 393–401
43. Novo S., Pernice C., Caruso R., Tantillo R., Longo B. Influence of risk factors and ageing on asymptomatic carotid lesions. In: Advances in Vascular Pathology 1997. Nicolaides A.N and Novo S. (Eds). Elsevier Excerpta Medica, Amsterdam, 1997. In press.
44. Novo S., Abrignani M.G., Barbagallo M., Putignano E., Liquori M., Corda M., Pinto A., Barbagallo Sangiorgi G., Strano A. Haemodynamic changes during physiological aging. Intern Assoc Biomed Gerontol 1991; 29: 7 (Abstract)
45. Novo S., Abrignani M.G., Barbagallo M., Liquori M., Longo B., Corda M., Pinto A., Strano A. Risk factors and vascular aging. Intern Assoc Biomed Gerontol 1991; 188: 128
46. Van Bortel L.M.A.B., Kool M.J.F., Spek J.J. Disparate effects of antihypertensive drugs on large arteries distensibility and compliance in hypertension. Am J Cardiol 1995; 76 (Suppl. E): 46E-49E.

8

OXIDATIVE STRESS AND ADVANCING AGE

Impact on Blood Pressure

Giuseppe Paolisso,* Maria Rosaria Tagliamonte, Maria Rosaria Rizzo, Daniela Manzella, Sabrina Manduca, Giuseppina Petrella, Michelangela Barbieri, and Michele Varricchio

Department of Geriatric Medicine and Metabolic Diseases
II University of Naples
Naples, Italy

Free radicals are highly reactive atoms or molecules that have one or more unpaired electrons in their atomic structure. Oxidative damage inflicted by reactive oxygen species is also referred to as "oxidative stress" (1). The susceptibility of a given organ or system to the oxidative stress is function of the balance between pro-oxidant factors and those scavenging them (1). The nonenzymatic, free radicals mediated oxidation of biological molecules, membranes and tissue is associated with a variety of pathological events such as cancer, aging and, diabetes mellitus (1). In this latter disease, oxidative stress seems mainly due to both an increased production of plasma free radical concentrations and a sharp reduction of antioxidant defenses (1).

OXIDATIVE STRESS AND ADVANCING AGE

The relationship between oxidative stress and advancing age has been widely addressed and investigated. Briefly, it has been demonstrated that aging per se and age-related degenerative diseases may induce changes that favor a systemic antioxidant/pro-oxidant imbalance (2), which results in oxidative stress. With regards to the age investigated, previous studies have enrolled as participants octo-nonagenarians (2), while no data on healthy centenarians have been provided. Previous studies have outlined that centenarians have an immunologic profile (3), endocrinological and metabolic characteristics (4) and nutritional status (5) better than aged subjects. Thus, it is not surprising that also the so called "oxidative stress", a complex web made by anti- and pro-oxidant factors, is lower in centenarians than in aged subjects. Several hypotheses can be suggested to explain the difference in degree of

* Address for correspondence: Giuseppe Paolisso, MD, Dept. of Geriatric Medicine and Metabolic Diseases, Servizio di Astanteria Medica, I-80138 Napoli (Italy). Tel: +38-81-5665016. Fax: +39-81-5665051. E-mail: gpaoliss@tin.it

Recent Advances in Geriatrics, edited by Barbagallo, Licata, and Sowers.
Plenum Press, New York, 1998.

oxidative stress between centenarians and aged subjects. Environmental and genetic factors, in a separate or combined fashion, might play a role. With regard to the environmental factors, centenarians have demonstrated to have an elevated daily protein intake, mainly made by vegetables, (6). Since vegetables are the main natural source of antioxidants (for example, Vitamins C and E), one can suppose the difference in anti-oxidant defense between aged subjects and centenarians due to the difference in diet composition. The role of metabolic factors should be evaluated. In fact, in multivariate analysis fasting plasma glucose and FFA concentrations and insulin action were significant determinants of the degree of oxidative stress. Lastly, centenarians have low fasting plasma glucose and FFA concentrations and better insulin action than aged subjects.

The negative impact of a rise in plasma glucose upon oxidative stress is widely known. There are many ways by which hyperglycemia may increase the generation of free radicals. The terms "autoxidative glycosylation" describes the capability of glucose to enolize, thereby reducing molecular oxygen and yielding oxidizing intermediates (7). The reduced oxygen products formed in the autoxidative reaction are superoxide anion (O_2^-), the hydroxyl radical (OH^-) and hydrogen peroxide (H_2O_2). All can damage proteins through crosslinking, fragmentation and lipid oxidation (7).

As far as fasting plasma FFA is concerned, Toborek and Hennig (8) showed that fatty acids cause an increase in oxidative stress in cultured endothelial cells and an initial decrease in reduced glutathione concentrations after 6-hour exposure in the incubation medium. Among the 18-carbon-fatty acids used, 18:2 (linoleic acid) was the most effective in vivo. Intralipid infusion rose plasma FFA concentrations with a secondary increase in plasma TBARS and LPO concentrations and decrease in the plasma GSH/GSSG ratio (9). The effects of FFA on degree of oxidative stress was time- and dose-dependent and partially also explained the inhibitory effect of FFA upon insulin action (9). Such findings strengthened the hypothesis that a relationship between plasma FFA and oxidative stress occurs.

Hyperinsulinemia/insulin resistance should be also taken into account. Several lines of evidence seem to indicate a relationship between hyperinsulinemia and free radicals production. In intact human fat cells exposure to insulin leads to a time-and dose-dependent accumulation of hydrogen peroxidase in the suspension medium (10). This effect, which was related to the presence of a membrane bound NADPH oxidase, persisted after cell disruption and did not require ATP, indicating that the receptor kinase step was bypassed (10). In rats increased insulin concentrations following intraperitoneal injection of dextrose have been found associated with increased free radical production (11). Since fasting hyperinsulinemia is considered a hallmark of insulin resistance (12) a relationship between insulin resistance and plasma free radical concentrations cannot be excluded. The genesis of free radical concentrations in insulin resistant conditions might be also due to an insulin-mediated overdrive of the sympathetic nervous system activity (12–13). In diabetics animals, cathecolamine may increase free radical production through induction of the metabolic rate and auto-oxidation (14). Whether oxidative stress precedes or follows hyperinsulinemia/insulin resistance is still an open question. Only a longitudinal study designed to address this specific point will clear up the sequence of events linking hyperinsulinemia and oxidative stress.

HYPERGLYCEMIA AND ENDOTHELIAL FUNCTION

Endothelial cells play an important role in arterial relaxation because they produce nitric oxide, a potent endogenous vasodilator that modulates vascular tone by increasing the production of cyclic guanosine monophosphate. The development of atherosclerosis based on metabolic disorders is accompained by a smoothed response of morphologically unaltered blood vessels to endothelium dependent vasodilators like acetylcholine and bradykinin. This reduced vasodilator response that precedes overt atherosclerosis is called endothelium dysfunction. And is thought to depend upon reduced synthesis, effect or availability of endogenous nitric oxide (NO). If endothelial dysfunction has a role in promoting atherosclerosis, it may be a link between hyperglycemia and diabetic macroangiopathy. In isolated aortic rings from normal rabbits exposed to elevated glucose levels, the attenuation of endothelium-dependent relaxation can be prevented by treatment with superoxide dismutase (SOD, a scavenger of superoxide anion) or catalase (a scavenger of hydrogen peroxide). It has been demonstrated that mesenteric arterioles from normal rats exposed to high glucose exhibited endothelial dysfunction which can also be prevented by treatment with SOD or catalase. Similarly, in the mesenteric arterioles from streptozotocin-induced diabetic rats, it has been showed that SOD or 1,3-dimethyl-2-thiourea (a scavenger of hydroxyl radicals) completely restored the impaired endothelium dependent relaxation to the level observed in non-diabetic rats. In analogous experiments in the aorta from diabetic rats, other investigators have also reported that the impaired endothelium dependent relaxation can be normalized after treatment with SOD. Thus studies in animal models of diabetes support nitric oxide inactivation by oxygen-derived free radicals as a cause of endothelial dysfunction. Superoxide anion is implicated in the physiological inactivation of NO. The reaction between O_2^- and NO yields peroxinitrite (–OONO), which is by itself a powerful oxidizing agent. Besides quenching NO, thus limiting its availability to vascular smooth muscle cells, O_2^- may activate the prostaglandin H_2/thromboxane A_2 receptor, thus directly contributing to vasoconstriction. As a consequence, removal of O_2^- by SOD enhances NO biological activity and probably play a major role in counteracting the negative effect of high glucose on endothelial cell function. It is still unclear whether the acute changes in oxidative balance induced by high glucose *in vitro* and *in vivo* in animal models of diabetes also occur in humans. We recently found that acute elevation of plasma in glucose levels to 15 mmol/l (270 mg/dl) in normal subjects produced a significant increase in systolic and diastolic blood pressure and a decreased blood flow through the femoral artery, suggesting vasoconstriction. These haemodynamic changes were unlikely to be mediated by the simultaneous increase in plasma insulin, with a consequent stimulation of sympathetic noradrenergic activity, since blocking insulin secretion with the somatostatin analogue octreotide did not influence the vascular effects of hyperglycemia. On the other hand, a parallel glutathione infusion completely prevented the haemodynamic changes brought about by hyperglycemia, suggesting that acute hyperglycemia may increase the generation of free radicals that in turn will quench NO, reducing its availability to target cells. This interpretation was further supported by the finding that intravenous infusion of L-arginine (1 g/min) — natural precursor of NO — superimposed to hyperglycemia in normal subjects, completely normalized both the increases in blood pressure and the decrease in leg blood flow. Moreover, the infusion of the arginine analogue L-NMMA (NG-monomethyl-L-arginine) which inhibits the endothelial constitutive NO-synthase, produced vascular effects similar to those brought about by hyperglycemia.

MECHANISMS OF ENDOTHELIAL DYSFUNCTION IN HUMAN DIABETES

Endothelium-dependent relaxation may be impaired in human diabetes. Many, though not all, studies have shown that endothelium-dependent vasodilatation as assessed by forearm venous plethysmography, may be abnormal in diabetic patients. Part of the variability of the results so far obtained may be explained by the use of different muscarinic agonists (acetylcholine, metacholine, carbachol) and by differences in forearm lenght accounting for about 60% of divergent responses between sexes. Also, factors such as the ambient glucose concentration during the endothelial function tests and microalbuminuria might be confounding variables in human studies. In any case, more recent studies have consistently shown endothelial dysfunction in diabetic patients — both IDDM and NIDDM — in comparison with non diabetic subjects. Among the mechanisms proposed as explanations for this endothelial dysfunction in diabetic patients there are decreased synthesis or release of NO by endothelial cells, decreased responsiveness of vascular smooth muscle cells to endothelium derived NO, and increased inactivation of NO by oxygen-derived free radicals. In patients with NIDDM and no evidence of vascular complications, acute intra-arterial administration of vitamin C (24 mg/min) improves endothelium-dependent vasodilatation responses to methacholine, whereas the endothelium-independent vasodilator responses to nitroprusside (an exogenous nitric oxide donor) and to verapamil (a direct smooth muscle relaxant) are not significantly altered. This confirms previous data showing an acute blood-pressure lowering effect of three structurally unaltered antioxidants — vitamin C, thiopronine (a substrate for glutathione synthesis) and glutathione — in diabetic patients whether or not they were hypertensives. The vasodilating effects of these agents are probably mediated by their ability to directly or indirectly scavenge excess superoxide anions, decreasing NO inactivation. Another pathway to account for endothelial dysfunction in diabetic subjects is the high levels of glycosylated haemoglobin. *In vitro* experiments with incubation of isolated aortic rings from normal rats with glycosylated hemoglobin resulted in impaired endothelium-dependent relaxation provided that its concentration was 9% or higher. This effect was abolished by SOD suggesting that the interaction of glycosylated hemoglobin with endothelial NO is mediated by superoxide anion production. Finally, hyperglycemia may enhance low density lipoprotein (LDL) oxidation. Oxidized LDL may promote endothelial dysfunction by several mechanisms, including damage to endothelial membrane receptors for vasodilating agonists, decreased synthesis or release of NO and inactivation of NO.

HYPERINSULINEMIA AND ATHEROSCLEROSIS

Resistance to the insulin action on muscle and fat tissues is found in the majority of NIDDM patients and aged subjects and is closely associated with fatness (15–16). Nevertheless, genetic abnormalities can not be excluded (17). It is generally believed that hyperinsulinemia is the motor which drives the other components of the insulin resistance syndrome, namely hypertension and dyslipidemia and it has been suggested that insulin resistance might be the main cause of coronary heart disease (CHD) in developed countries. Actually, the main evidence for a role of hyperinsulinemia as an independent risk factor for atherosclerosis comes from three large prospective studies carried out in healthy men, in which a positive relationship between insulin levels (mainly post challenge) and morbidity and mortality from CHD was found. However, more recent studies (three in Europe and four in the USA) on representative samples of the general population have not confirmed this association. In four prospective studies of patients with NIDDM or glucose intolerance, there was no association between endogenous insulin levels and CHD. Thus insulin is likely to be more a marker of other risk factors (central obesity) than a risk factor in itself.

HYPERGLYCEMIA AND ATHEROSCLEROSIS

Moderate increase in fasting plasma glucose concentration frequently occurs in advancing age; it is therefore reasonable to assume that the long-term vascular complications of elderly are a direct consequence of a modest but long-term chronic hyperglycemia. The acceptance of hyperglycemia as a risk factor for cardiovascular mortality and morbidity has been a matter of strenuous debate, perhaps because no strong relation between cardiovascular diseases (CVD) and glucose levels has been consistently found. However, recent prospective studies have shown that among NIDDM patients, glycaemic control, as measured by hemoglobin A_{1c} (HbA_{1c}), is an important predictor of cardiovascular mortality and morbidity. The results of the Framingham Study, which have long been used to deny any relationship between chronic hyperglycemia and CVD, also indicate that HbA_{1c} predicts cardiovascular mortality, at least in women. HbA_{1c} predicts not only the microvascular complications of diabetes, but some of the hard end points of diabetic macroangiopathy as well, including coronary mortality and lower-extremity amputations. There are several compelling reasons why hyperglycemia should be regarded as a cardiovascular risk factor: i) elevated glucose levels are related to abnormalities in lipoprotein composition; ii) increased susceptibility of LDL to oxidation; iii) alterations of the coagulation system; iv) accumulation of advanced glycosilation endproducts on vascular structures. We have put forward the hypothesis that enhanced free radical generation may be an important and presumably ultimate mechanism by which hyperglycemia exerts its toxic effects on the vasculature.

CAN ANTIOXIDANT ADMINISTRATION AFFECT BLOOD PRESSURE?

Vitamin E administration has been shown to decline plasma free radicals concentrations and degree of oxidative stress, to improve insulin action and to reduce the amount of oxidized LDL. Whether pharmacological doses of vitamin E may affect blood pressure is unknown. We performed a single blind, randomized vs placebo study in which 26 patients with light to moderate hypertensive patients were treated by 300 mg vitamin E (twice daily). After 4 week treatment, vitamin E vs placebo administration was associated with a significant decline in mean arterial blood pressure (141 ± 8.3 vs 122 ± 5.8 mmHg $p < 0.03$).

CONCLUSIONS

The rise of oxidative stress with advancing age is a well known phenomenon which can affect several metabolic and cardiovascular parameters. Hyperglycemia, hyperinsulinemia and elevated fasting plasma FFA concentration together with changes that favor a systemic antioxidant/pro-oxidant imbalance are responsible for the age-related rise in plasma free radicals concentrations. The excess of plasma free radicals might be responsible for endothelial dysfunction. From a clinical point of view such endothelial dysfunction might result in a more elevated arterial blood pressure. On the other hand, chronic vitamin E administration seems an useful tool to lower plasma free radicals concentration and arterial blood pressure. Thus, one can conclude that age-related increase in oxidative stress may play a role in pathophysiology of arterial blood pressure.

REFERENCES

1. Paolisso G and Giugliano D.: Oxidative stress and insulin action: is there a relationship? *Diabetologia* 1996; 39: 357–363
2. Mezzetti A., Lapenna D., Romeno F et al.: Systemic oxidative stress and its relationship with age and illness . *J.Am.Geriatric.Soc.* 1996;44: 823–827
3. Sansoni P., A. Cassarizza, V. Brianti, F. Fagnoni, G. Suelli, D. Monti, A. Mercato, G. Passeri, C. Ortolani, E. Forti, V. Fagiolo, M. Passeri, C. Franceschi: Lymphocyte subset and natural killer activity in healthy old people and centenarians. *Blood* 1993; 82: 2767–2773
4. Paolisso G., Gambardella A., Ammendola S. Varricchio M and D'Onofrio F.: Glucose tolerance and insulin action in healthy centenarians. *Am..J. Physiol (Endocrinol.Metab)* 1996; 270: E890–894
5. Paolisso G., Gambardella A., Balbi et al.: Body composition, body fat distribution and resting metabolic rate in healthy centenarians. *Am. J. Clin. Nutr.* 1995; 62: 746–750
6. Italian Multicenter Study on Centenarians. Ed. Pozzi - Roma- 1996 pp 1–104
7. Giugliano D., Ceriello A.and Paolisso G.:Oxidative stress and diabetic vascular complications. *Diabetes Care* 1996; 19: 257–263
8. Toborek M and Hennig B.: Fatty acid-mediated effects on the glutathione redox cycle in cultured endothelial cells. *Am.J.Clin.Nutr.* 1994 59: 60–65
9. Paolisso G., Gambardella A.,Tagliamonte MR.Varricchio M., D'Onofrio F and Howard BV.: Does free fatty acid infusion impair insulin action also through an increase in oxidative stress?. *J.Clin.Endocrinol.Metab.*1996; 81: 4244–4248
10. Krieger Brauer H. and Kather H.: Human fat cells possess a plasma membrane bound H_2O_2 generating system that is activated by insulin via a mechanism by passing the receptor kinase. *J. Clin. Invest.* 1992; 89: 1006–1013
11. Habib MP, Dickerson FD., Mooradian AD. Effect of diabetes, insulin and glucose load on lipid peroxidation in the rat. *Metabolism* 1994;43: 1442–1445
12. De Fronzo RA., Ferrannini E.:Insulin resistance: a multifaced syndrome responsible for NIDDM, obesity, hypertension, dyslipidemia and atherosclerotic cardiovascular disease. *Diabetes Care* 1991; 14: 173–191
13. Rowe JW., Young JB, Minaker KL., Stevens AL., Pallotta J., Landsberg L. Effect of insulin and glucose infusion on sympathetic nervous system activity in normal men. *Diabetes* 1981; 30: 219–225
14. Singal PK, Beamish RE, Dhalla NS. Potential oxidative pathways of cathecolamines in the formation of lipid peroxides and genesis of heart disease. *Adv. Exp. Med. Biol* 1983;161: 391–401
15. Paolisso G., Scheen AS., and Lefebvre P.: Glucose handling, diabetes and ageing. *Horm.Res.* 1995; 43:52–57
16. Ferrannini E., Vichi S., Beck-Nielsen, Paolisso G., Laakso M .: Insulin action and age. *Diabetes* 1996; 45: 947–953
17. Liang P., Hughes V and Fukagawa N.K.: Increased prevalence of mithocondrial DNA deletions in skeletal muscle of older individuals with impaired glucose tolerance. A possible marker of glycemic stress. *Diabetes* 1997; 46: 920–923

9

HYPERTENSION IN THE ELDERLY

Hormonal and Therapeutic Aspects

Haralambos Gavras and Irene Gavras

Hypertension and Atherosclerosis Section
Department of Medicine
Boston University School of Medicine
715 Albany Street
Boston, Massachusetts 02118

1. INTRODUCTION

Progressive elevation of blood pressure (BP) is a fact of life in acculturated societies, so that beyond age 65 about one in two individuals reaches hypertensive levels, i.e., systolic BP over 160 mmHg, with or without diastolic elevation over 95 mmHg. Systolic BP tends to rise slowly during childhood, adolescence and the early adult years, with a steeper rise after age 40, continuing through the eighth decade of life. Diastolic BP rises steadily until age 60, but tends to decline in later years. This accounts for the high prevalence in older people of isolated systolic BP elevation.

It is now well established that hypertension is strongly associated with disability and death from coronary heart disease, congestive heart failure, stroke and renal failure in every age group and risk gradients do not wane with advancing age, on the contrary, they become steeper.[1] Moreover, systolic BP predicts better than diastolic for every major cardiovascular event. It is also now well documented by recent studies in elderly populations, that lowering of BP by use of both pharmacologic and non-pharmacologic interventions produces unequivocal benefits in terms of decreased cardiovascular morbidity and mortality in all types of hypertension, including isolated systolic hypertension.[2–4] (Although lifestyle changes may be more stressful and difficult to implement in this age group). Nevertheless, two issues bear particular scrutiny: 1) All of these interventional pharmacologic trials, like trials in younger hypertensive populations, have produced a far greater reduction in the incidence of strokes and other hypertensive complications than in the incidence of heart attacks; unlike trials in younger patients, however, there was no significant reduction in overall mortality rates in the EPWHE[2] and SHEP[4] trials, suggesting that non-cardiovascular causes of death might have been increased by the treatment. 2) Some British publications have reported the phenomenon of the J shaped curve, i.e., a lowest point of mortality at diastolic BPs of 85–90 mmHg, with higher rates of ischemic cerebrovascu-

Recent Advances in Geriatrics, edited by Barbagallo, Licata, and Sowers.
Plenum Press, New York, 1998.

lar and cardiovascular events at BPs below that range.[5] Although not specifically related to age (indeed it was not observed in the SHEP trial), this phenomenon, if true, would be more likely to occur in subjects with widespread atherosclerotic vascular disease and impaired autoregulatory mechanisms. Both of these issues may be relevant to the choice of antihypertensive medications in the elderly. Knowledge of age-related changes in the anatomy and physiology of the cardiovascular system is also relevant to the choice of appropriate drugs.

2. PATHOPHYSIOLOGY OF AGING

2.1. Anatomical Aspects

The myocardium undergoes degenerative changes with increase in the size of myocytes, lipid and lipofuscin deposition, diminished numbers of myocytes, widespread fat and amyloid deposits and increase in fibrous tissues, all of which are characteristic of the cardiomyopathy of aging. The number of pacemaker cells and the density of conduction fibers decrease, whereas fibrosis and calcification increase throughout the sinus node, conduction system (causing propensity to dysrhythmias) and valves. Arteries lose their elasticity, lengthen, thicken, dilate and become tortuous. Endothelial cells change in size and shape, the subendothelial layer contains more lipids, connective tissue and calcium deposits, the smooth muscle layer thickens and contains polyploid cells.[6] Cardiac output tends to decline and fails to rise appropriately during exercise, due to impaired ventricular filling, tendency to diminished contractile capacity, inadequate heart rate rise in response to stimuli and increased peripheral vascular resistance. These changes may lead to systolic and diastolic dysfunction of the myocardium and left ventricular hypertrophy even in the absence of established hypertension. They are further accentuated by the increased aortic stiffness (causing increased systolic stress) and loss of recoil capacity (causing low perfusion pressure during diastole), which also attenuate the baroreflex sensitivity.[7] Left ventricular hypertrophy is an independent risk factor for myocardial ischemia and heart failure.[8]

Other age-related anatomical changes relevant to blood pressure regulation and to antihypertensive drug treatment include diminished body water content—especially intravascular fluid volume and increased percentage of body fat—which affect the volume of distribution of hydrophilic and lipophilic drugs.[1] Renal function also diminishes with aging, due to decrease in renal blood flow and glomerular filtration rate.[9,10] As a result, there is a physiological decline of creatinine clearance by about 1% annually. This, in addition to the diminished enzymatic activity in the liver, leads to decreased metabolic clearance rates for various substances, and hence relatively prolonged action of drugs.

2.2. Neurohormonal Aspects

Aging is associated with a diminished responsiveness of the usual regulatory mechanisms that maintain circulatory homeostasis.[11] There is generally reduced baroreceptor sensitivity, decreased responsiveness of β-adrenergic receptors, reduced resting vagal activity and blunted heart rate response to increased blood pressure.[12–14] These changes indicate a "physiological" degree of autonomic insufficiency, which, in conjunction with the decreased intravascular fluid volume and loss of arterial wall elasticity, predispose elderly subjects to orthostatic hypotension. The normal circadian variation of blood pressure is maintained in older subjects, although younger subjects have a greater nocturnal fall in arterial pressure ("night dipping").

Aging is also associated with a number of changes in normal levels of vasoactive hormones at rest and after stimulation.[14–17] Plasma renin activity and plasma aldosterone levels are generally suppressed and fail to increase appropriately when stimulated by dehydration, hypotension, etc. On the contrary, plasma levels of catecholamines tend to rise with age, so that the normal level for a 70-year-old is about twice that of the average 20-year-old. However, old age is not characterized by a hyperadrenergic state, but rather by diminished overall adrenergic activity, evidently due to diminished numbers and overall activity of α- and β-adrenergic receptors.[13,14,18,19] Plasma vasopressin levels tend to be higher in older subjects, and are significantly more elevated in black hypertensives. Vasopressin plays a more important role in the maintenance of arterial pressure in older and in black subjects, as shown by the greater fall in blood pressure in response to specific vasopressin antagonists.[20,21] In the elderly, this may be explained by the fact that the other two major pressor systems (i.e., the renin-angiotensin and the sympathetic system) are hyporesponsive, and therefore blood pressure maintenance depends to a greater extent on the pressor contribution of vasopressin. In support of this interpretation is the fact that diabetics who, regardless of age, tend to have some degree of autonomic insufficiency as well as hyporeninemic hypoaldosteronism, tend also to rely much more on the pressor effect of vasopressin for blood pressure maintenance.[22]

Another important consideration is the tendency to develop some degree of insulin resistance with aging. Essential hypertension is already a state of diminished insulin sensitivity, even in younger and nonobese subjects.[23,24] Both advancing age and the attendant weight gain tend to further accentuate this metabolic characteristic, so that elderly hypertensives are more likely to present the "metabolic syndrome X": the coexistence of insulin resistance, hyperglycemia, hyperinsulinemia, hyperlipidemia and hypertension. This syndrome is associated with abdominal adiposity (the "apple shape"), characterized by a high waist-to-hip ratio, rather than generalized obesity.[25] Patients exhibiting these characteristics are more prone to develop type II diabetes mellitus.

3. CHOOSING ANTIHYPERTENSIVE MEDICATIONS

Choice of the most appropriate BP-lowering drug for a particular patient should be an individualized decision, taking into account medical factors such as the type of hypertension, coexisting diseases or hypertensive complications, that might be beneficially or adversely affected by the drug, side-effect profile of the drug, potential for interaction with concurrent medications, as well as psychosocial considerations, such as independent or assisted living, family situation, level of activity, convenience, compliance and cost of medication.[26]

In general, drug doses should be lower and dosing intervals longer in elderly frail patients. The Joint National Commission on Hypertension in its fifth report[27] has recommended thiazide diuretics and beta-adrenergic blockers as first choice for all hypertensives who have no special indication for other therapy. For elderly patients, this recommendation was based on the SHEP trial,[4] whose subjects were carefully selected and otherwise healthy. Although generally safe, effective, convenient and available as inexpensive generics, both of these classes have a number of limitations. Following is a brief overview of the advantages and disadvantages of each class of drugs, as described in more detail elsewhere.[28]

Thiazides accentuate the tendency to orthostatic intolerance, cause metabolic abnormalities such as hypokalemia (arrhythmias), insulin resistance (hyperglycemia that may precipitate or aggravate type II diabetes mellitus), hyperuricemia (gout attacks), dyslipidemias (whose importance as a coronary risk factor in this population remains debatable) and are associated with a high rate of sexual dysfunction. Thus, their low initial cost may be negated by the need for frequent monitoring and additional medications (potassium supplements, urate suppressants, etc.).

Beta-adrenoceptor blockers are particularly suitable for patients with coexisting angina or certain arrhythmias and are the preferred mode of treatment for patients with orthostatic intolerance. Agents with intrinsic sympathomimetic activity may minimize some of the side-effects of beta-blockade, such as bronchoconstriction or excessive bradycardia, but are contraindicated in the presence of coronary insufficiency or post-myocardial infarction. Beta-blockers are absolutely contraindicated in patients with chronic obstructive pulmonary disease and relatively contraindicated in a number of other conditions, such as congestive heart failure (with systolic dysfunction, though possibly helpful in diastolic dysfunction), sick sinus syndrome and other bradyarrhythmias, peripheral obstructive arterial disease, diabetes treated with insulin or oral hypoglycemic agents, mental depression. They also tend to cause sluggishness, fatigue and sexual dysfunction, although these effects are probably dose-related and are less likely to occur with small doses.

Centrally acting sympatholytic agents such as clonidine, methyldopa and reserpine are probably not a good first choice for elderly patients, as they are commonly associated with mental depression, lethargy, cognitive impairment, loss of memory and general psychosocial difficulties. Peripheral $alpha_1$-adrenoceptor antagonists carry the real risk of orthostatic intolerance, although they have otherwise a good efficacy and metabolic profile, and are especially helpful in men with dysuric symptoms resulting from benign prostatic hypertrophy and in patients with chronic obstructive pulmonary disease.

Calcium channel blockers are generally safe and effective, provided they are well tolerated. They are particularly suitable for patients with concurrent coronary disease, but not after a heart attack, especially in the presence of systolic dysfunction. They have a neutral metabolic profile and usually do not interact with other drugs—except for verapamil, which interferes with elimination of digoxin and which accentuates the negative inotropic and proarrhythmic effect of beta-blockers. Most common causes of intolerance are constipation and peripheral edema, the latter being most pronounced with dihydropyridine derivatives (nifedipine, amlodipine, felodipine etc.), which have a more pronounced vasodilatory action. The long-term safety of calcium channel blockers has recently come under scrutiny and remains a matter of controversy.

Angiotensin-converting enzyme (ACE) inhibitors are an excellent first choice both in terms of efficacy and of side-effect profile. Despite earlier speculation that elderly low-renin patients might be less responsive to ACE inhibition, in fact they are equally or more responsive and require smaller doses.[29] ACE inhibitors have a beneficial metabolic profile (they tend to attentuate insulin resistance and related metabolic aberrations)[30] and generally do not interact with concurrent medications except, possibly, non-steroidal anti-inflammatory drugs. They are particularly suitable for patients with coexisting coronary heart disease, prior myocardial infarct, cardiomyopathies, congestive heart failure, type I or II diabetes mellitus, diabetic nephropathy or hypertensive nephrosclerosis. Because of preferential vasodilation of the cerebral, cardiac and renal vasculature, ACE inhibitors preserve or enhance blood flow to vital organs, even when systemic blood pressure is decreased. Several comparative studies have shown that ACE inhibitors have the least impact on the patient's quality of life. The main side-effects limiting their tolerability are cough, whose incidence tends to increase with advancing age, and tendency to hyperkalemia in the presence of renal insufficiency. These and the very rare angioedema are "class effects" likely to recur with every ACE inhibitor, whereas allergic reactions are less common with the second generation of ACE inhibitors, which also have the great advantage of once-daily dosing unrelated to meals.

The latest class of antihypertensive agents is the antagonists of angiotensin II at the level of the AT_1 receptor. The prototype of Ang II antagonists is losartan,[31] but several others are already at various stages of clinical development. Comparative studies have shown that monotherapy with losartan is at least as effective as monotherapy with any other agent for all age groups, and presents all the advantages of ACE inhibition without the nuisance of cough.[32] It is particularly suitable for older hypertensives with coexisting diabetes, renal insufficiency or chronic heart failure. A surprising recent development was the report[33] that in older subjects with congestive heart failure, losartan decreased the mortality rates more than captopril (surprising because ACE inhibition has been so far the only treatment shown to prolong life in such patients and is now the standard treatment for congestive heart failure). If this is confirmed by other studies, it would suggest that for older hypertensives, Ang II antagonists are not just an alternative to ACE inhibitors when the latter cause cough, but are in fact preferable to ACE inhibition.

In conclusion, cardiovascular disease remains the most frequent cause of morbidity and mortality in people over age 65. However, this group includes a wide range of subjects at different stages of chronologic and biologic aging, with different expectations from specific treatments. The choice of the most suitable antihypertensive agent(s) is guided by the specific goals set for each individual, but the general principles are the same: to offer the most benefit with the fewest disadvantages, keep drug regimens simple, choose agents that will not impair psychosocial performance and quality of life, and that have the best potential to prolong life.

REFERENCES

1. Gavras H, Gavras I: *Hypertension in the elderly*. Publishers: John Wright PS Inc., Littleton, Massachusetts and Bristol, England; pp 1–240, 1983.
2. Amery A, Birkenhager W, Brixko R, Bulpitt C, Clement D, Derayttere M, et al. Efficacy of antihypertensive drug treatment according to age, sex, blood pressure and previous cardiovascular disease in patients over the age of 60. Lancet 2:589–592, 1986.
3. Dahlof B, Lundholm L, Hansson L, Schersten B, Ekbom T, Wester PO: Morbidity and Mortality in the Swedish Trial in Old Patients with Hypertension (STOP-Hypertension). Lancet 338:1281–1285, 1991.
4. SHEP Coorperative Research Group. Prevention of stroke by antihypertensive drug treatment in older persons with isolated systolic hypertensin: final results of the systolic hypertension in the Elderly Program (SHEP). JAMA 265:3255–3264, 1991.
5. Cruickshank JM, Thorp JM, Zacharias FJ: Benefits and potential harm of lowering high blood pressure. Lancet i:581–584, 1987.
6. Wei JY: Age and the cardiovascular system. N Engl J Med 327:1735–1739, 1992.
7. Folkow B, Svanborg A. Physiology of cardiovascular aging. Physiological Reviews 73:725–764, 1993.
8. Levy D, Garrison RJ, Savage DD, Kannel WB, Castelli WP. Left ventricular mass and incidence of coronary heart disease in an elderly cohort: the Framingham Heart Study. Am Int Med 110:101–107, 1989.
9. Hollenberg NK, Adams DF, Solomon HS, et al: Senescence and the renal vasculature in normal man. Circ Res 1974;34:309–316.
10. Epstein M: Effects of aging on the kidney. Fed Proc 1979;38:168–179.
11. Lipsitz LA: Abnormalities in blood pressure homeostasis associated with aging and hypertension. In: Blood Pressure Regulation and Aging (Horan MJ, Steinberg GM, Dunbar JB, Hadley EL, eds) Biomedical Info, Corp., New York, NY 1986. pp 201–212.

12. Kawanamoto A, Shimada K, Matsubayashi K, et al: Cardiovascular regulatory functions in elderly patients with hypertension. Hypertension 1989;13:401–407.
13. Lakatta EG: Age-related alterations in the cardiovascular response to adrenergic mediated stress. Fed Proc 1980;39:3173–3177.
14. Rowe JW, Troen BR: Sympathetic nervous system and aging in man. Endocr Rev 1980;1:167–179.
15. Crane MG, Harris JJ: Effect of aging on renin activity and aldosterone excretion. J Lab Clin Med 1976;86:947–959.
16. Stern N, Beahm E, McGinty D, et al: Dissociation of 24-hour catecholamine levels from blood pressure in older men. Hypertension 1985;7:1023–1029.
17. Gavras I, Gavras H, Chobanian AV, Tifft CP, Melby JC, Jick H: Hypertension and age: clinical and biochemical correlates. Clin Exper Hyper Theory and Practice A4(7):1097–1106, 1982.
18. Bursztyn M, Bresnahan M, Gavras I, Gavras H: Pressor Hormones in Elderly Hypertensive Persons Racial Difference. Hypertension 15:(Suppl I) I-88-I-92, 1990.
19. Bursztyn M, Bresnahan M, Gavras I, Gavras H: Effect of Aging on Vasopressin, Catecholamines, and Alpha$_2$ -Adrenergic Receptors. Amer Geriatr Soc 38:628–632, 1990.
20. De Paula RB, Plavnik FL, Rodrigues CIS, De Assis Rocha Neves F, Kohlmann O Jr, Ribeiro AB, Gavras I, Gavras H: Contribution of vasopressin to orthostatic blood pressure maintenance in essential hypertension. Am J Hypertens 6:794–798, 1993.
21. De Paula RB, Plavnik FL, Rodrigues CIS, De Assis Rocha Neves F, Kohlmann O Jr, Ribeiro AB, Gavras I, Gavras H: Age and race determine vasopressin participation in upright blood pressure control in essential hypertension. Ann NY Acad Sci 689:534–536, 1993.
22. Saad CI, Ribeiro AB, Zanella MT, Mulinari RA, Gavras I, Gavras H: The role of vasopressin in blood pressure maintenance in diabetic orthostatic hypotension. Hypertension 11(Suppl 1):I-217-I-221, 1988.
23. Reaven GM. Role of insulin resistance in human disease. Diabetes 37:1595–1607, 1988.
24. Rocchini AP. Insulin resistance and blood pressure regulation in obese and nonobese subjects. Hypertension 17:837–842, 1991.
25. Bjŏrntorp P. Abdominal obesity and risk. Clin and Exper Hypertens A12:783–794, 1990.
26. Bursztyn M, Gavras I, Gavras H: Hypertension in the Aging Patients Implications for the Selection of Drug Therapy. J Am Geriatr Soc 37:814–818, 1989.
27. Fifth Report of the Joint National Committee on Detection, Evaluation and Treatment of High Blood Pressure. Arch Int Med 153:154–184, 1993.
28. Gavras I, Manolis AJ, Gavras H: Drug Therapy for Hypertension. American Family Physician 55:1823–1834, 1997.
29. Mulinari R, Gavras I, Gavras H: Efficacy and tolerability of enalapril monotherapy in mild-to-moderate hypertension in older patients compared to younger patients. Clin Ther 9(6):678–692, 1987.
30. Pollare T, Lithell H, Berne C: A comparison of the effects of hydrochlorothiazide and captopril on glucose and lipid metabolism in patients with hypertension. New Eng J Med 321:868–873, 1989.
31. Goodfriend TL, Elliott ME, Catt KJ: Angiotensin receptors and their antagonists. New Eng J Med 334:1649–1654, 1996.
32. Tikkanen I, Omvik P, Jensen HA: Comparison of the angiotensin II antagonist losartan with the angiotensin converting enzyme inhibitor enalapril in patients with essential hypertension. J Hypertens 13:1343–1351, 1995.
33. Pitt B, Segal R, Martinez FA et al. Randomized trial of losartan versus captopril in patients over 65 with heart failure (ELITE study). Lancet 349:747–752, 1997.

METABOLIC AND CARDIOVASCULAR MANIFESTATIONS OF HYPERTENSION IN THE ELDERLY

V. Rajkumar, Luis C. Afonso, Joel Steinberg, Stephen L. Farrow, and James R. Sowers*

Wayne State University School of Medicine
Detroit, Michigan 48201

Aging in industrialized societies is associated with an increasing prevalence of hypertension, type II diabetes mellitus, renal disease and atherosclerotic vascular disease. This increase in chronic disease processes in industrialized societies is related, in part, to increasing obesity, reduced physical activity, medications such as non-steroidal anti-inflammatory agents, and other environmental influences. Hypertension in the elderly is characterized by high peripheral vascular resistance, reduced baroreflex sensitivity, a low renin state with reduced cardiac output / increased hypertrophy, reduced intravascular volume, and an increased propensity to salt-sensitivity. Type II diabetes commonly accompanies hypertension in the elderly, in part related to reduction in lean body mass and relative increase in adiposity. Lipid abnormalities are also relatively common in the elderly and should generally be treated in a similar fashion to those in the middle-aged individual.

1. INTRODUCTION

The incidence and prevalence of cardiovascular heart disease, the principal cause of morbidity and mortality in industrialized countries,[1] is highest in persons over age 65, and most coronary events occur after 65 years of age.[2–8] Although coronary heart disease (CHD) is less common in women than men,[2] CHD, including heart disease and stroke, is the leading cause of death in women older than 50 years.[2] Over 200,000 women between the ages of 50 and 79 years die of CHD in the U.S. each year.[2] Thus, CHD is the leading cause of death in both elderly men and women. The potential for reduction of CHD-related mortality in the elderly through primary prevention seems promising because of the high attributable risk in the elderly.[6,8,9] This review discusses major risk factors for CHD, including hypertension, diabetes and dyslipidemia in the elderly.

* Correspondence to: James R. Sowers, MD, Professor of Medicine and Physiology, Director, Division of Endocrinology, Metabolism and Hypertension, Wayne State University School of Medicine, 4201 St. Antoine, UHC-4H, Detroit, MI 48201. Tel: 313/745-4008. Fax: 313/993-0903. E-mail: sowers@oncgate.roc.wayne.edu

Recent Advances in Geriatrics, edited by Barbagallo, Licata, and Sowers.
Plenum Press, New York, 1998.

2. HYPERTENSION IN THE ELDERLY

Diastolic blood pressure (DBP) levels rise with advancing years until age 55, while systolic blood pressure (SBP) increases throughout life.[1,10–13] Isolated systolic hypertension ISH was present in 11.7% of patients older than 60 years enrolled in the Systolic Hypertension in the Elderly Program SHEP.[14] ISH has been observed in 30% of the Japanese population at age 90 years.[15] Data from non-industrialized societies fail to show similar-age related increases, suggesting that this age-associated elevation in blood pressure phenomenon, seen primarily in industrialized societies, may be caused by environmental factors, such as diet, obesity and sedentary lifestyles Table 1.[16–18]

Atherosclerotic vascular disease morbidity and mortality—including CHD, stroke, renal disease, and mortality from all causes—increase progressively with higher levels of both SBP and DBP; these relationships are strong, continuous, independent, predictable, and clinically significant.[13] Epidemiologic studies have shown that a modest increase in blood pressure is associated with an increased risk for cardiovascular disease. Patients with SBP levels ranging from 140 to 160 mm Hg or DBP levels of 85 to 89 mm Hg still incur a modest risk. Systolic blood pressure is a greater risk factor for cardiovascular morbidity and mortality than DBP, especially in the elderly.[10–13] Data from the Multiple Risk Factor Intervention Trial have shown SBP elevation to be a more potent risk factor than DBP elevation.[11,19] In this study, SBP of 160 mm Hg was found to be a more significant correlate of mortality than a DBP of 95 mm Hg.[19]

3. PATHOPHYSIOLOGICAL FACTORS IN HYPERTENSION IN THE ELDERLY

Aging in industrialized societies is often associated with functional and structural alterations of the cardiovascular system (Table 2). The central factor in the genesis of hy-

Table 1. Pathophysiological factors in age-related hypertension

- Industrialization, which is associated with increased salt, decreased calcium, potassium, and magnesium consumption; physical inactivity; and stress.
- Increased obesity with aging, which is associated with hyperinsulinemia and insulin resistance, and enhances sympathetic activity and increases peripheral vascular resistance.
- Decreased ability to handle sodium, which involves a genetic decrease in the ability of the senescent kidney to excrete sodium genetic salt sensitivity and decreased ability of the kidney to generate natriuretic substances like dopamine and prostaglandins.
- Increased intracellular free calcium, which increases peripheral vascular resistance.
- Increased sympathetic nervous system activity, with increased norepinephrine levels, particularly with exercise, sleep, and upright posture.
- Decreased vascular beta-adrenergic vasodilatation function, leaving unopposed alpha-adrenergic receptor vasoconstriction in response to elevated norepinephrine levels.
- Decreased endothelium vasorelaxation function.
- Vascular structural alterations:
  - Increased rigidity and decreased compliance of large vessels.
  - Hyaline degeneration within media of precapillary arterioles, resulting in decreased wall-to-lumen ratio and increased vascular resistance.
  - Atherosclerosis and other aging effects on the carotid and aortic baroreceptor sensitivity, resulting in enhanced sympathetic activity, increased blood pressure lability, and increased tendency to orthostatic hypotension.

Table 2. Changes in the cardiovascular system of the elderly

Cardiovascular hemodynamics
• Tendency to contracted intravascular volume
• Increased peripheral vascular resistance.
• Tendency to lowered cardiac output.
• Decreased baroreceptor sensitivity.
• Increased blood pressure variability.
• Tendency to reduced renal blood flow.
• Suppressed plasma renin activity.
• Decreased vascular endothelium production of nitric oxide.
Renal factors
• Salt retention.
• Decreased renal prostaglandin production.
• Decreased production of other renal natriuretic factors.
• Increased renovascular resistance.
• Decreased renin production.

pertension in the elderly is the increase in smooth muscle tone along with a concomitant increase in systemic vascular resistance. Increased rigidity and decreased elasticity and compliance of the aorta and other large vessels is caused by progressive muscle hypertrophy, fracturing and uncoiling of the elastic fibers in large vessels, and deposition of calcium and collagen within vessel walls.[15–20] Because of the reduced vascular compliance, the pulse wave generated during systole is not effectively dampened in transit through the aorta and its tributaries, leading to a rapid rise in intraarterial pressure and sustained peak pressures with cardiac ejection. Aging is also associated with decreases in cardiac compliance and circulating blood volume, an increase in cardiac wall thickness and an attenuation of the renin-angiotensin responses to various physiologic stimuli (Table 2).

Structural changes associated with aging contribute to cardiovascular baroreflex dysfunction[15–20] and associated lability of blood pressure,[21] as well as a propensity toward orthostatic hypotension.[22] Clinically significant reductions in blood pressure on assuming the erect posture occur frequently in the elderly, making them prone to orthostatic hypotension as well as asymptomatic hypotension, both of which often accompany and complicate antihypertensive therapy.[18,20] There are also age-related physiological alterations in the vascular system that contribute to increases in peripheral vascular resistance,[16] the hallmark of hypertension in the elderly.[23] There is loss of β-adrenergic responsiveness in various tissues, including those of the cardiovascular system, with increasing age.[24] There is, however, no such clear cut diminution in the alpha-adrenergic responsiveness with aging. Thus, for a given release of norepinephrine at adrenergic nerve terminals, there is a greater vasoconstrictor response from these age-related alterations in adrenergic receptor responsiveness.[18]

Changes in renal function also contribute to age-related increases in blood pressure. Advancing age is associated with progressive decrement in functioning nephron units and renal blood flow resulting in a reduced glomerular filtration rate (GFR). Further, microcirculatory adaptive changes occur after a critical loss of renal mass; preglomerular vasodilatation or impaired autoregulation is associated with structural and functional hypertrophy of the residual intact nephrons.[27] The aging kidney's diminished functional reserve and microcirculatory maladaption places it at greater risk for the progression of hypertensive arteriolar nephrosclerosis and also renders it vulnerable to critical reductions in tissue blood delivery from relatively modest short term declines in mean arterial pressure. The high prevalence of salt sensitivity in the elderly may be associated with senescent renal changes and consequent reduced ability to excrete a salt load.[28–30] An age-related decrease in the natriuretic response to increased dietary salt may result from a reduced ability to generate natriuretic substances, such as dopamine and prostaglandins.[30]

4. CHANGES IN BODY COMPOSITION IN THE ELDERLY

Advancing age is generally associated with a loss of lean body mass and an increase in adipose tissue, particularly central body fat.[31–36] In women there appears to be an accelerated accumulation of total body fat in the postmenopausal years.[35,37] The age-related increase in fat mass and central adiposity is greater in women than men.[37] Studies[37,38] suggest that regularly performed endurance exercise partially protects, but does not abolish, the increase in body "fatness" with aging. One report indicated that even when master athletes maintain optimal exercise volume and intensity, body fat increased by approximately 2% over a 10-year period. However, physically active men and women have less central adiposity than their sedentary counterparts.[39,40] Exercise intervention studies [38,41] have demonstrated that endurance training selectively reduces body fat centrally. These observations are important in that central adiposity has been observed to be strongly and positively associated with CHD mortality.[36,42]

5. DIABETES MELLITUS IN THE ELDERLY — ROLE IN CHD

In industrialized societies, glucose intolerance increases with age and type II diabetes is especially prevalent in the geriatric population.[43] However, our understanding of basis for the increase in prevalence of type II diabetes with increasing age is not complete. Type II diabetes is generally considered to develop if the level of insulin secretion is inadequate to maintain euglycemia under prevailing conditions of insulin resistance.[44] Studies have shown that maximum glucose-induced insulin secretion per beta-cell declines progressively as rats age.[45] However, those rats maintain euglycemia as they age, as a result of an approximate four-fold increase in pancreatic beta cell mass.[45]. Although there is evidence that beta-cell mass can increase in the aging person, the magnitude of the change is much less than that seen in rodents.[46] Despite the limitations of beta-cell hyperplasia in elderly humans, the plasma insulin concentrations in response to an oral glucose load are relatively normal with only subtle abnormalities in insulin secretion.[47–50] The increased insulin resistance in aging appears to relate to attenuated insulin-induced mobilization of the GLUT 4 transporter to the target cell membrane[49] as well as body composition changes. Regardless of the mechanisms involved, fasting plasma glucose levels have been observed to rise 1 to 2 mg/dl for each decade past 40 years.[51,52] CHD is the leading cause of mortality in type II diabetes, including elderly subpopulations where CHD is independently prevalent.[53,54] Observations from the Rancho Bernardo Study of elderly community-dwelling persons indicate that asymptomatic ischemic heart disease documented by resting electrocardiograms was 1.80 times more common in women with type II diabetes and 1.75 times more common in men with type II diabetes than in an age-matched control population.[54] Diabetes also increases the likelihood of stroke in the elderly, and mortality is substantially higher in diabetic individuals who suffer from myocardial infarction or stroke compared to nondiabetic persons.

6. COEXISTENT DIABETES AND HYPERTENSION

Diabetes and hypertension are interrelated diseases that increase with age in industrialized societies.[55,56] Data gained from death certificates show that hypertensive disease has been implicated in 4.4% of deaths coded to diabetes, and diabetes was involved in 10% of deaths coded to hypertensive disease. Indeed, an estimated 35% to 75% of diabetic cardiovascular and renal complications can be attributed to hypertension.[55] Hypertension also contributes to diabetic retinopathy, which is the leading cause of newly diagnosed blindness in the U.S.[55,56] For all these reasons, hypertension and diabetes should be recognized and treated early and aggressively.

Both diabetes and hypertension increase CHD risk via a number of mechanisms. As recently reviewed,[1,56] these disorders are individually associated with increased platelet aggregation, a procoagulant state, and atherogenic lipoprotein profiles. Further, all of these co-existing conditions contribute to endothelial dysfunction and increased vascular activity, which are the hallmarks of hypertension in diabetics, particularly elderly diabetic persons.[55,56] Further, it appears that hyperglycemia, per se, may exacerbate the vascular and renal disease associated with hypertension and diabetes mellitus.[56]

7. DYSLIPIDEMIA AND AGING

Pooled data from 22 cohort studies has shown that total cholesterol and low density lipoprotein cholesterol levels were significantly related to fatal CHD in both men and women across a broad age range and into older populations >65 years; however, relative risk decreased with increasing age[58]. This is probably a result of a selective survivor effect (i.e. individuals without risk factors are likely outlive those with)[59,60]. A recent analysis of the Framingham Study identified total serum cholesterol as an independent risk factor for CHD and confirmed that while relative risk for CHD associated with high cholesterol decreases with age, attributable risk increases with age[61]. Cardiovascular comorbidity such as hypertension and diabetes may increase the risk for CHD with hypercholesterolemia among elderly patients[62]. Since CHD is more prevalent among older persons as well as in those with diabetes and hypertension, the cholesterol treatment panel[63] have indicated that age is not a contraindication to cholesterol-lowering therapy . A meta-analysis of cholesterol reduction intervention studies describes a 19% decrease in CHD risk for each 10% reduction of serum cholesterol among 75–84 year olds[64]. Further, one small study in Italy[61] indicates that 1 year of therapy with an HMG-CoA reductase inhibitor was associated with either arrest or regression of atherosclerotic plaques in elderly patients with hypercholesterolemia. Nevertheless, primary prevention trials in elderly men suggest that at least 2 years are required before a reduction in CHD becomes manifest.[65] In elderly diabetic hypertensive patients with a prior CHD event, the benefits may be manifested earlier, however controlled trials in this population are yet to be performed.

The CHD rates in elderly women are comparable to those in men and of note is the fact that women comprise about 75% of the population over 65 years of age[66]. Lipoprotein profiles consisting of low density lipoprotein, high density lipoproteins and triglyceride levels have been demonstrated to be predictors of CHD death in elderly women.[57]

Estrogen replacement therapy (ERT) is believed to have cardioprotective effects and has been recommended as an intermediate step between diet and drug therapy of hyperlipidemia in older women[67].The cardioprotective effects of ERT cannot be explained by modest changes (increase in HDL and decrease in LDL) lipid levels alone. Estrogen appears to have a stabilizing effect on the vasculature making it less susceptible to atherogenesis. Additionally, estrogen has been demonstrated to have antiplatelet and antioxidant effects, to increase endothelial nitric oxide release, inhibit vascular smooth muscle mitogenesis, decrease insulin resistance, and favorably influence the clotting profile. The addition of progestins does not significantly reduce the cardioprotective benefits of ERT[68]. However no clinical trials of ERT with CHD end points have been completed to strongly support its use in women over 65. Data from ongoing trials should provide useful data in this regard in the near future.

ACKNOWLEDGMENTS

The authors wish to thank Paddy McGowan for her excellent work in preparing and editing this review. Our work is supported by a VA research grant, NIH RO1-HD24497 and the American Heart Association.

REFERENCES

1. Sowers JR, Farrow SL. Treatment of elderly hypertensive patients with diabetes, renal disease, and coronary heart disease. Am J Geriatr Cardiol 1996;5:57–70.
2. Bush TL. The epidemiology of cardiovascular disease in postmenopausal women. *Ann NY Acad Sci* 1990;592:262–271.
3. Stuck SE, Siu AL, Wieland GD, Adams J, Rubenstein LZ. Comprehensive geriatric assessment: a meta-analysis of controlled trials. *Lancet* 1993;342:1032–1036.
4. Robinson JG, Leon AS. The prevention of cardiovascular disease: emphasis on secondary prevention. *Med Clin North Am* 1994;78:69.
5. Scott M, Owen P, Porter P, et al. Prevalence of adults with no known risk factors for coronary heart disease. Behavioral risk factor surveillance system, 1992. *MMWR* 1994;43:61
6. Stamler J, Wentworth D, Neaton JD. Is the relationship between serum cholesterol and risk of premature death from coronary Heart disease continuous and graded? Findings in 356,222 primary screenees of the Multiple Risk Factor Intervention Trial MRFIT *JAMA* 1986;256:2823–8.
7. Lau J, Antman EM, Jimenez-Silva J, et al. Cumulative meta-analysis of therapeutic trials for myocardial infarction. *N Engl J Med* 1992;327:248.
8. Adult Treatment Panel II: Second report of the Expert Panel on Detection, Evaluation, and Treatment of High Blood Cholesterol in Adults. *Circulation* 1994;89:1336.
9. Malenka DJ, Baron JA. Cholesterol and coronary heart disease: the importance of patient-specific attributable risk. *Arch Intern Med* 1988;148:2247–2252.
10. Vokonas PS, Kannel WB, Cupples LA: Epidemiology and risk of hypertension in the elderly: The Framingham study. *J Hypertens* 1988;6 suppl I :S3-S9.
11. Whelton PK, Klag MJ: Epidemiology of high blood pressure. *Clin Geriatr Med* 1989;5:639–655.
12. Sowers JR, Khoury S, Imam K, et al: Therapeutic approach to hypertension in the elderly. *Primary Care* 1991;18:593–604.
13. The fifth report of the Joint National Committee on Detection, Evaluation, and Treatment of High Blood Pressure JNC-V . *Arch Intern Med* 1993;153:154–183.
14. Perry HM, Smith WM, McDonald RH, et al. Morbidity and mortality in the Systolic Hypertension in the Elderly Program SHEP pilot study. *Stroke* 1989;20:4–13.
15. Kuramato K, Matsushito S, Kuwajimi I. The pathogenetic role of elderly hypertension. *Jpn Circ J* 1981;45:833–843.
16. Sowers JR. Hypertension in the elderly. *Am J Med* 1987;82:1–8.
17. Sowers JR, Mohanty PK. Effects of advancing age on cardiopulmonary baroreceptor function in hypertensive men. *Hypertension* 1987;10:274–279.
18. Sowers JR, Mohanty PK. Norepinephrine and forearm vascular resistance responses to tilt and cold pressor test in essential hypertension: Effects of aging. *Angiology* 1989;40 10 :872–879.
19. Fleich JH, Hooker CS. The relationship between age and relaxation of vascular smooth muscle in the rabbit and rat. *Circ Res* 1976;38:243–249.

20. Shimada K, Kitazumi T, Sadakane N, Ogura H, Ozawa T. Age-related changes of baroreflex function, plasma norepinephrine, and blood pressure. *Hypertension* 1985:7:113–117.
21. Khoury S, Yarows S, O'Brian T, Sowers JR. Ambulatory blood pressure monitoring in a nonacademic setting: Effects of age and sex. *Am J Hypertens* 1992;5:616–623.
22. Sowers JR, Rubenstein LZ, Stern N. Plasma norepinephrine responses to posture and isometric exercise with age in the absence of obesity. *J Gerontol* 1983;38:315–317.
23. Gambert SR, Duthie EH. Effect of age on red cell membrane sodium-potassium dependent adenosine triphosphatase activity in healthy men. *J Gerontol* 1983;38:23–28.
24. Van Brummelen P, Buhler FR, Kiowski W, et al. Age-related increase in cardiac and peripheral vascular responses to isoproterenol: studies in normal subjects. *Clin Sci* 1981;60:571–577.
25. Lindeman RD, Tobin JD, Shock NW. Association between blood pressure and the rate of decline in renal function with age. *Kidney Int* 1984;26:861–868.
26. Brown WW, Davis BB, Spry LA, et al. Aging and the kidney. *Arch Intern Med* 1986;146:1790–96.
27. Anderson S, Brenner BM. Effects of aging on the renal glomerulus. *Am J Med* 1986;80:435–442.
28. Weinberger MH, Fineberg NS. Sodium and volume sensitivity of blood pressure: Age and pressure change over time. *Hypertension* 1991;18:67–72.
29. Zemel MB, Sowers JR. Salt-sensitivity and hypertension in the elderly. *Am J Cardiol* 1988;61:7H-12H.
30. Sowers JR, Zemel MB, Zemel P, Beck FWJ, Walsh MF, Zawada ET. Salt sensitivity in blacks: salt intake and natriuretic substances. *Hypertension* 1988;12:485–90.
31. Borkan GA, Norris AH. Fat redistribution and the changing body dimensions of the adult male. *Hum Biol* 1977;49:495–514.
32. Flynn MA, Nolph GB, Baker AS, Martin WM, Krause G. Total body potassium in aging humans: a longitudinal study. *Am J Clin Nutr* 1989;50:713–717.
33. Durning J, Womerskly J. Body fat assessed from total body density and its estimation from skin fold thickness: Measurements in 481 men and women aged from 16 to 72 years. *Br J Nutr* 1974;32:77–97.
34. Sowers JR, Standley PR, Ram JL, et al. Insulin resistance, carbohydrate metabolism, and hypertension. *Am J Hypertens* 1991;4:466S-472S.
35. Fukagawa NK, Bandini LG, Young JB. Effect of age on body composition and resting metabolic rate. *Am J Physiol* 1990;259:E233-E238.
36. Flack JM, Sowers Jr. Epidemiologic and clinical aspects of insulin resistance and hyperinsulinemia. *Am J Med* 1991;91 suppl 1A:11S-21S.
37. Poelman ET, Toth MJ, Bunyard LB, Gardner AW, Donalson KE, Colman E, Fonong T, Ades PA. Physiological predictions of increasing total and central adiposity in aging men and women. *Arch Int Med* 1995;155:2443–48.
38. Kohrt WM, Obert KA, Holloszy JO. Exercise training improves fat distribution patterns in 60- to 70-year-old men and women. *J Gerontol* 1992;47:M99-M105.
39. Troisi RJ, Heinold JW, Vokonas PS, Weiss ST. Cigarette smoking, dietary intake, and physical activity: effects on body fat distribution: the Normative Aging Study. *Am J Clin Nutr* 1991;53:1104–1111.
40. Wing RR, Matthews KA, Kuller LH, Meilahn EN, Plantinga P. Waist to hip ratio in middle-aged women: associations with behavioral and psychological factors and with changes in cardiovascular risk factors. *Arterioscler Thromb* 1991;11:1250–1257.
41. Schwartz RS, Shuman WP, Larson V, et al. The effect of intensive endurance exercise training on body fat distribution in young and older men. *Metabolism* 1991;40:545–551.
42. Folsom AR, Kaye SA, Sellers TA, et al. Body fat distribution and 5-year risk of death in older women. *JAMA* 1993;269:483–487.
43. Harris MI, Hades WC, Knowler WC, Bennet PH. Prevalence of diabetes and impaired glucose tolerance and plasma glucose levels in US population aged 2–74 years. *Diabetes* 1987;36:423–434.
44. Saad MF, Pettit DJ, Mott DM, Knowler WC, Nelson RG, Bennett PH. Sequential changes in serum insulin concentration during development of non-insulin-dependent diabetes. *Lancet* 1989;1:1356–1359.
45. Reaven EP, Curry DL, Reaven GM. Effect of age and sex on rat endocrine pancreas. *Diabetes* 1987;36:1397–4000.
46. Maclean N, Ogilvie RF. Quantitative estimation of the pancreatic islet tissue in diabetic subjects. *Diabetes* 1955;4:367–376.
47. Reaven GM, Reaven E. Age, glucose intolerance, and non-insulin-dependent diabetes mellitus. *J Am Geriatr Soc* 1985;33:286–290.
48. Rowe JW, Minnaker KL, Pallotta JA, Flier JS. Characterization of the insulin resistance of aging. *J Clin Invest* 1983;71:1581–1587.
49. Fink RI, Wallace P, Olefsky JM. Effects of aging on glucose-mediated glucose disposal and glucose transport. *J Clin Invest* 1986;77:2034–2041.

50. Reaven GM, Chen N, Hollenbeck C, Chen Y-DI. Effects of age on glucose tolerance and glucose uptake in healthy individuals. *J Am Geriatr Soc* 1989;37:735–740.
51. Wilson PWF, Anderson KM, Kannel WB. Epidemiology of diabetes mellitus in the elderly. *Am J Med* 1986;80(suppl 5A):3–9.
52. Goldberg AP, Coon PJ. Non-insulin-dependent diabetes mellitus in the elderly. Influence of obesity and physical inactivity. *Endocrinol Metab Clin North Am* 1987;16(4):843–865.
53. Aronow WS, Herzig AH, Etienne F, D'Alba P, Ronquillo J. 41 Month follow-up risk factors correlated with new coronary events in 708 elderly patients. *J Am Geriatr Soc* 1989;37:501–506.
54. Barrett-Connor EL, Cohn BA, Wingard DL, Edelstein SL. Why is diabetes mellitus a stronger risk factor for fatal ischemic heart disease in women than in men? The Rancho Bernardo Study. *JAMA* 1991;265:627–631.
55. The National High Blood Pressure Education Program Working Group. National High Blood Pressure Education program Working Group report on hypertension in diabetes. *Hypertension* 1994;23:145–158.
56. Sowers JR, Epstein M. Diabetes mellitus and hypertension: an update. *Hypertension* 1995;26(part 1):869–879.
57. Bass KM, Newschaffer CJ, Klag MJ, Bush TL. Plasma lipoprotein levels as predictors of cardiovascular death in women. *Arch Intern Med* 1993;153:2209–15.
58. Manolio TA, Pearson TA, Wenger NK, Barrett-Connor E, Payne GH, Harlan WR. Cholesterol and heart disease in older persons and women. Review of an NHLBI workshop. *Ann Epidemiol* 1992;2:161–176.
59. Benfante R. Is elevated cholesterol level a risk factor for coronary artery disease in the elderly? JAMA 1990; 263 : 393.
60. Mukerji V, Holman AJ, Artis AK, et al. Risk factors for coronary atherosclerosis in the elderly. Angiology 1989; 40:88.
61. Castelli WP, Wilson PW, Levy D, Anderson K. Cardiovascular risk factors in the elderly. Am J Cardiology 1989; 63: 12H-19H.
62. Aronow WP, Starling I, Etienne F et al. Risk factors for coronary artery disease in persons older than 62 in a long term care facility. Am J Cardiology 1986; 57: 518–520.
63. Terranova R, Luca S. Effects of treatment with Simvastatin in elderly patients with primary hypercholesterolemia. *Rivista Europea Per Le Scienze Mediche e Farmacologiche* 1993; 15 (3–4):163–170.
64. Law MR, Wald NJ, Thopson SG. By how much and how quickly does reduction in serum cholesterol concentrations lowerrisk of ischewmic heart disease? Br Med J 1994; 308:367–372.
65. Davenport J, Whittaker K. Secondary prevention in elderly survivors of heart attacks. *AFP* 1988;38 (1):216–224.
66. La Rosa JC. Dyslipoproteinemia in women and the elderly. Med Clin North Am.1994;78:163.
67. Expert Panel on Detection, Evaluation and Treatment of High Blood cholesterol in Adults: Summary of the second report of the National Cholesterol Education program (NCEP) expert panel . JAMA.1993; 269:3015.
68. The writing group for the PEPI Trial: Effects of estrogen or estrogen/progestin regimens on heart disease risk factors in postmenopausal women: The postmenopausal Estrogen/Progestin Intervention(PEPI) Trial. JAMA.1995; 273:199.

11

EFFECTS OF DIABETES AND HYPERTENSION ON THE AGING KIDNEY

Konstantinos Makrilakis[1] and George L. Bakris[1,2*]

[1]Rush University Hypertension Center
Rush Presbyterian/St. Luke's Medical Center
Chicago, Illinois
[2]Division of Nephrology
University of Illinois Medical Center at Chicago
Chicago, Illinois 60612

INTRODUCTION

As the body ages a number of physiologic changes occur that affect both arterial compliance and renal function. These factors are listed in Table 1. Perhaps one of the most important of these factors is a reduction in muscle mass. Reduction in muscle mass directly correlates to a reduced production in creatinine. Under normal circumstances this would lead to a reduction in serum creatinine levels. However, GFR slowly decreases as well with the aging process and hence serum creatinine remains normal (1,2). Consequently, when one sees a patient greater than 65 years of age with a normal serum creatinine, they should *not* assume that their GFR is 100–120 ml/min, Figure 1 (3).

The average range of glomerular filtration rate (GFR) for someone who is age 70 with a serum creatinine of 1.0 mg/dl is between 60 and 75 ml/min, Figure 1. Moreover, this baseline level of reduced renal function has major implications with regard to susceptibility for renal injury in such individuals. These age related changes may increase the susceptibility of the aged kidney to ischemic injury and accelerate progression of renal failure in the elderly individuals with renal disease (4). Additionally, this reduced level of renal function has major implications with regard to drug dosing as well as any other therapeutic intervention that may effect renal function (5). Lastly, it should be kept in mind that elderly patients have a diminished ability to conserve sodium (6). Thus, one of the most common causes of acute renal insufficiency in elderly patients is *volume depletion* (6). Therefore, especially in the elderly patients, one must insure adequate hydration prior to any pharmacologic intervention, especially diuretics.

* Address for correspondence: George L. Bakris, MD, Rush Presbyterian/St. Luke's Medical Center, 1725 W. Harrison St., Suite 117, Chicago, IL 60612. Tel: (312)563-2195; fax: (312)942-4464

Recent Advances in Geriatrics, edited by Barbagallo, Licata, and Sowers.
Plenum Press, New York, 1998.

Table 1. The renal, cardiovascular, and endocrine alterations associated with the aging process (heart rate remains unchanged)

Increased	Decreased
• Peripheral vascular resistance • Arterial rigidity • Serum catecholamines	• Muscle mass • Renal blood flow • Glomerular filtration rate • Plasma renin activity • Sodium conservation • Renal mass • Cardiac stroke index • Cardiac output • β-adrenoreceptor sensitivity • Baroreceptor sensitivity

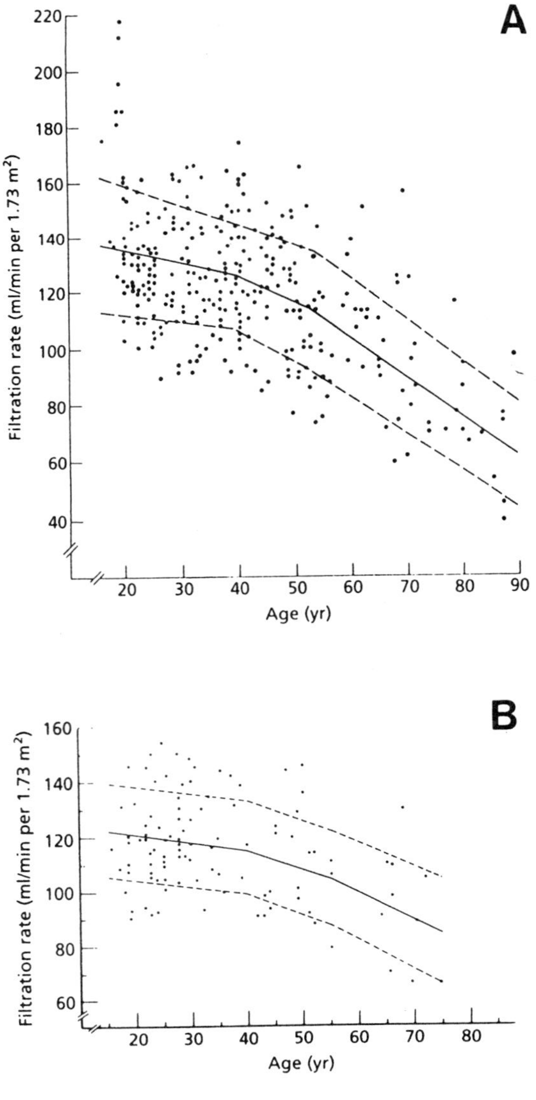

Figure 1. (A) Glomerular filtration rates (inulin clearances) corrected for body surface areas in normal men versus age collected from 38 studies. The solid and broken lines represent the means plus one standard deviation. (B) Glomerular filtration rates (inulin clearances) corrected for body surface areas in normal women versus age collected from 38 studies. The solid and broken lines represent the means plus one standard deviation.

This paper will discuss the natural history of the aging kidney in the context of two very common diseases, hypertension and diabetes. We will focus on how the rate of decline in renal function is altered by these diseases and how lowering arterial pressure with certain classes of antihypertensive medications may provide unique benefits to the kidney beyond simply reducing arterial pressure.

DETERIORATION OF RENAL FUNCTION: AGING VERSUS DISEASE

The normal rate of GFR loss with aging is, on average, 1 ml/min/year, after the age of 35 years (2). This is largely derived from the Baltimore Longitudinal Study that evaluated over 500 normal healthy males for a period of over 40 years, Figure 2 (7). More recent studies have documented, however, that GFR (as measured by inulin clearance) is only modestly lower in healthy elderly compared to young healthy individuals. Moreover, other cardiovascular confounding factors, such as hypertension and heart failure, have a major adverse effect on renal hemodynamics and other aspects of renal function (8). This is exemplified by the fact that effective renal plasma flow is lower in the elderly and filtration fraction and renovascular resistance higher compared to young subjects (8).

The average rate of renal function loss is between 10–12 ml/min/year in the absence of blood pressure control for patients with insulin dependent diabetes mellitus (IDDM) and 6–8 ml/min/year for noninsulin dependent diabetes mellitus (NIDDM) patients (9,10). There have been a number of therapeutic trials that have assessed both blood pressure control and renal function in patients over the age of 55 years with essential hypertension and/or diabetes. In general, when blood pressure is reduced to levels between 125–145/80–95 mmHg, these studies demonstrate a reduction in the rate of GFR decline ranging from 1.2–4 ml/min/year depending on the point of intervention in the natural history of a given renal disease. The antihypertensive medication chosen for intervention also plays an important role in determining the degree of renal disease progression.

One of the earliest studies to examine progression of renal disease in elderly patients as a function of blood pressure control was the SHEP Study (11). This study followed 4,736 patients (10% with diabetes), ≥ 60 years old, with isolated systolic hypertension (systolic blood pressure 160–219 mmHg and diastolic blood pressure ≤ 90 mmHg), randomized to either a diuretic (plus a β-blocker if needed) or placebo for its therapy, and evaluated cardiovascular events. These patients all had normal renal function entering the study and none of them demonstrated any degree of renal insufficiency at study end. Simi-

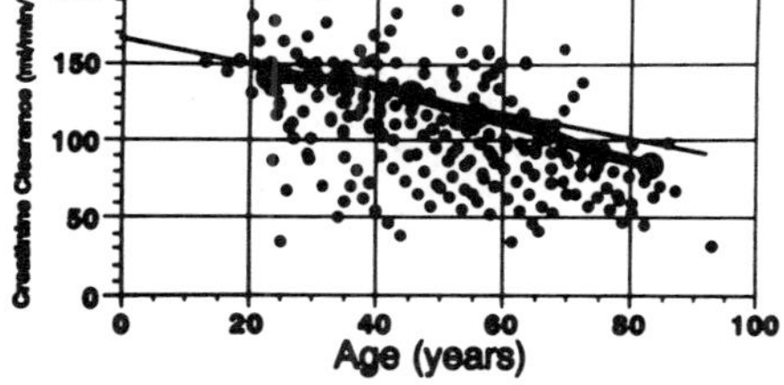

Figure 2. The creatinine clearance of 548 men with normal renal function followed for an average of 30 years.

lar results were obtained in the MRC Trial, which evaluated 4,396 elderly patients (65–74 years of age) with essential hypertension, treated again with diuretics and/or β-blockers, and looking at cardiovascular events (12). This trial, which excluded patients with diabetes showed no adverse renal effects over the 5.8 years of follow-up.

A review of six randomized trials of treatment of hypertension in the elderly, using diuretics and/or β-blockers exclusively, corroborates the previous findings. Specifically, antihypertensive treatment with these agents did not have any untoward renal effects on elderly patients with essential hypertension (13). Taken together, these studies indicate that adequate control of blood pressure (< 160/90 mmHg) in elderly Caucasian patients contributes to the stabilization of renal function, in addition to the well established cardiac and cerebrovascular benefits.

In recent years there has been a dramatic increase, of almost epidemic proportions, in the incidence of patients with NIDDM who reach end-stage renal disease and enter dialysis programs (14). Apart from the undoubted role of hyperglycemia and the importance of genetic predisposition, there is no question that elevated blood pressure is a significant determinant of the risk for the appearance of nephropathy as well as its progression (15–17). A summary of the most important risks factors that correlate with progression of diabetic nephropathy are listed in table 2.

More recently there have been a number of long term studies in patients with NIDDM associated nephropathy that have evaluated control of blood pressure on progression of renal disease. One study compared 74 patients with a mean age of 63 years, randomized in a double-blinded manner to either a thiazide diuretic or an ACE inhibitor. This study demonstrated that both drugs slowed progression of renal disease. The ACE inhibitor, however, slowed progression to a greater extent than the thiazide diuretic (18). The results of this study are further corroborated by a recently completed randomized six year follow-up study in patients with NIDDM associated nephropathy and a mean age of 62 years. This study demonstrated that ACE inhibitors and nondihydropyridine calcium channel antagonist, i.e., sustained release verapamil or diltiazem, slowed renal disease progression to levels of between 1.2 and 1.6 ml/min/year, whereas the beta blocker, atenolol reduced progression by 3.4 ml/min/year (19). Additionally, in a recently published randomized, prospective five year follow-up study in African-Americans with NIDDM associated nephropathy (mean age 61 years), the non-dihydropyridine calcium channel antagonist, sustained release verapamil, slowed renal disease progression by 1.7 ml/min/year, whereas β blockade with atenolol slowed progression by 3.7 ml/min/year (20). Taken together these studies demonstrate that, given similar levels of blood pressure reduction, certain classes of antihypertensive agents slow renal disease progression to a greater extent than others (21).

Table 2. Risk factors that predict reductions in glomerular filtration rate in order of decline importance*

Diastolic blood pressure	(r = 0.70)
Systolic blood pressure	(r = 0.64)
Mean arterial pressure	(r = 0.59)
Protein/creatinine ratio	(r = 0.45)
Serum cholesterol	(r = 0.38)
Age	(r = 0.29)

*Note all these factors were statistically significant. Adapted from references 16, 17.

One must, however, put progression of renal disease into proper perspective. The most common cause of death in anyone with renal disease results from cardiovascular events (22–23). In hypertensive patients without renal disease, all randomized, prospective, long term, multicenter trials clearly demonstrate that thiazide diuretics and β blockers reduce these events, especially strokes (24,25). While there are no such data for persons with renal disease, however, it is clear that older patients i.e., age > 60 years, also benefit with regard to decline in renal function (19). Data from a study in which elderly patients with essential hypertension were randomized to either a β blocker or diuretic versus other forms of blood pressure lowering therapy illustrates this point. Obese patients given either a β blocker or diuretic had a 2.2-fold greater risk of developing new onset diabetes compared to other patients (27). These medications, however, are not without an increased metabolic risk. Thus, it appears that antihypertensive agents shown to have the best overall profile on renal disease progression, like ACE inhibitors and non-dihydropyridine calcium channel antagonists have not been tested, as yet in this context.

ACE inhibitors and non-dihydropyridine calcium channel antagonists have been shown, however, to reduce cardiovascular events and improve survival in both post-MI and heart failure patients (28–31). A new class of antihypertensive medications, the angiotensin II (AT_1) receptor antagonists, show great promise in the context of renal disease progression as well. A recently completed 48 week trial, comparing the AT_1 receptor antagonist, losartan, with captopril in 722 elderly (mean age = 74 years) heart failure patients, showed no significant difference in renal disease progression between the two groups (11.4% for both). Losartan was found to be better tolerated than captopril and was noted to have a lower overall mortality compared to the ACE inhibitor (32). Thus, one could claim, based on the available data, that if only diuretics or β blockers were used alone to control arterial pressure in a patient greater than 60 years of age with pre-existing renal impairment (serum creatinine > 2.0 mg/dl), one might keep them alive long enough to go on dialysis.

Thus, given this information it is clear that blood pressure control is critically important for preservation of renal function. An ACE inhibitor or a non-dihydropyridine calcium channel antagonist (verapamil or diltiazem) appear to have unique benefits not only to preserve renal function but to reduce mortality. Moreover, a recent consensus panel of the National Institutes of Health on the treatment of blood pressure in patients with renal insufficiency suggests that these classes of agents have unique benefits to preserve renal function (33). The AT_1 receptor antagonists also show promising results with regard to cardiorenal preservations in the elderly, although more studies are need with this class of agents. One must remember, however, regardless of drugs used to lower arterial pressure, if blood pressure is not adequately reduced to levels of < 130/85 mmHg, optimal cardiovascular or renal effects will not be observed (31).

CONCLUSIONS

The major messages of this paper include the following:

- Both isolated systolic and elevated diastolic hypertension are risk factors for renal disease progression in the elderly.
- Adequate control of arterial pressure to levels of < 130/85 mmHg will slow progression of renal disease and preserve renal function in the elderly. Ideally, ACE inhibitors or nondihydropyridine calcium antagonists with or without a thiazide diuretic should be used initially to achieve this goal.

- Patients in whom creatinine increases more than 50% within two weeks of ACE inhibitor initiation should first be evaluated for volume status; if euvolemic, they should then be assessed for bilateral renal artery stenosis.

REFERENCES

1. Fliser D, Ritz E. Renal hemodynamics in the elderly. Nephrol Dial Transplant 1996;11(suppl 9):2–8.
2. Rowe JW, Andres RA, Tobin JD, Norris AH, Shock NW. The effect of age on creatinine clearance in man: a cross-sectional and longitudinal study. J Gerontol 1976;31:155–163.
3. Hadj-Aissa A, Dumarest C, Maue P, Pazt N. Renal function in the elderly. Nephron 1990;54:365–369.
4. Meyer BR. Renal function in aging. J Am Geriatr Soc. 1989;37:791–800.
5. Brater DC. Pharmacokinetics of renal and antihypertensive drugs in the elderly.
6. Rowe JN, Minaker KL and Len M. Pathophysiology and management of electrolyte disturbances in elderly In: Hypertension and Renal Disease in the Elderly. Manuel Martinez-Maldonado (ed). Blackwell Scientific Publications 1992; 115–126.)
7. Lindeman RD, Tobin J, Shock NW. Longitudinal studies on the rate of decline in renal function with age. J Am Geriatr Soc 1985;33:278–285.
8. Fliser D, Franek E, Joest M, Block S, Mutschler E, Ritz E. Renal function in the elderly: impact of hypertension and cardiac function. Kidney Int 1997;51:1196–1204.
9. Parving HH, Smidt UM, Hommel E. Effective antihypertensive treatment postpones renal insufficiency in diabetic nephropathy. Am J Kidney Dis 1993;22:188–195.
10. Myers BD, Nelson RG, Tan M, Beck GJ, Bennett PH, Knowler WC, Blouch K, Mitch WE. Progression of overt nephropathy in non-insulin-dependent diabetes. Kidney Int 1995;47(6):1781–1789
11. SHEP Cooperative Research Group. Prevention of stroke by antihypertensive drug treatment in older persons with isolated systolic hypertension. Final results of the Systolic Hypertension in the Elderly Program (SHEP). JAMA 1991;265:3255–3264.
12. MRC Working Party. Medical Research Council Trial of treatment of hypertension in older adults: principal results. BMJ 1992;304:405–412.
13. Beard K, Bulpitt H, Mascie-Taylor H, O'Malley K, Sever P, Webb S. Management of elderly patients with sustained hypertension. BMJ 1992;304:412–416.
14. Ritz E, Keller C, Bergis KH. Nephropathy in type II diabetes mellitus. Nephrol Dial Transplant 1996;11(suppl 9):38–44.
15. Nelson RG, Pettitt DJ, Baird GR, Charles MA, Liu QZ, Bennett PH, Knowler WC. Pre-diabetic blood pressure predicts urinary albumin excretion after the onset of type 2 (non-insulin dependent) diabetes mellitus in Pima Indians. Diabetologia 1993;36:998–1001.
16. Dillion JJ, The quantitative relationship between treated blood pressure and progression of diabetic renal disease. Am J Kidney Dis 1993:22:798–802.
17. Perry HM, Miller JP, Fornoff JR. Early predictors of 15-year end-stage renal disease in hypertensive patients. Hypertension 1995;25:587–594.
18. Walker WG, Hermann JA, Anderson JE. Randomized doubly blinded trial of enalapril vs. hydrochlorothiazide on GFR in diabetic nephropathy. Hypertension 1993;22:410 (abstract).
19. Bakris GL, Copley JB, Vicknair N, Sadler R, Leurgans S. Calcium channel blockers versus other antihypertensive therapies on progression of NIDDM associated nephropathy: Kidney Int. 1996;50:1641–1650.
20. Bakris GL, Mangrum A, Copley JB, Vicknair N, Sadler R. Effect of calcium channel or beta blockade on the progression of diabetic nephropathy in African Americans. Hypertension 1997;29:744–750.
21. Tarif N and Bakris GL Preservation of renal function: the spectrum of effects by calcium channel blockers. Nephrol Dial Transpl, In press.
22. Raine AEG. Epidemiology, development and treatment of end-stage renal failure in non-insulin dependent diabetic patients in Europe. Diabetologia 1993;36:1099–1104.
23. United States Renal Data System. USRDS 1993 Annual Data Report. US Department of Health and Human Services. The National Institutes of Health, National Institute of Diabetes and Digestive and Kidney Diseases, Bethesda, MD, August 1993.
24. Hypertension Detection and Follow-up Program Cooperative Group. Five year findings of the Hypertension Detection and Follow-up Program. II. Mortality by race, sex and age. JAMA 1979;242:2572–2577.
25. National High Blood Pressure Education Program Working Group. National high blood pressure education program working group report on hypertension in the elderly. Hypertension 1994;23:275–285.

26. Sowers JR, Farrow SL. Treatment of elderly hypertensive patients with diabetes, renal disease, and coronary heart disease. Am J Geriat Cardiol 1996;5:57–70.
27. Mykkanen L, Kuusisto J, Pyorala K, Laakso M, Haffner SM Increased risk of non-insulin dependent diabetes mellitus in elderly hypertensive subjects. J Hypertens 1994;12:1425–1432.
28. Pffefer MA, Braunwald E, Moye L, et. al. on behalf of the SAVE Investigators. Effect of captopril on mortality and morbidity in patients with left ventricular dysfunction after myocardial infarction. Results of the Survival and Ventricular Enlargement Trial. N Engl J Med 1992;327:669–677.
29. The Danish Study Group on Verapamil in Myocardial Infarction. Effect of verapamil on mortality and major events after acute myocardial infarction (The Danish Verapamil Infarction Trial II - DAVIT II) Am J Cardiol 1990;66:779–785.
30. SOLVD Investigators. Effect of enalapril on mortality and the development of heart failure in asymptomatic patients with reduced left ventricular ejection fractions. N Engl J Med 1992;327:685–691.
31. Hansen JF, Hagerup L, Sigurd B, Pedersen F, Mellemgaard K, Bjergaard OP, Mortensen LS for the Danish Verapamil Infarction Trial Study Group. Cardiac Event Rates after acute myocardial infarction in patients treated with verapamil and trandolapril versus trandolapril alone. Am J Cardiol 1997, 79:738–741.
32. Pitt B, Segal R, Martinez FA, Meurers G, et. al. on behalf of ELITE Study Investigators. Randomized trial of losartan versus captopril in patients over 65 with heart failure (Evaluation of Losartan in the Elderly Study, ELITE) Lancet 1997;349:747–752.
33. National High Blood Pressure Education Program Working Group. 1995 update of the Working Group reports on chronic renal failure and renovascular hypertension. Arch Intern Med 1996;156:1938–1947.

12

CLINICAL FEATURES OF HYPERTENSION IN THE ELDERLY

G. Abate, M. Zito, and A. Di Iorio

Department of Medicine and Aging
University of Chieti
Italy

In the last decades, further research developments regarding hypertension in the elderly, including both epidemiologic and clinical trial data, have answered a number of important issues for the clinician. The purpose of this review will be to focus on those features, which are peculiar to senile hypertension, and have clinical relevance for the prognosis and pharmacological treatment.

ISOLATED SYSTOLIC HYPERTENSION

The average systolic blood pressure (SBP) increases with advancing age, the average diastolic blood pressure (DBP) decreases concomitantly, and the prevalence of isolated systolic hypertension (ISH) increases as the population ages (1,2). Data from the screnees for the pilot study in the Systolic Hypertension in the Elderly Program (SHEP), for example, showed that 8% of those aged 60 to 69 had ISH, defined as SBP greater than 160 mmHg and DBP below 90 mmHg; 11% of those aged 70 to 79 and 22% of those over age 80 were classified as having ISH (3).

Several studies have reported that, far from being a physiological and harmless concomitant of aging, this condition represents an important risk factor for cardiovascular complications, such as stroke, congestive heart failure and coronary heart disease (4,5).

Ambulatory Blood Pressure Monitoring (ABPM) studies have shown that in ISH of the elderly day-time mean systolic blood pressure is much lower than clinic systolic blood pressure. However it is not a specific feature of ISH, because it involves patients with a systo-diastolic hypertension as well. Although much lower than the clinical values, day-time average systolic blood pressure of ISH patients is considerably higher than that seen in normotensive controls. This is the case also for the night-time and the 24 hour mean systolic blood pressure. Therefore, the hypothesis that ISH may be due to an hyperreactivity of elderly individuals to stressful stimuli, reflecting a pronounced "white coat" phenomenon, cannot be accepted (6,7).

Epidemiological studies have shown that about 16% of incident cases of ISH had previous diastolic hypertension (8); moreover, the values of diastolic blood pressure have

Recent Advances in Geriatrics, edited by Barbagallo, Licata, and Sowers.
Plenum Press, New York, 1998.

been found higher in ISH patients than in normotensive subjects (6); these results suggest that ISH can be, at least in some cases, a "burned out" systo-diastolic hypertension.

BLOOD PRESSURE VARIABILITY, ORTHOSTATIC HYPOTENSION, AND POSTPRANDIAL HYPOTENSION

A number of ABPM studies, performed in subjects with hypertension of different age, have shown that systolic blood pressure variability (expressed as standard deviation or coefficient of variability) is increased in the elderly (9,10).

This finding has clinical relevance, because, as found in cross sectional and longitudinal observations, for comparable haemodinamic loads, an increased variability is associated to a greater risk of target organ damage (11).

The factors involved are a reduced sensitivity of baroceptors and an impairment of autonomic drive, with prevalence of sympathetic on parasympathetic control of the heart and vessels (9,12).

On the clinical ground, the failure of the mechanisms of homeostatic control accounts for an increased prevalence and incidence of orthostatic hypotension (OH) and postprandial hypotension (PPH) (13). In the Cardiovascular Health Study the prevalence of asymptomatic OH was 9.4% in age group 65–69 and 14.1% in age group 85 and over; the prevalence of symptomatic OH was 1.6% in age group 65–69 and 5% in age group 85 and over (14). Orthostatic hypotension was associated significantly with frequent falls, history of myocardial infarction and transient ischemic attacks.

The prevalence of PPH also increases in the elderly. This phenomenon has been reported to be due mainly to shift of blood to intestinal arteries and veins, which must be associated with failure of neural mechanisms to maintain the systemic blood pressure (15).

Thus OH and PPH appear to share a common mechanism though the times of appearance of the two phenomena are very different. As for OH the symptoms caused by PPH may range from feeling of apathy and lightheadedness to somnolence and syncope. These are probably dependent on the extent to which perfusion is impaired in different vascular regions. With carotid artery stenosis, for instance, even with a small fall in pressure, there may be a greater propensity to cerebral symptoms with the possibility of transient ischemic attacks and stroke.

DIPPERS VERSUS NON DIPPERS

Besides increased variability, ABPM studies have shown, in elderly patients with hypertension, a blunted nocturnal fall of blood pressure. Therefore the prevalence of non dippers (defined as subjects whose SBP decreases during sleep less 10% of awake values) is higher in old people (16,17).

This finding may have rational explanations. In the course of aging the structure of sleep is disrupted, with frequent nocturnal awakenings and increased non REM/REM sleep ratio; the autonomic drive is impaired; the distensibility of the resistance vessels is reduced by cause of aging or atherosclerosis (18,19). Moreover the level of physical activity decreases in the elderly, minimizing the effects of an elevated cardiac output in the aroused state, which partly accounts for the day-night blood pressure changes (20).

Cardiovascular events have been reported more frequently in non dippers than in dippers (21). Cerebrovascular events also have been found to be more frequent in non dippers (22,23), but this conclusion has been partly challenged by recent studies. Kario et al., in patients free from clinical cerebrovascular complications, observed the highest prevalence of lacunar lesions, detected by brain magnetic resonance imaging, not only in non dippers, but also in subjects with extreme dipping of BP values (24). The increased prevalence of lacunas in overdippers was attributed to hypotensive crises, spontaneous or induced by treatment, leading to critical ischemia in the deep watershed area, mainly in subjects with impaired autoregulation of blood flow. Others observed that the nocturnal blood pressure decline is reduced only in certain subgroups of cerebrovascular diseases, mainly those involving subcortical areas, and is relatively well preserved in patients with wide cortical infarctions (25,26). Subcortical lesions could lead to specific injury of the central autonomic nervous system, which throughout the night reduces sympathetic activity and increases parasympathetic activity (27). Therefore the blunted nocturnal fall could be a consequence of cerebrovascular complications rather than a cause.

In conclusion non dipping is frequent in elderly subjects with hypertension; further research however is needed to establish whether this condition may have a negative prognostic relevance for cerebrovascular events, as for cardiovascular complications.

COGNITIVE FUNCTIONS IN ELDERLY SUBJECTS WITH HYPERTENSION

The relationship between hypertension and cognitive decline is an issue of great relevance in the elderly. It is quite obvious that hypertension is the major risk factor for stroke and therefore for multi-infarct dementia.

Recent studies have shown that hypertension may be also associated with cerebral small lacunar infarctions or white matter periventricular hypodensities. These lesions are frequently asymptomatic, but are detected with increasing frequency by neuroradiologic evaluation in elderly subjects. Lacunae are defined as small cerebral infarcts that lie in the deeper non cortical parts of the brain and result from occlusion of penetrating branches of large cerebral arteries. White matter lesions are ill defined, patchy or diffuse hypodensities in the frontal and occipital horns and trigones of the lateral ventricles, medial cells of the lateral ventricles and semioval centre.

Hypertension has been recognized as a major risk factor for subcortical lesions, but some studies suggest that also hypotensive crises may be a causative factor, inducing ischemia in the deep watershed area, which is particularly vulnerable to sudden decrease of cerebral blood flow.

Both lacunar lesions and leukoaraiosis can be associated to cognitive abnormalities and can lead, in case of severe damage, to a subcortical form of vascular dementia.

Besides anatomical lesions, hypertension may influence cognitive function by means of other different pathogenetic mechanisms. Some authors suggest that a hypertension related reduction in cerebral blood flow or dysfunctions in autoregolatory mechanisms might adversely affect neuropsychological functioning (28–30). According to other studies, neurochemical alterations in prefrontal, limbic or hypothalamic regions could be responsible for both the development of hypertension and the impairment of a variety of neuropsychological functions (31,32). Finally, according to Kuusisto et al. (33), hyperinsulinemia seems to identify a subgroup of hypertensive subjects with a particularly poor performance in neuropsychological tests requiring complex cognition, such as semantic memory, problem solving, and abstraction.

On the basis of these findings hypertension therefore must be regarded as a significant risk factor for cognitive decline in the elderly.

HYPERTENSION AND MORTALITY IN THE VERY OLD

Epidemiological studies in younger and middle-aged subjects have consistently shown the lowest coronary heart disease or cardiovascular mortality in subjects with the lowest levels of both systolic and diastolic blood pressure (34). However, a variety of studies have suggested that this positive relationship between blood pressure and cardiovascular mortality is weakened, or indeed reversed in the very old. The mortality and morbidity rates were grater for the highest and lowest values of SBP, both in cross sectional and longitudinal observations (35–38). Moreover in clinical trials an excessive fall in blood pressure with use of antihypertensive medication was found associated with increased mortality (39,40).

However in these studies the lower levels of blood pressure were frequently associated to prior cardiac disease, or poor general conditions. Actually when subjects with atrial fibrillation, atrioventricular heart block, heart failure, previous myocardial infarction, bronchial asthma, diabetes, recent weight loss, anemia, malignancies or any serious disease were excluded, the increased mortality at lower pressures virtually disappeared.

Therefore there is strong evidence that J-shaped curves of survival are secondary rather than causal.

THERAPEUTICAL IMPLICATIONS

Randomized trials establish that treating healthy older persons with hypertension is highly efficacious, preventing both CHD and cerebrovascular morbid and mortal events. Existing trial data also suggest that 5-year (short-term) morbidity and mortality benefits of antihypertensive therapy are greater for older than younger adults (3,39).

However actual estimates of benefits and risks of treating elderly persons with hypertension derived from trials with highly selected subjects are not readily generalizable to clinical practice. In SHEP trial, for example on 447,921 subjects selected for inclusion only 4736 were considered eligible for the study.

In practice clinicians offer treatment to patients who may not have been eligible for a trial or who, if eligible, would have refused participation. Every generalization therefore should be approached with forethought. Without the individual attention and extra visits provided in many trials, even clinic patients who technically would be eligible for studies may be less compliant than trial partecipants. Patients with significant comorbidities and complicated medical regimens may also have poorer compliance, less benefit, and more adverse effects than trial partecipants. On the other hand, clinicians should not always assume that less benefit will be seen in "real-life" clinical setting. A person who is at high immediate risk of suffering a cardiovascular event and does not have other competing illnesses, (e.g. an 80-year-old woman with systolic hypertension and hystory of stroke and dyslipidemia) may have a higher benefit-to-risk ratio than a trial partecipant.

In conclusion, despite differences between characteristics of trial participants and the general population, the evidence of the effectiveness of antihypertensive treatment in the elderly is strong, consistent, and convincing.

Notwithstanding, the optimal blood pressure values to be reached in the elderly in order to prevent cardiovascular complications have not been defined. A clinical trial (Hypertension Optimal Treatment = HOT Study) yet in progress, will give more definite answers. At present, clinical and physiopathological considerations suggest caution in lowering too much and too rapidly blood pressure, mainly in patients with critical arterial stenoses and/or diffuse vascular lesions.

REFERENCES

1. Kannel W.B., Dawbe T.R., Mcgee D.L.: Perspective in systolic hypertension: the Framingham Study. Circulation 1980; 61: 1179
2. Colandrea M.A., Friedman G.D., Nichman M.Z., Lund C.N.: Systolic hypertension in the elderly. Circulation 1970; 41: 239
3. SHEP Cooperative Research Group: Prevention of stroke by antihypertensive drug treatment in older persons with isolated systolic hypertension: final results of the Systolic Hypertension in the Elderly Program (SHEP). JAMA 1991; 265: 3255
4. Gerland C., Barret-Connor E., Suarez L., Criqui M.H.: Isolated systolic hypertension and mortality after age 60 years. Am.J.Epidemiol. 1983; 118:365
5. Dustan H.P.: Isolated systolic hypertension: a long-neglet cause of cardiovascular complications. Am.J.Med. 1989; 86: 368
6. Zito M., Cervone C., Piersante P., Benighi D.M., Parati G., Puddu G.M., Abate G., Mancia G.: Ambulatory blood pressure monitoring in elderly subjects with isolated systolic hypertension, essential hypertension and normotension. High Blood Pressure 1994; 3: 97
7. Thijs L., Amery A., Clement D., Cox J., De Cort P., Fagard R., Fowler G., Guo C., Mancia G., Marin R., O'Brien E., O'Malley K., Palatini P., Parati G., Petrie J., Ravogli A., Rosenfeld J., Staessen J., Webster J.: Ambulatory blood pressure monitoring in elderly patients with isolated systolic hypertension. J.Hypertens. 1992; 10: 693
8. Bulpitt C.J., Fletcher A.E.: Aging, blood pressure and mortality. J.Hypertens. 1992; 10(suppl.7): S45
9. Mancia G., Ferrari A.U., Gregorini L., Parati G., Pomidossi G., Bertinieri G., Grassi G., Di Rienzo M., Pedotti A., Zanchetti A.: Blood pressure and heart rate variabilities in normotensive and hypertensive human beings. Circ.Res. 1983; 53: 96
10. Zito M., Parati G., Omboni S., Cervone C. Ulina L., D'Aviero M., Abate G., Mancia G.: Effects of aging on blood pressure variability. J. Hypertens. 1991; 9 (suppl.6). S328
11. Frattola A., Parati G., Cuspidi C., Albini F., Mancia G.: Prognostic value of 24-hour blood pressure variability. J. Hypertension 1993; 11: 1133
12. Zito M., Cervone C., Cavoni M.A., Guglielmi M.D., Mezzetti A., D'Aviero M.: Monitoraggio della pressione arteriosa e rischio cardiovascolare. Giorn. Geront. 1989; 10: 869 (abstr.)
13. Lipsitz L.A.: Orthostatic hypotension in the elderly. N.Engl.J.Med. 1989; 321: 952
14. Rutan G.H., Hermanson B., Bild D.E., Kittner S.J., Labaw F., Tell G.S.: Orthostatic hypotension in older adults. The Cardiovascular Health Study. Hypertension 1992; 19: 508
15. Mathias C.J.: Postprandial hypotension. Pathophysiological mechanisms and clinical implications in different disorders. Hypertension 1991; 18: 694
16. Abate G., Zito M., Lamanna P., Paci L., Volikas K., Puddu G.M.: Physiopathological risk factors of hypertension in the elderly. 2nd European Congress on Geriatric treatment, Catania 1995; pag.36 (abstr.).
17. Lagi A., Tamburini C., Colzi L.: Age and future vascular events in hypertensives with blunted or absent blood pressure nocturnal fall. 7th Europ.Meeting on Hypertension, Milan 1995; 438: 101
18. Nystrom F.H., Ohman K.P., Karlberg B.E.: White coat blood pressure increases with age and non-dipping phenomenon is common in a population based ambulatory blood pressure reference material. 7th Europ.Meeting on Hypertension, Milan 1995; 593:135
19. Biston P., Van Cauter E., Linkowski P., Degaute J.P.: Aging and sleep quality impairment are associated with dampening of the 24-hour blood pressure profile. 7th Europ.Meeting on Hypertension, Milan 1995; 92: 23
20. Munakata A., Imai Y., Abe K., Saaki S., Minami N., Hashimoto J., Ichijo T., Yochizawa M., Sekino H., Yoshinaga K.: Assessment of age-dependent changes in circadian blood pressure rhythm in patients with essential hypertension. J. Hypertension 1991; 9: 407
21. Verdecchia P., Schillaci G., Guerrieri M., Gatteschi C., Benemio G., Boldrini F., Porcellati C.: Circadian blood pressure changes and left ventricular hypertrophy in essential hypertension. Circulation 1990; 81: 528
22. O'Brien E., Sheridan J., O'Malley K.: Dippers and non dippers. Lancet 1988; 13: 397 Letter.
23. Kobrin J., Oigman W., Kumar A., Ventura H.O., Messerli F.H., Frohlich E.D., Dunn F.G.: Diurnal variation of blood pressure in elderly patients with essential hypertension. J. Am. Ger. Soc. 1984; 32: 896
24. Kario K., Shimada K.: Change in diurnal blood pressure rhythm due to small lacunar infarct. Lancet. 1994; 344: 200 Letter.
25. Yamamoto Y., Akiguchi I., Oiwa K., Satoi H., Kimura J.: Diminished nocturnal blood pressure decline and lesion site in cerebrovascular disease. Stroke 1995; 26: 829

26. Furlan R., Guzzetti S., Crivellaro W., Dassi S., Tinelli M., Basselli G., Cerutti S., Lombardi F., Pagani M., Malliani A.: Continous 24-hour assessment of the neural regulation of systemic arterial pressure and RR variabilities in ambulant subjects. Circulation 1990; 81: 537
27. Pickering T.G., James G.D.: Determinants and consequences of the diurnal rhythm of blood pressure. Am.J.Hypertens. 1993; 6:1665
28. Rodriguez G., Arvigo F., Marenco S., Nobili F., Romano P., Sandini G., Rosadini G.: Regional cerebral blood flow in essential hypertension. Data evaluation by a mapping system. Stroke 1987; 18: 13.
29. Baumbach G.L., Heistad D.D.: Cerebral circulation in chronic arterial hypertension. Hypertension 1988;12: 89.
30. Mentis M.J., Salerno I., Horwits B., Grady C., Shapiro M.B., Murphy D.G., Rapaport S.I.: Reduction of functional neuronal connectivity in long-term treated hypertension. Stroke 1994; 25: 601.
31. Brody M.J., O'Neill T.P., Porter J.P.: Role of central catecholaminergic systems in pathogenesis and treatment of hypertension. J. Cardiovasc. Pharmacol. 1984; 9 (suppl.5): 727.
32. Kruglikov R.I.: Basic trends in research into the neurochemical mechanisms of learning and memory. Neuroscience and Behavioral Physiology 1987;17: 192.
33. Kuusisto J., Koivisto K., Mykkanen L., Helkala E.L., Vanhanen M., Hanninen T., Pyorala K., Riekkinen P., Laakso M.: Essential hypertension and cognitive function. The role of hyperinsulinemia. Hypertension 1993; 22: 771.
34. Kannel W.B., Wolf P.A., McGree D.L., Dawber T.R., McNamara P., Castelli W.P.: Systolic blood pressure, arterial rigidity, and risk of stroke. JAMA 1981; 245: 1225
35. Fletcher A.E., Bulpitt C.J.: Epidemiological aspects of cardiovascular disease in the elderly. J.Hypertension 1992; 10 (suppl.2): S51
36. Bots M.L., Grobbee D.E., Hofman A.: High blood pressure in the elderly. Epidemiol.Res. 1991; 13: 294
37. Zito M., Corneli M., Cervone C., D'Aviero M., Santicchia S., Amatetti M., Guarino F., Fici F., Abate G.: Hypertension in the elderly. A retrospective study in istitutionalized subjects. Eur. Rev. Med. Pharmacol. Sci. 1987; 9: 185
38. Mattila K., Haavisto M., Rajala S., Heikinheimo R.: Blood pressure and five year survival in the very old. BMJ 1988; 296: 887
39. Coope J., Warrender T.S., Mcpherson K.: The prognostic significance of blood pressure in the elderly. J.Hum.Hypertens. 1988; 2; 79
40. Staessen J., Bulpitt C., Clement D., De Loeuw P., Fagard R., Fletcher A., Forette F., Leonetti G., Nissinen A., O'Malley K., Tuomilehto J., Webster J., Williams B.O.: Relation between mortality and treated blood pressure in elderly patients with hypertension: report of the European Working Party on High Blood Pressure in the Elderly. BMJ 1989; 298: 1552

13

THE AGING HEART

M. Varricchio, M. R. Tagliamonte, M. R. Rizzo, G. Varricchio,* and A. Gambardella

Department of Geriatric Medicine and Metabolic Diseases
Second University of Naples
Naples, Italy

INTRODUCTION

It is often difficult to study the alterations of aging heart because there is a very large spectrum of cardiovascular function among elderly population. Aging is associated to an increase in prevalence and incidence of coronary disease. In fact, the 50% of aging subjects have a known or latent coronary artery disease and only few of them underwent invasive studies to exclude coronary heart failure. Furthermore, a decline in cardiac performance can be related also to an age-related reduction in daily physical activity with a secondary deconditioning. For all these reasons it is not so easy to clarify what is "normal heart" in the elderly people. In our opinion interactions among aging, disease, and life-style could be considered in interpreting age-associated changes in cardiovascular structure and function (1).

AGE-RELATED CHANGES IN VASCULAR STRUCTURE AND FUNCTION

Aging is associated to arterial stiffening. This can be due both to changes in vascular media and possibly to increased arterial tonus secondary to an alteration in adrenergic modulation. The vascular media shows an increase in the amount of collagen and changes in cross-linking of collagen, characteristics of collagen, and nature of elastin.

On the other hand, aging is associated to a deterioration of the "communication" between the nervous system and the heart and vasculature in both healthy humans and animals (2). The vascular dilatory response to β-adrenergic stimulation declines, but the response to α-agonists remains unchanged; for this reason in elderly population there is an imbalance of α–β-adrenergic co-modulation that could lead to inappropriately exaggerated arterial stiff-

* Corresponding author: Prof. M. Varricchio, Dept. Geriatric Medicine, II University of Naples, P.zza Miraglia 2, 80138 Naples, Italy.

Recent Advances in Geriatrics, edited by Barbagallo, Licata, and Sowers.
Plenum Press, New York, 1998.

ness, but conclusive evidence for this hypothesis remains to be shown. Plasma catecholamine levels increase with age, particulary during stress (3), probably because of exaggerated central nervous system adrenergic discharge secondary to diminished baroreceptor sensitivity. However, this exaggerated level of plasma catecholamines is associated with a decrease in postsynaptic β-adrenergic response in the heart and vasculature.

AGING CHANGES IN CARDIAC STRUCTURE AND FUNCTION

Not all the authors are in agreement to consider the cardiac weight modifications as physiologically related to aging or secondary to a pathological conditions like hypertension and coronary artery disease.

The most important age-related myocardial alterations are:

- increase in adipose tissue
- increase in collagen content
- basofilic degeneration of mithocondria
- increase in lipofucsin content
- increase in left ventricular wall thickness
- increase in the number of collateral coronay circles

Age-related abnormalities in aortic distensibility cause the characteristic aortic impedance modulus to increase with age, creating a mismatch between ventricular ejection and aortic flow energies (4). Thus, peripheral vascular resistance, characteristic aortic impedance, and pulse wave reflection characterize the total arterial load on the left ventricle. In order to sustain a normal ventricular pattern at rest in these conditions there are two primary cardiac adaptation: the left ventricular wall thickens modestly, mainly because of an increase in cardiac myocyte size, and myocardium maintains a greater contractile force later in systole (5). Although prolonged contractile activation (and possibly structural changes in the heart) results in a reduced left ventricular early diastolic filling rate in healthy elderly persons, atrial enlargement and an enhanced atrial contribution to ventricular filling, which is the cause of the audible fourth heart sound in the elderly, prevents a reduction of the end diastolic volume in most persons. The end diastolic volume, in fact, increase slightly with advanced age in healthy men. Neither the end systolic volume nor the ejection fraction at rest are age-related.

MECHANISMS OF ALTERED CONTRACTILE FUNCTION WITH AGING

Age-related changes in myocardial wall thickness and contractile force in healthy elderly humans suggest underlying alterations in cellular biochemistry, structure and function. In order to study these modifications the best characterized model is that of the aging rat. In this model there are changes in individual cardiac myocytes and characteristic alterations in many aspects of cardiac muscle excitation-contraction coupling mechanisms have been identified at cellular level in the normotensive aging rat compared with the younger adult rat (6–12). During isometric contraction, the transmembrane action potential is prolonged in the senescent animal (6). Small increases in the peak sarcolemmal L-type Ca^{++}-channel current density, combined with a reduction in its inactivation rate, and changes in other insufficiently characterized membrane currents appear to produce the major prolongation of action potential. The transient cytosolic calcium concentration (partly derived from the overall decreased rate of sarcoplasmic reticulum Ca^{++} reuptake) that initiates contraction and the resultant contraction are prolonged in isolated cardiac muscle from senescent rats (6–7). The myofilament force responce to Ca^{++}, however, is not altered with aging. The myosin heavy-chain isozyme composition shifts from predominantly V1 (rapid adenosine triphosphate hydrolytic isozyme) to predominantly V3 (slower hydrolytic isozyme), and the myosin Ca^{++} adenosine triphosphate activity decrease consequentely with senescence (10). This could partially account for the reduction in speed and extent of isotonic shortening in muscle from senescent rats compared with that from younger adults (13). The recovery period of the excitation-contraction coupling cycle is prolonged in senescent muscle.

Probably same of these alterations may be adaptive rather then degenerative in nature. Thus, the prolonged time course of the Ca_i transient in senescent heart prolongs myofilament force development and cardiac contraction after excitation (6), enabling the continued ejection of blood during late systole. This mechanism probably serves as a beneficial adaptation to the concurrent age-associated increase (and prolongation) in left ventricular afterload because of increased aortic impedance. However, the aging heart is also more susceptible to Ca^{++} overload and to Ca^{++} oscillations. Under conditions that enhance cell Ca^{++} loading, cardiac muscle of senescent heart is more prone to develop electrical manifestations of spontaneous sarcoplasmic reticulum Ca^{++} release, i.e., diastolic after-depolarizations. Furthermore, the threshold for Ca^{++} dependent ventricular fibrillation is reduced in the senescent heart.

The underlying molecular basis of the long-term modulation of exitation-contraction mechanisms during aging involves also an alterated expression of genes that code for proteins governing these processes. The espression of the β-myosin heavy-chain gene increases with advancing age while the α-myosin heavy-chain decreases. This "switching" of genes is one factor that underlies the reduction in shortening velocity with aging. It could be also speculate that changes in expression of genes regulating sarcolemmal ionic channels may underlie the prolonged action potential in the senescent heart.

ABILITY OF THE AGING HEART TO CHRONIC HAEMODYNAMIC OVERLOAD

The prevalence of congestive heart failure increases in older person (14). An hypothesis is that the substrate on which specific disease is superimposed becomes altered with age. According to this hypothesis, the biochemical and physiologic capacity of the heart in response to long-term increases in haemodynamic load may become reduced (15).

The heart's functional reserve capacity may be viewed as the combined ability to rapidly recruit functional contractile units to augment cardiac output in response to short-term changes in circulatory demand and to positively regulate the intrinsic capacity of individual functional contractile units to better handle long-term haemodynamic load or stress. Thus, the reduction of both the hypertrophic growth response and its functional adaptations in response to mechanical stresses may be viewed as the age-associated loss of elements of intrinsic functional reserve capacity of the heart (1,7,8,11). This reduced capacity of response may be related to a deficiency of activation of genes or of post-transcriptional processes that ordinarily result in an increase in protein synthesis (16–17). A progressive age-associated loss of myocyte number occurs in both ventricles and is accompanied by increased cardiac myocyte size (18) that may be compromised by this progressive decline in turnover of contractile and other protein constituents. This cellular loss also occurs dramatically in the sinus node (19), and this loss of pacemaker cells probably contributes to the high prevalence of atrial dysrhythmias, especially sick sinus syndrome in elderly persons (20).

CARDIOVASCULAR FUNCTION DURING STRESS

The heart rate augmentation during vigorous exercise is less in healthy elderly persons compared with younger persons, and compensatory cardiac dilatation at end diastole occurs in older patients (21) to maintain appropriate cardiac output. Despite the maintenance or augmentation of stroke volume through end-diastolic dilatation, the proportionate reduction of end-systolic volume during vigorous exercise is less in elderly then in younger persons, thus accounting for the apparent smaller increase in ejection fraction seen in older persons (21). The increase in end-diastolic (and end-systolic) volume tends to compensate (Frank-Starling's law) for the blunted augmentation of heart rate, end-systolic volume and ejection fraction. These changes can be due in elderly population to:

- A deficit in intrinsic myocardial excitation-contraction mechanisms
- A diminished β-adrenergic modulation
- An age-related increase in characteristic aortic impedance
- A large end-diastolic dimension

β-ADRENERGIC MODULATION OF CARDIOVASCULAR PERFORMANCE

One of the most notable age-related changes that occurs in cardiovascular system is the diminished responsiveness to β-adrenergic modulation. During moderate exercise, characteristic aortic impedance does not increase in younger men (22) despite increasing aortic pressure, essentially because the aorta in these young persons reversibly dilates. In contrast, characteristic aortic impedance does increase during exercise in both senescent and β-adrenergically blocked young dog (23). Thus, it has been suggested that a deficient β-adrenergic relaxant effect on aortic smooth muscle in the senescent dog is at least partly responsible for the increase in characteristic aortic impedance during exercise (23). In the same way, it has been demonstrated a reduction in the effectiveness of β-adrenergic stimulation to relax arteries and veins in humans (24,25) and in isolated aortic muscles from senescent animals (26) compared with younger ones. In isolated cardiac muscle or perfused myocardium of aging rats, the β-adrenergic enhancement of the contractile state is diminished compared with that in the muscle of myocardium from younger adult rats (1). It has been also demonstrated that the contractile response to norepinephrine is diminished as is the phosphorilation of the contractile protein, troponin I (27,28).

β-adrenergic modulation of cardiac pacemaker cells accounts in part for the increase in heart rate during exercise. The effect of bolus infusion of β-adrenergic agonists results in a diminished heart rate response in elderly persons compared with younger persons (29).

CONCLUSIONS

Overall cardiovascular function at rest in healty elderly persons meets the body's needs for pressure and flow. The basal heart rate is unchanged. Left ventricular volume increases slightly in older men, and heart wall thickness increases modestly, largely because of an increase in myocyte size. Although the early diastolic filling rate is reduced, an enhanced atrial contribution to ventricular filling in older persons maintains filling volume at a normal level. Although systolic pressure at rest increases with age, the resting and-systolic volume and ejection fraction are not altered, partly because of the increase in left ventricular thickness. The increase in exercise heart rate is smaller in older persons, but cardiac dilatation maintains stroke volume, and thus cardiac output adequate. In these persons, the exercise-induced reduction in end-systolic volume and increase in ejection fraction are less than those in younger persons. These age-associated alterations in haemodynamic responses to physical stress may be due in part to diminished responsiveness to β-adrenergic stimulation of the heart and vasculature.

REFERENCES

1. Lakatta EG: Heart and Circulation. *In* Handbook of the Biology of Aging, edn. 3. Edited by Schneider EL, Rowe J. New York: Academy press; 1990: 181–216.
2. Xia RP, Lakatta EG: Mechanisms of altered b-adrenergic modulation of th Cardiovascular system with aging. *Rev. Clin. Gerontol* 1991; 1:309–322.
3. Fleg JL, Tzankoff SP, Lakatta EG: Age-related augmentation of plasma catecholamines during dynamic exercise in healthy males. *J. Appl. Phisiol* 1985; 59:1033–1039.
4. Nichols WW, O'Rourke MF, Avolio AP et al.: Age-related changes in left ventricular/arterial coupling. *In* Ventricular vascular coupling: clinical Physiological, and Engineering aspects. Edited by Yin FCP. New York: Springer-Verlag; 1987: 79–114.
5. Lakatta EG: Normal changes of aging. *In* Merck Manual of Geriatrics. Edited by Abrams WB, Berkow R. Rahway: Merck Sharp & Dohme Research Laboratories; 1990: 310–325.
6. Wei JY, Spurgeon HA, Lakatta EC: Exitation-contraction in rat myocardium: alterations with adult aging. *Am. J. Physiol.* 1984; 246:H784-H791.
7. Lakatta EG: Do hypertensionand aging have a similar effect on the myocardium? *Circulation* 1987; 75 (supplI): I69-I77.
8. Lakatta EG: Regulation of cardiac muscle function in the hypertensive heart. *In* Cellular and Molecular mechanisms of hypertension. Edited by Cox RH. New York: Plenum; 1991: 149–173.
9. Froehlich JP, Lakatta EG, Beard E, et al: Studies of sarcoplasmic reticulum function and contraction duration in young and aged rat myocardium. *J. Mol. Cell Cardiol* 1978; 10: 427–438.
10. Effron MB, Bhatnager GM, Spurgeon HA et al: Changes in myosin isoenzymes, ATPase activity and contraction duration in rat cardiac muscle with aging can be modulated by thyroxine *Circ Res* 1987; 60: 238–245.
11. Schwartz K, Lompre AM, De La Bastie D et al: Mechano-genic transduction in the hypertrophied heart. *J Mol Cell Cardiol* 1989; 21 (suppl III): S24.
12. Weisfeldt ML, Lakatta EG, Gerstenblith G: Aging and the heart. *In* Heart Disease; a textbook of cardiovascular medicine,vol.2, edn. 4. Edited by Braunwald E. Philadelphia: WB Saunders; 1992: 1656–1669.
13. Capasso Jmm Malhotra A, Remily RM et al: Effects of age on mechanical and electrical performance of rat myocardium. *Am J Physiol* 1983: 245: H72-H81.
14. McFee PA, sCastelli WP, McNamara PM et al: The natural hystory of congestive heart failure: the Framingham Study. *N Engl J Med* 1971; 285:1441–1446.
15. Lakatta EG: Cardiovascular reserve capacity in healthy older humans. *Aging Clin. Exp. Res.* 1994; 6: 213–223.
16. Isoyama S, Grossman W, Wei JY et al: Effect of age on myocardial adaptation to volume overload in the rat. *J Clin Invest* 1988; 81:1850–1857.
17. Takahashi T, Schunkert H, Isoyama S et al: Age-related differences in the expression of proto-oncogene and contractile protein genes in response to pressure overload in the rat myocardium. *J Clin Invest* 1992; 89:939–946.
18. Olivetti G, Melissari M Capasso Jm et al: Cardiomyopathy of the aging human heart: myocyte loss and reactive cellular hypertrophy. *Circ Res* 1991; 68: 1560–1568.
19. Davies MJ: Pathology of tha conduction system. *In* Cardiology in old age. Edited by Caird FL, Dalle JLC, Kennedy RD; New York : Plenum press; 1976:57–59.

20. Wei JY, Gersh BJ: Heart disease in the elderly. *Curr Probl Cardiol* 1987; 12:1–65.
21. Rodeheffer RJ, Gerstenblith G, Becker Lc et al: Exercise cardiac output is maintained with advancing age in healthy human subjects: Cardiac dilatation and increased stroke volume compensate for diminished heart rate. *Circulation* 1984; 69: 203–213.
22. Murgo JP, Westerhof N, Giolma JP et al: Effect of exercise on aortic input umpedance and pressure wave forms in normal human. *Circ Res* 1981;48:334–343.
23. Yin FCP, Weisfeldt ML, Milnor WR: Role of aortic input impedance in the decreased cardiovascular response to exercise with aging in dogs. *J Clin Invest* 1981; 68: 28–38.
24. Pan HYM, Hoffman BB, Pershi RA: Decline in beta adrenergic receptor-mediated vascular ralexastion with aging in man. *J Pharmacol Exp Ther* 1986; 228: 802–807.
25. Van Brummelen P, Buhler FR, Kiowski W et al.: Age-related decrease in cardiac and peripheral vascular responsiveness to Isoprenaline: Studies in Normal Subjects. *Clin Sci* 1981; 60: 571–577.
26. Godfraiṅd T: Alternative mechanisms for the potentiation of the realxation evoked by Isoprenaline in aortae from young and aged rats. *Eur J Pharmacol* 1979; 53: 273–279.
27. Sakai M, Danziger RS, Staddon JM, et al: Contractile response of individul cardiac myocytes to norepinephrine decreases with senescence. *Am J Phisiol* 1992; 262: H184-H189.
28. Danziger RS, Sakai M, Lakatta EG et al: Interactive a- and b-adrenergic actions of norepinephrine in rat cardiac myocytes. *J Mol Cell Cardiol* 1992; 22: 111–123.
29. Yin FCP, Spurgeon HA, Raizes GS et al: Age-associated decrease in chronotropic response to Isoproterenol. *Circulation* 1976; 54 (suppl II): 11.

14

EARLY MARKERS OF CARDIOVASCULAR DAMAGE

Giuseppe Licata*

Cattedra di Medicina Interna
Istituto di Clinica Medica
Università di Palermo

INTRODUCTION

Cardiovascular (CV) disease represents at present one of the most frequent causes of morbidity and mortality in western industrialized countries. The prevalence of CV disease is increased in subjects with hypertension (HTN), diabetes mellitus (DM), dyslipidemia and central obesity. In these conditions, it is possible to detect early alterations of metabolic, hormonal, hemostatic, genetic and hemodynamic parameters, frequently associated with morphological and functional modifications of the left ventricle (LV) and the vascular system. Since these changes generally precede and are closely related to the occurrence of CV events, they may be considered early markers of CV disease. In recent years, the study of these parameters as prognostic factors has been facilitated by the introduction of new sensitive laboratory and image methods that allow their accurate quantification. In fact, several studies have investigated specific markers to document the early involvement of the CV system.

On the basis of epidemiological, pathophysiological and clinical data, we have proposed several markers, some of them *direct expression of CV injury,* such as LV hypertrophy (LVH), pre-clinical alterations of systolic and diastolic LV function, microalbuminuria, carotid lesions and endothelial dysfunction. Other parameters, such as alterations in 24-h blood pressure (BP), renin profile, LP(a), coagulation-fibrinolysis factors and insulin and homocysteine metabolism, may be considered only *associated and/or correlated with CV injury*, and clinical events.

In this review we will examine briefly the direct and indirect markers, as well as other factors proposed as early markers of CV disease, the role of which is not yet established (Table 1).

* Correspondence to: Prof. Giuseppe Licata, Istituto di Clinica Medica, Piazza delle Cliniche 2, 90127 Palermo, Italy. Tel: 091/6552151; fax: 091/6552153.

Recent Advances in Geriatrics, edited by Barbagallo, Licata, and Sowers.
Plenum Press, New York, 1998.

Table 1. Early markers of cardiovascular damage

Direct markers
- Left ventricular hypertrophy
- Preclinical alterations of left ventricular function
- Microalbuminuria
- Carotid lesion
- Endothelial dysfunction

Indirect markers
- 24 h BP
- Renin profile
- Insulin resistance
- Lp(a)
- Homocysteine
- Coagulation and fibrinolysis factors

Other markers
- Atrial natriuretic peptide
- C-Reactive protein
- Fibrinopeptide A
- C3

DIRECT MARKERS OF CARDIOVASCULAR INJURY

Direct markers of *early CV damage* include: LVH, pre-clinical alterations of LV systolic and diastolic function, microalbuminuria, carotid lesions and endothelial dysfunction (ED).

Left Ventricular Hypertrophy

LVH is an increment in myocardial mass, either idiopatic or secondary to altered LV function, produced by an increased pre- or after-load. Although the presence of LVH may represent a compensatory phenomenon to the chronic volume and/or pressure overload, it is hard to recognize when LVH is not adequate to maintain a normal LV function. LVH may be associated with BP, race, salt intake, BMI[1], and with hormonal factors, such as catecolamines, renin-angiotensin system and growth factors.

The introduction and development of echocardiography have permitted accurate measurements of LV mass (LVM). Indeed, a greater number of subjects with LVH are now identified, respect to former years when the diagnosis was based on EKG criteria[2,3]. Studies comparing echocardiographic measurements of LVM ante-mortem with direct post-mortem measurements, have demonstrated the high sensitivity and specificity of this method.

LVH is independently associated with an increased frequency of CV events[4,5] and its regression is followed by a higher survival in both hypertensives and subjects with ischemic heart disease[1,3]. This is probably due to the fact that chronic LVH impairs LV function[6], reduces coronary reserve[7], and it is associated with cardiac arrhythmias and adrenergic nervous system dysfunction, including reduced β-adrenergic receptors[8].

Additionally, Devereux et al.[9] recently reported that in hypertensives different adaptative changes in LV geometry occur in response to the increased post-load, such as eccentric or concentric hypertrophy, concentric remodeling or normal LV geometry. These structural modifications lead to diverse hemodynamic changes with different frequency of CV events. As such, subjects with concentric hypertrophy and remodeling are at higher risk, therefore should be followed up closely and treated aggressively.

Left Ventricular Function

In the past, the study of LV function was classically referred to systolic function The development of non-invasive and accurate methods, such as radioisotopic angiography and echocardiography, consent the evaluation of both systolic and diastolic phases, in basal conditions and after exercise. The recognition of the diastolic phase of the cycle as an active phenomenon lead to consider the diastolic function involvement as an important component of the altered LV function, occasionally representing the earliest marker of dysfunction[10–13]. In fact, at least in some CV diseases, the only dysfunction corresponds to an altered ventricular filling[10].

Systolic Function (SF). In the evaluation of the systolic phase of cardiac cycle, the most frequently and easiest parameter measured is the ejection fraction (EF), that determines the efficiency of systolic function in normal and pathologic conditions.

Several studies have demonstrated that EF is decreased in HTN even in the absence of LVH or clinical signs of LV dysfunction[14]. As such, an inverse relation between EF and 24-h BP has been demonstrated[15]. In central obesity an early modification of EF has been documented, both in resting conditions and after stress-test[16–18]. We demonstrated that in addition to the severity, the duration of obesity is an important determinant of LV systolic function even in the absence of clinical signs of cardiac involvement. Subjects with more than 20 years of obesity had decreased or clearly negative response of EF to stress-test[18]. These data are of extreme interest, since an increased EF response to stress is considered a parameter of a competent LV performance[19], in addition to the risk classification.

Therefore, the determination of basal and stress-test EF may represent a useful tool in the identification of systolic LV dysfunction that is followed in a variable length of time by clinically evident cardiopathy.

Diastolic Function (DF). The diastole is characterized by an active loss of tension with ATP consumption, regulated by intrinsic and extrinsic factors. Intrinsic factors include passive elastic ventricular properties (wall thickness and composition, consistency characteristics ("stress relaxation" or permanent deformation"), diastolic negative pressure, endothelial factors and contractile state. Among the extrinsic factors the most important are related to the pericardium, atrial contraction, circulating volume, and right ventricle state. DF was initially studied in experimental models, and in the last years it has been explored in human hearts by hemodynamic studies, angiography, echocardiography and radio-isotopic studies.

The clinical conditions most frequently associated with altered ventricular relaxation are myocardial ischemia, cardiomyopathies and congestive heart failure. More recently the study of DF has been directed to subjects with HTN, DM and central obesity. Regarding HTN, several studies have shown a negative correlation between 24-h BP and peak filling rate (PFR), both at rest and after stress, independently of the presence of systolic alterations or clinical signs of LV dysfunction[15,20], and enhanced in the presence of LVH[13]. The mechanism of the early involvement of DF in HTN is not yet clarified, however, the fact that diastolic alterations are more severe in hypertensives with LVH suggests that increased rigidity with a consequent reduced diastolic compliance may contribute[12,13]. In fact, regression of LVH is associated with an improvement in PFR[13].

In recent years our group has investigated the behavior of DF in obese subjects, particularly in relation to central fat distribution. We demonstrated that modifications of PFR, measured by radioisotopes and echocardiography, are present early in subjects with central obesity and are closely related to the degree and duration of obesity. Further, PFR is inversely related to waist/hip ratio (WHR) in these subjects[21]. PFR alterations in these subjects are more evident in the presence of other CV risk factors, such as microalbuminuria, elevated Lp(a) or a family history of stroke[22].

Although the mechanisms of early diastolic dysfunction in obesity are not completely understood, it is possible that not only hemodynamic modifications, but also genetically determined neuro-hormonal changes, such as adrenergic hyperactivity, insulin resistance or alterations in sodium balance regulation, may contribute.

Microalbuminuria

Microalbuminuria is an increased urinary albumin excretion (UAE) in a range below the measurable levels with traditional methods[23]. Since physiological UAE in a normal individual is 1–22 mg/24h, values of 30–300 mg/24h or 20–200 μg/min are considered pathologic microalbuminuria. Numerous studies have demonstrated that microalbuminuria may predict the emergence of overt proteinuria, chronic renal failure and CV mortality in diabetic patients[23–26].

Epidemiological data have also demonstrated that microalbuminuria is closely related to the prevalence of CV disease in HTN and central obesity[25,26,29]. In both populations, this parameter has been associated with the expression of other early markers of CV injury[22,25–28]. Interestingly, the incidence of coronary artery disease (CAD) and peripheral vasculopathy is significantly greater in subjects with microalbuminuria, independently of BP, the co-existance of DM or the presence of other risk factors.

It is possible that in HTN and in obesity, hemodynamic and renal modifications may favor the presence of microalbuminuria. As such, Yoshida et al.[30] reported that rats submitted to subtotal nephrectomy, have albuminuria even with only mild structural glomerular alterations. In humans, Bigazzi et al.[31] demonstrated that the presence of microalbuminuria is expression of unfavorable renal hemodynamic changes that may induce or worsen the hypertensive renal injury. In other study, Pedrinelli et al.[32] demonstrated a significant relation of microalbuminuria and endothelial dysfunction in HTN, suggesting that microalbuminuria may be the expression of a generalized endothelial dysfunction, not limited exclusively to the kidney.

In regards to obesity, we have recently demonstrated that microalbuminaria is present almost exclusively in central obese subjects. In these individuals microalbuminuria is associated with reduced renal blood flow and increased renal resistance. We observed a direct positive relation between microalbuminuria and Lp(a), cardiac morphologic parameters, mean 24h BP and family history of CV events. We conclude that in some central obese subjects, microalbuminuria is early associated with other markers of CV damage[33] (see Figs. 1 and 2).

Carotid Lesion

The carotid atherosclerotic lesion, as any other vascular lesion, evolves from a minimal endothelial damage that progresses to endothelial thickness and media layer involvement. The abnormal accumulation of cells in the endothelial space determine the true neo-endothelial lesion, which depends on modifications of cellular growth/death ratio. Among the numerous growth factors involved, PDGF and angiotensin II (AII) appear to play a particularly important role[34]. Recent studies suggest that attenuated apoptosis contribute substantially to the genesis of the atherosclerotic lesion[35]. It appears that PDGF and

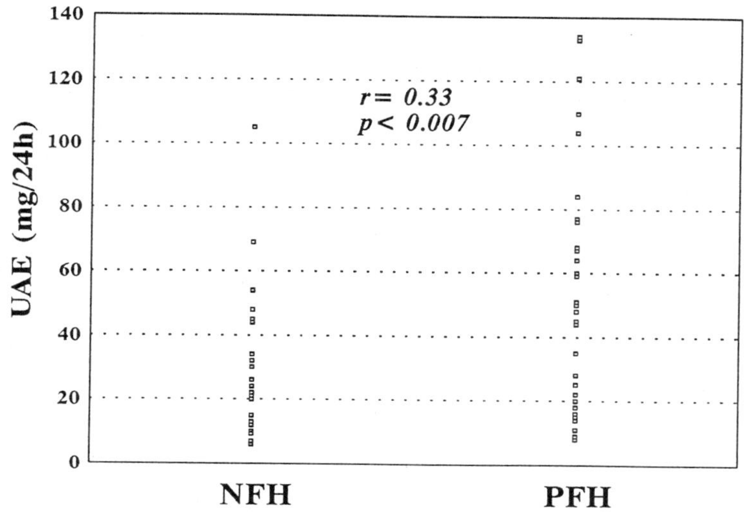

Figure 1. Relation between microalbuminuria and family history of stroke in young central obese subjects (factorial analysis of variance). UAE: urinary albumin excretion; NFH: negative family history; PFH: positive family history.

AII have anti-apoptotic effects on vascular smooth muscle cells (VSMC), in addition to the growth stimulating action. The transduction systems that mediate this anti-apoptotic effects remain unknown. However, alterations in the cellular redox status modulating the activation of apoptotic programs and some integrins may play a relevant role in the survival of vascular cells[36].

VSMC present in endothelial lesions belong to a cellular population with altered phenotypic characteristics, with altered expression of transcription and growth factors, apoptosis regulating genes, integrins, proteases, and matrix proteins, controlled by the expression of Bax-Bcl-2 family and the protease Interleukin Converting Enzyme[35–37]. The result is a population of VSMC with an increased tendency to proliferate, migrate and elaborate extracellular matrix proteins. Although the molecular mechanisms of these alterations are net yet clarified, the activation of such genetic program may be similar to that operating during fetal development[34].

From a clinical point of view, although the atherosclerotic lesion is in constant evolution with angiogenesis and frequent hemorragic and lipidic infiltration, there is a long

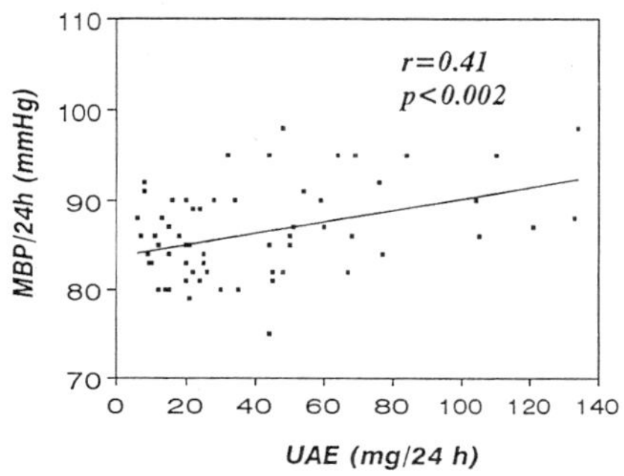

Figure 2. Relation of microalbuminuria (UAE) and 24h blood pressure in young central obese subjects.

asymptomatic phase (the CV event frequently opens the clinical scene). Therefore, for primary prevention it is essential to identify the initial lesion the earliest possible. To that purpose the use of ultrasound have allowed the visualization of the plaque, and further, to identify early endothelial-media thickness[38–40]. In hypertensives, we have demonstrated a close relationship between the degree of HTN and the popliteal endothelial-media thickness[41]. In other study from our group, the frequency of carotid plaques was independent of cholesterol levels in patients with familial heterozigote hypercholesterolemia, while it was greater in patients with associated HTN[42].

In former studies performed in autopsies, an association between carotid and coronary atherosclerotic lesions was observed as well as between the presence of these lesions and CAD morbidity and mortality[43]. This association has been recently confirmed with ultrasonographic methods in subjects over 50 years; as such, subjects with severe carotid lesions, have ten times greater probability to present three vessel CAD[44–46]. Conversely, severe CAD associated with hypercholesterolemia is a strong predictor of carotid plaque progression[47]. Therefore, carotid lesions may be markers of systemic atherosclerotic disease, even in the asymptomatic patient.

Finally, the presence of carotid atherosclerotic lesions is associated with alterations in coagulation and fibrinolytic profiles. This hemostatic alterations are worsen in subjects with contemporaneous CAD, confirming that the activation of coagulation factors and depression of fibrinolytic system may play a major role in both the pathogenesis of atherosclerotic vasculopathy and the manifestation of thromboembolic events[48].

Endothelial Dysfunction (ED)

The endothelium is a monocellular layer between the blood and VSMC. In contrast to the former view of endothelium as a mechanical barrier, at present it is recognized an important paracrine organ, that produces numerous regulatory substances in physiologic and pathologic states, that modulate platelet function and VSMC proliferative/contractile state[49]. In physiologic conditions the endothelium produces predominantly vasodilating substances, with anti-aggregative and anti-proliferative actions, suggesting that the main function is to assure and adequate blood supply depending on tissular metabolic demand. However, in some pathologic conditions (i.e. atherosclerosis and HTN), the production of endothelial substances with vasoconstrictive properties increases, which along with a reduced production of vasodilating substances, may result in a substantially altered regional blood supply.

In CAD, regardless the mechanism leading to myocardial ischemia, the abnormal endothelial responsiveness may be a common denominator. In fact, endothelial-dependent vasodilation is altered in human atherosclerotic arteries and results in a paradoxical vasoconstriction in response to vasodilating substances such as acethylcholine, or in increased responses to vasoconstrictor agents[49,50]. In the last years several studies have documented the presence of ED in different forms of ischemic cardiopathy and also in conditions that precede CAD, such as hypercholesterolemia and HTN[51].

Regarding HTN, experimental data suggest that ED is a consequence more than a cause of hypertension, and progresses in parallel with the disease. ED appears to be intimately connected with the degree of HTN, such that normalization of BP is able to regress ED in 8 weeks[49]. In humans, ED may be evaluated by forearm blood flow response to the administration of endothelial-dependent (acetylcholine or methacholine) and endothelial-independent agonists (sodium nitroprusiate)[49,51]. With this method, several studies have demonstrated a decreased endothelium-dependent vasodilation in essential hypertensive respect to normotensive subjects, particularly those with LVH[49,51]. Therefore, it is at present accepted that human HTN is associated with ED and the mechanisms involved may include endothelium derived cyclo-oxigenase-dependent contracting factors (EDCFs) and a defect in L-arginine metabolism, responsible for endothelial nitric oxide (NO) synthesis. This relation has been supported by two evidences: 1) in essential hypertensives, but not in normotensives, NO inhibitors do not modify the vasodilatory effect of acetylcholine; 2) the infusion of NO inhibitors produces a vasoconstriction that is correlated with basal NO release, effect that is lower in hypertensives compared to normotensives, suggesting a decreased delivery of NO in these patients. Therefore, ED may be the consequence of an alteration in NO synthesis and/or NO difusibility, or in the production of EDCFs.

It has been demonstrated that ED associated with experimental HTN is present in early stages of the disease and may contribute to elevate BP and/or to the development of complications. Additionally, in young normotensives with genetic predisposition to the development of HTN, a reduced vasodilatatory response to acethylcholine has been documented, suggesting that ED may precede the development of hypertension and not only be a consequence but also a genetically determined cause of the disease[52].

Besides the evaluation of endothelium-dependent vasodilatory activity, endothelial function may be evaluated by the analysis of endothelial cell products, which may be direct or indirect expression of endothelial damage. Among them, of particular relevance are endothelins and adhesion molecules that we will review in the following paragraphs.

Endothelins

Endothelins are autacoids produced by the endothelium which pathogenetic role in CAD and HTN is still argued. Elevated plasmatic levels of endothelin have been reported after myocardial infarction (MI) both in experimental animals and in humans and IV infusion of endothelin has been shown to reduce coronary blood flow by more than 90%[53] Moreover, the infusion of an endothelin receptor antagonist is able to reduce MI extension in dogs[53,54]. A study by Brunner[55] demonstrated that endothelin release is increased in rats during reperfusion phase, suggesting a relevant role in the genesis of subsequent myocardial damage. The one year mortality in patients who suffer a MI strongly correlates to the plasma endothelin-1 concentrations determined three days after infarction[56]. Another study demonstrated an important role of endothelin in the emergence of neo-intimal lesions after angioplasty in rats. Those lesions were reduced with the administration of an endothelin receptor antagonist[57].

Concerning the role of endothelin in HTN, the available data are still controversial: while some studies report elevated endothelin levels in hypertensives respect to normotensives[58,59], other studies do not show any difference[61]. In humans, endothelin infusion produce vasoconstriction that is greater in hypertensive respect to normotensive subjects, potentiating sympathetic venoconstriction that follows a deep inspiration[62] and that is positively correlated with mean BP[63]. Also, several studies have documented a positive relation between endothelin levels and LVM and a negative relation with parameters of LV function[53,63,64].

Few studies have evaluated the behavior of endothelin in subjects with central obesity. Data from our group have demonstrated that circulating levels of endothelin are elevated in central obese subjects with respect to non-obese controls; endothelin is further elevated in these subjects if they have HTN or other CV risk factors[22]. Also, in a group of obese hypertensives, we found that endothelin levels are positively related to mean 24-h BP and LVM and inversely related to PFR[58]. This suggests that in hypertensives with central obesity, endothelin may play an important role in the maintenance of high BP as well as in the development of CV damage.

Adhesion Molecules

The early stages of atheromatous lesion involve the adhesion of circulating monocytes to and altered endothelium with subsequent monocyte transmigration[34]. This adhesion is mediated by the interaction of receptor couples in both adherent cells. These receptors, called adhesion molecules, are able to activate signal transduction systems inside the adherent cell. Multiple adhesion molecules have been identified, including member of several receptor families:

1. *Selectin* family include three main molecules: a) L-Selectin (LECAM-1, LAM-1, CD62L) expressed in all circulating leukocytes. b) P-Selectin (PADGEM, GMP-140, CD62P), secreted in response to thrombin and histamine. c) E-Selectin (ELAM-1, CD62E) which expression is induced by pro-inflamatory cytokines in endothelial cells.
2. *Mucines* are proteins that interact with selectin. This group includes GLYCAM-1 (glycosilation-dependent cell adhesion molecule) and CD34, which is a sialomucine expressed in stem-multipotential cells and endothelial cells.
3. *Integrins* are perhaps some of the most versatile adhesion molecules. Among the numerous integrins recently described, at least five are important in the interaction of leukocytes and endothelial cells.
4. Several members of the *immunoglobulin* superfamily expressed in the endothelium are related to integrins expressed in leukocytes. Those include ICAMs (ICAM-1, 2, 3), VCAM-1, MadCAM-1.

Among the adhesion molecules mentioned, E-selectin may be considered an early marker of ED. The soluble form of E-selectin is found in healthy subjects, and elevated levels have been reported in several pathologies that involve directly or indirectly the endothelium, such as HTN and DM. Our preliminary data indicate that E-selectin levels increase in response to immunologically mediated endothelial damage induced by anti-endothelium antibodies. Recently, we evaluated the behavior of soluble E-selectin in 45 young subjects (mean age 37±6 y) with central obesity and 26 non-obese control subjects, all without mayor CV risk factors. We identified 11 subjects from the obese group with elevated levels of E-selectin (>80 ng/ml). Obese subjects with the highest levels of E-selectin had the highest BMI and WHR together with a significative reduction in EF. In the same group MVS and total peripheral resistance was incremented, although this increase did not reach statistical significance. E-Selectin was directly related to BMI and inversely related to EF. This may support the notion that some central obese subjects have an early ED related to pre-clinical systolic LV dysfunction (see Fig. 3).

INDIRECT MARKERS OF CARDIOVASCULAR DAMAGE (ASSOCIATED OR CORRELATED TO CV DISEASE)

24-hour BP

Ambulatory BP monitoring (ABPM) has evolved in the last twenty years and currently an extensive literature concerning its validity and utilization is available. The current ABPM devices are completely automated, small in size and easy to operate and allow

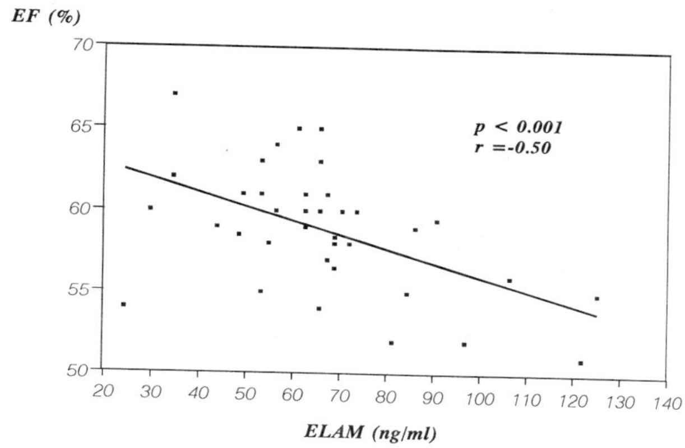

Figure 3. Relation of plasmatic levels of Selectin-E (ELAM) and left ventricle ejection fraction (EF) in a group of central obese subjects.

BP measurements at standard schedules (every 15 min or less), during day and night time, with the patient following normal daily activities. With ABPM, it is also possible to analyze BP variability.

The relevance of ABPM comes from the evidence of a more significant relationship to HTN-induced CV damage in any vascular bed (cardiac, renal, brain, retina, lower limbs), respect to casual measurements. Accordingly, several investigators agree with the notion that in hypertensive subjects, 24-hour BP correlates positively with LVM and negatively with parameters of LV function[15,65,66]. We have demonstrated that in recently diagnosed hypertensives without treatment, 24-hour BP is inversely correlated with PFR, even in the absence of clinically evident LV dysfunction[20]. In a group of central obese individuals we demonstrated a direct and significant correlation between 24-hour BP, WHR, Lp(a), microalbuminuria and family history of CV events. These data may allow the identification of subgroups of obese at higher risk, with several associated markers of CV damage[67,68].

Most hypertensive subjects are considered "dippers", referred to a 10 to 20% BP reduction during night-time, related to sleeping and awaking periods. "Non-dippers" are subjects in whom the night reduction is absent or diminished. In this regard, Verdecchia et al.[71] demonstrated that non-dipper hypertensives, particularly female subjects, are characterized by an increased frequency of CV events respect to dippers. However, the importance of nocturnal BP effects on CV risk has been argued by some authors advocating that the definition of dippers and non dippers is arbitrary, and that the times considered as sleeping and awaking periods (8–22h and 22–8h) hardly reflect what really happens in the single patient[72,73]. In an attempt to solve these discrepancies, our group proposed an original technique to analyze ABPM with a mathematical model (polynomial analysis by a third grade cubic function). With this method we demonstrated that the presence of target organ damage (LVH or ischemia) was higher in hypertensives with absence or inversion in BP circadian rhythm respect to hypertensives with preserved BP circadian rhythm[74].

In conclusion, 24-h BP analysis may be important in the early detection of hypertensive subjects with higher risk of CV damage and events.

Renin Profile and ACE Gene Polymorphism

The negative effect of elevated renin levels on CV morbidity and mortality in hypertension was proposed in the '60s by Laragh et al.[75,76] Since then, numerous experimental observations have described alterations in the renin-angiotensin system (RAS) that may contribute to the acceleration of atherosclerosis and the occurrence of cardiac or cerebrovascular events in hypertensive, diabetic and central obese populations. Among these observation the following are particularly pertinent:

1. Renin excess is associated with cardiac, renal and cerebral lesions in experimental models [77].
2. Elevated AII levels, even at lower concentrations than those producing BP increases, favor the development of CV lesions in several districts[77].
3. Inability to suppress renin responses to a salt load precedes the development of HTN and vascular lesion in stroke prone-SHR[78,79]. Similar evidence has been reported in Zucker rats[80], central obese subjects[81] and offsprings of subjects with precous CV events[82].
4. CV damage and fatal ischemic events have been reduced in experimental models under therapy with ACE- inhibitors[83].
5. In humans, the fenotype characterized by elevated renin levels exhibits an incidence of MI seven fold higher respect to hypertensive with normal or low renin, independently of cholesterol, fasting glucose, smoking and the presence of LVH[84].

These considerations support the hypothesis that early dysregulation of RAS may contribute to the risk of future CV events both in hypertensive and central obese subjects. Regarding the mechanism by which these alterations may affect the myocardium, is pertinent to consider that AII stimulates the expression of vasoactive peptides and a variety of growth factors that results in VSMC and cardiomyocytes growth. Several investigators have directed their research to explore the mechanisms by which this hormone is produced. In the human myocardium, ACE is responsible for a small portion of the AII produced; conversely in the vascular wall, ACE is responsible for most AII produced, particularly in the endothelium where this enzyme is ubiquitous. ACE gene clonation has allowed its transfection into rat VSMC in culture. With these technique it has been demonstrated that renin and ACE are rate-limiting in AII formation at the vascular wall; its co-transfection stimulate DNA and RNA synthesis through a mechanism inhibited by losartan-induced AT-1 receptor blockade[85].

ACE gene cloning has also permitted to identify the somatic and endothelial forms, that are codified by two different alleles differentiated by D/I polymorphism. This refers to an insertion (allele I) or deletion (allele D) of 287 base pairs correspondent to a repetitive sequence ALU in the intron 16. In humans, the phenotype DD is associated with ACE plasmatic levels that are twice the value of those present in subjects with phenotype II.

There is a growing interest in the study of the relationship between ACE gene polymorphism and CV risk, although there are contrasting reports. For example, a retrospective analysis by Cambien et al. demonstrated that the loose of ACE gene polymorphism was associated with an increased frequency of MI, particularly in subjects with low CV risk profiles[86]. Also, the DD phenotype has a high frequency among relatives of subjects with CV events[87], hypertensives with LVH, and patients with re-stenosis after coronary angioplasty[88]. In contrast, a recent study conducted in American physicians did not demonstrate any association between MI incidence and ACE DD phenotype[89]. However, it is possible that differences in selection criteria and race among the participants may explain the different results in these studies.

Thus, molecular genetic studies may permit in the future the detection of other markers of CV damage, consenting the use of simple genetic tests to identify subjects with predictable CV disease for an effective prevention and/or the use of genetic therapy (see Fig. 4).

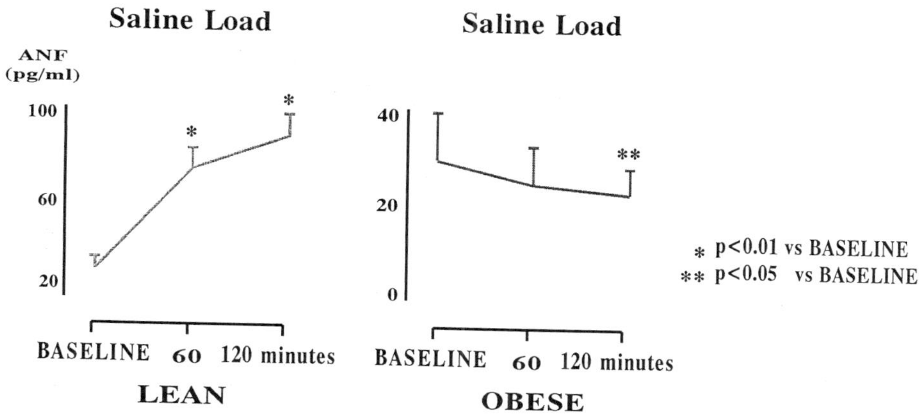

Figure 4. Atrial natriuretic factor (ANF) response to a saline load in lean and obese subjects.

Insulin Resistance (IR)

The hypothesis that elevated insulin levels may contribute to the development of atherosclerosis or its complications is not new and epidemiological studies have documented the association of insulin levels and incidence of CAD[90,91]. Also, Ducimetiere reported that fasting insulin and insulin/glucose ratio may predict future coronary events[92]. IR is not only present in conditions with an elevated frequency of CAD such as HTN, DM, dyslipidemia and obesity, but may also accelerate the progress of atherosclerotic lesions[93–95]. This is probably due to the stimulating effects of insulin on cellular proliferation, that render it a true growth factor[96,97].

The mitogenic action of insulin on VSMC is mediated by specific insulin receptors or insulin like growth factor-I (IGF-I) receptors. Insulin also may potentiate other mitogenic factors (PDGF and FGF), or may modulate their effects (AII). Hyperinsulinemia and/or IR, may induce sympathetic nervous system activation[98], fibrinolytic activity decrease[99], and ED by the reduction in NO production[100]. Insulin also induces sodium retention, that chronically affects CV efficiency (increased peripheral resistance, intravascular and cardiac volume, LV dysfunction). This effect is mediated directly by an increase in tubular sodium reabsortion[101], and indirectly by sympathetic stimulation[102], AII-related increase in aldosterone production[103] and a reduction in atrial natriuretic hormone release[104].

Thus, in recent analysis, the association of hyperinsulinemia and/or IR and CV events through accelerated development of atherosclerosis, appears strongly significant.

Lp(a)

Lp(a), described by Berg in 1963[105], contains one or more APO A molecules bound to APO B-100 by disulfide bounds. Numerous epidemiological studies have demonstrated that plasmatic concentrations of Lp(a) > 30 mg% are associated with an increased risk of CAD and other complications of atherosclerotic disease[106–108]. Also, an interesting study by Bailleul et al.[109] demonstrated that Lp(a) levels are higher in offsprings from subjects with diverse CV risk factors, and Watts et al.[110] reported a significant relationship of Lp(a) and carotid atherosclerosis demonstrated angiographycally. From a biological point of view, the analogy of a portion of Lp(a) with plasminogen and the presence of the lipoprotein in the atheromatous lesion, suggest a possible double pathogenic role, since it may affect thrombosis-fibrinolysis mechanisms as well as contribute to the formation of atheroma. Additionally, the Familial Atherosclerosis Treatment Study demonstrated that reductions in Lp(a) are associated with regression of atherosclerotic lesions[111]. More recently, several subtypes of Lp(a) have been identified, with a correlation to atherogenic risk dependent on their molecular weight (MW)[112–113]. As such, subtypes with the lowest MW are associated with the highest atherogenic risk. Recently, data from Pozza et al.[114] revealed the existence of a direct relation between low MW Lp(a) levels and total Lp(a) levels in subjects with precous CAD. Dividing the subjects according to the Lp(a) subtype, coronary patients with low MW Lp(a) presented the highest levels of total Lp(a). Thus, in addition to the demonstration of the atherogenic role of low MW Lp(a) subtype, this study confirms the utility of total Lp(a) measurement for the screening of CV risk and events.

In subjects with central obesity our group has demonstrated a significant relation between Lp(a) levels and both, ABPM and LVM. Further, these relations remained significant when other factors that affect Lp(a), such as age, plasmatic insulin and total cholesterol, were considered[115]. In summary, at present epidemiological and physiopathologic data indicate that Lp(a) is a marker that help identify subjects with susceptibility to develop CAD.

Homocysteine

Homocysteine is an intermediary product of metionin metabolism which elevated plasmatic levels are the diagnostic basis for the autosomic recessive disease homocystinuria that is frequently associated with vascular complication of small and large arteries[116]. Genetic factors, age, gender, complex B vitamins and some medicaments may negatively affect homocystein metabolism[117–118].

Clinical and experimental studies have documented that elevated concentrations of homocysteine may be responsible for atherogenic and thrombotic manifestations, through a still unknown mechanism. It seems possible that hyperhomocystinemia has deleterious effects on the endothelium[119], on platelet aggregability and on coagulation events[120–121].

The presence of hyperhomocystinemia is associated with an increased severity of carotid stenosis and a positive correlation between homocysteine levels and the number of critique stenotic lesions has been demonstrated[117]. Finally, epidemiological studies have reported that homocystinemia is correlated with an increased frequency of MI[122,123]. Therefore, it is plausible to consider hyperhomocystinemia an early marker of atherosclerosis[117].

Coagulation and Fibrinolytic Factors

Atherosclerosis and its complications are associated with an increased frequency of hemostatic alterations. Numerous studies have been conducted with the purpose of detecting markers that may explain the involvement of hemostatic system in atherosclerosis. Coagulation factors that have been demonstrated to be highly predictive of CV events by epidemiological data include fibrinogen and factor VII; fibrinolysis factors include plasminogen activator inhibitor (PAI)-1 and tPA. As such, the Northwick Park Heart Study[124] demonstrated that elevated levels of factor VII and fibrinogen are associated with an elevated risk of ischemic cardiopathy and CV mortality.

In the ECAT Angina Pectoris Study[125] the development of CAD documented by angiography was associated with elevated levels of fibrinogen, factor VII, PAI-1 and tPA. Increased levels of PAI-1 were also found in subjects with vasospastic angina, confirming the possible role of fibrinolytic system depression in the genesis of CAD[126].

We have documented that in subjects with central obesity, increased thrombogenic activity and decreased fibrinolytic activity without other CV risk factors, there is a significant association between these parameters and asymptomatic LV dysfunction and LV morphology modifications. Thus, hemostatic modifications early present in subjects with central obesity as well as other parameters described by us previously[128], may be responsible for the frequent development of CAD in these subjects.

OTHER MARKERS

Other factors, in particular conditions, seem to be associated with the future development of CV disease, but this association is not yet clearly established. We'll review briefly some of those that appear more relevant:

Atrial Natriuretic Peptide (ANP). It is at present recognized that ANP has a pathophysiological role in HTN, heart failure and CAD[129,130]. As such, alterations in ANP secretion, correlated with cardiac necrosis enzymes, have been documented in MI. Additionally, a decreased ANP response to a saline load has been reported in relatives from subjects with a CV event, in subjects with dilatative cardiomyopathy, initial stages of heart failure and in subjects with central obesity[82,130].

Regarding brain natriuretic peptide (BNP), structurally similar to ANP, some studies have recently reported that these peptide has a role in the prognosis of MI and heart failure[131,132].

C-Reactive Protein and Amyloid A. It has been demonstrated that both C-reactive protein and amyloid A are significantly correlated with the development of MI in patients with unstable angina[133]. However, it is not yet known whether the elevation of C-reactive protein depends on the type of inflammatory stimulus or on the intensity of the individual response; it is not either clear whether the inflammatory stimulus is originated in the heart or at systemic level.

Fibrinopeptide A. Also this peptide may represent a marker of the evolution of unstable angina towards MI. In this regard, Neri Serneri et al. demonstrated that patients with unstable angina and endoventricular thrombosis have higher levels of fibrinopeptide A respect to healthy controls and subjects with stable angina. In the same study and only in patients with unstable angina, it was documented that monocytes have a pro-coagulant activity modulated by lymphocytes[134].

Complement. In a retrospective study, Puddu et al.[135] demonstrated that elevated serum levels of C_3 in subjects without precedent cardiac events are associated with a high prevalence of MI. They suggest that complement system may intervene in the genesis of CAD, however, prospective data are needed to evaluate more accurately this original finding.

CONCLUSIONS

Laboratory and image techniques currently available permit an early and accurate evaluation of CV damage induced by several pathologic conditions. Data from the literature and from our own experience confirm that it is possible to identify markers which are direct expression of CV damage, as well as other factors associated or correlated with it.

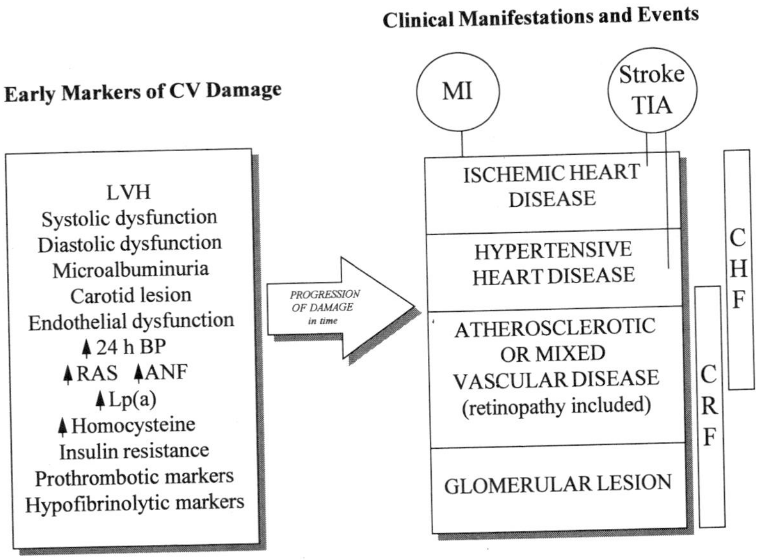

Figure 5. Early markers of cardiovascular damage and progression to clinical manifestations and cardiovascular events. LVH: left ventricular hypertrophy; RAS: renin angiotensin system; ANF: atrial natriuretic factor; MI: miocardial infarction; TIA: transit ischemic attack; CRF: chronic renal failure; CHF: congestive heart failure.

It is known that in diverse cardiac diseases diastolic dysfunction may precede the clinical expression of cardiopathy, as well as LVH represents one of the first manifestations of cardiac involvement in HTN, visceral obesity and DM. Also, particular attention has been devoted to the relationship between carotid atherosclerosis and CAD. This association may be more frequent than reported, since an invasive angiographic procedure is not performed in many patients with carotid lesions.

Regarding diabetes, microalbuminuria represents the first evidence of renal damage, that may evolve to overt nephropathy and chronic renal failure. In HTN and visceral obesity, microalbuminuria has been proposed as expression of both renal damage and systemic vascular involvement. Another expression of early physiopathological events is endothelial dysfunction, which association with risk and CV diseases has been confirmed in numerous studies.

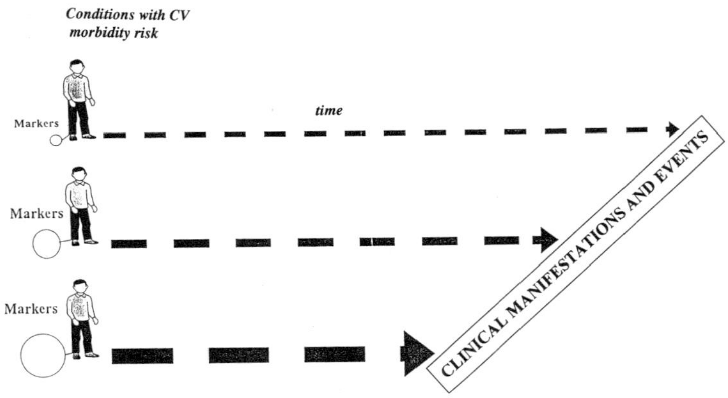

Figure 6. Markers of cardiovascular damage and risk classification.

Other markers associated or correlated with CV injury or events include 24h BP variablility, insulin resistance, elevated levels of Lp(a), renin, fibrinogen, factor VII, homocysteine, PAI-1 and tPA_1 and reduction of tPA_2. Finally, proposed parameters but not yet established include C-reactive protein, fibrinopeptide A and complement factors, of which C_3 and C_4, may indicate the evolution of unstable angina to MI.

The field that appears more promising is genetic research, that perhaps will allow to identify phenotypes with high frequency of CV events, therefore to characterize better the subjects who should be followed up closely to accomplish primary prevention.

At present, there is sufficient scientific evidence to recommend the use of markers mentioned in this review in the clinical practice, although the costs may limit their use. This approach may allow to identify early and accurately the possible candidates for CV events, therefore to conduct prompt preventive measures (see Figs. 5 and 6).

REFERENCES

1. Aronow WS. Left ventricular hypertrophy : significance in cardiac morbidity and mortality. Postgrad Med 1990; 87 (4): 147–158.
2. Levy D. Left ventricular hypertrophy: epidemiological insights from the Framingham Heart Study. Drugs 1988; 35 (Suppl. 5): 1–5.
3. Devereux RB, Reichek. Echocardiographic determination of left ventricular mass in man: anatomic validation of the method. Circulation 1977; 55: 613–618.
4. Aronow WS, Ahn C, Kronzon I, Koenigsberg M. Congestive heart failure, coronary events and atherothrombotic brain infarction in elderly blacks and whites with systemic hypertension and with and without echocardiographic and electrocardiographic evidence of left ventricular hypertrophy. Am J Cardiol 1991; 67: 295–299.
5. Casale PN, Devereux RB, Milner M, et al. Value of echocardiographic measurement of left ventricular mass in predicting cardiovascular morbid events in hypertensive men. Ann Int Med 1986; 105: 173–178.
6. Granger CB, Karimeddini MK, Smith VE, et al. Rapid ventricular filling in left ventricular hypertrophy. I. Physiologic hypertrophy. JACC 1985; 5 (4): 862–867.
7. Marcus ML, Koyanayi S, Harison DG, et al. Abnormality in the coronary circulation that occur as a consequence of cardiac hypertrophy. Am J Med 1983; 75 (Suppl. 3A): 62–66.
8. Diegel D, Cheitlin MD, Black DM, et al. Risk of ventricular arrhythmias in hypertensive men with left ventricular hypertrophy. Am J Cardiol 1990; 65: 742–747.
9. Koren MJ, Devereux RB, Casale PN, et al. Relation of left ventricular mass and geometry to morbidity and mortality in uncomplicated essential hypertension. Ann Int Med 1991; 114: 345–352.
10. Bonow RO, Bacharach SL, Green MV. Impaired left ventricular diastolic filling in patients with coronary artery disease: Assessment with radionuclide angiography. Circulation 1981; 64: 315–323.
11. Chiddo A, Gaglione A, Locuratolo N, et al. Funzione diastolica e danno anatomico del miocardio nella cardiomiopatia primitiva di tipo dilatativo. Cardiologia 1988; 33(7): 691–696.
12. Caponnetto S, Perocchio N. La funzione diastolica: recenti acquisizioni fisiopatologiche. Cardiologia 1989; 34(10): 829–833.
13. Fouad FM, Slominsky JM, Tarazi RC. Left ventricular diastolic function in hypertension: Relation to left ventricular mass and systolic function. JACC 1984; 3: 1500–1506.
14. Christian TF, Zinsmeister AR, Miller TD, et al. Left ventricular systolic response to exercise in patients with systemic hypertension without left ventricular hypertrophy. Am J Cardiol 1990; 65: 1204–1208.
15. Zachariah PK, Krier JD. Hypertension and ambulatory blood pressure monitoring. Primary Care 1991; 18 (3): 651–662.
16. Corrao S, Paterna S, Arnone S, et al. Two-dimensional echocardiographic evaluation of left ventricular ejection fraction by the ellipsoid single-plane algorithm: A reliable method for assessing low or very low ejection fraction values? Cardiology 1995; 86: 503–507.
17. Licata G, Scaglione R, Barbagallo M, et al. Effect of obesity on left ventricular function studied by radionuclide angiocardiography. Int J Obesity 1991; 15: 295–302.
18. Licata G, Scaglione R, Paterna S, et al. Left ventricular function response to exercise in normotensive obese subjects: influence of degree and duration of obesity. Int J Cardiol 1992; 37: 223–230.

19. Bonow RO. Prognostic implications of exercise radionuclide angiography in patients with coronary artery disease. Mayo Clin Proc 1988; 63: 630–634.
20. Licata G, Scaglione R, Parrinello G, Corrao S. Rapid left ventricular filling in untreated hypertensive subjects with or without left ventricular hypertrophy. Chest 1992; 102: 1507–1511.
21. Scaglione R, Dichiara MA, Indovina A, et al. Left ventricular diastolic and systolic function in normotensive obese subjects: influence of degree and duration of obesity. Eur Heart J 1992; 13: 738–742.
22. Licata G, Corrao S, Parrinello G, Scaglione R. Obesity and cardiovascular diseases. Ann Ital Med Int 1994; 9:29–33.
23. Mogensen CE. Microalbuminuria predicts clinical proteinuria and early mortality in maturity-onset diabetes. N Engl J Med 1984; 310: 356–360.
24. Mogensen CE, Christensen CK. Predicting diabetic nephropathy in insulin-dependent patients. N Engl J Med 1984; 311: 89–93.
25. Yudkin JS, Forrest RD, Jackson CA. Microalbuminuria as predictor of vascular disease in non-diabetic subjects. Lancet 1988; 2: 530–533.
26. Haffner SM, Stern MP, Gruber MKK, et al. Microalbuminuria: potential marker for increased cardiovascular risk factor in non-diabetic subjects?. Arteriosclerosis 1990; 5: 727–731.
27. Fauvel JP, Hadj-Aissa A, Laville M, Fadat G, Labeeuw M, Zech P, Pozet N. Microalbuminuria in normotensive with genetic risk of hypertension. Nephron 1991; 57: 375–376.
28. Bigazzi R, Bianchi S, Campese VM, Baldari G. Prevalence of microalbuminuria in a large population of patients with mild to moderate essential hypertension. Nephron 1992; 61: 94–97.
29. Groop L, Ekstrand A, Forsblom C, et al. Insulin resistance, hypertension and microalbuminuria in patients with Type 2 (non-insulin-dependent) diabetes mellitus. Diabetologia 1993; 36: 642–647.
30. Yoshida Y, Fogo A, Ichikawa I. Glomerular haemodynamics changes vs hypertrophy in experimental glomerular sclerosis. Kidney Int 1989; 25: 654–660.
31. Bigazzi R, Bianchi S, Baldari D, et al. Microalbuminuria in salt-sensitive patients: A marker for renal and cardiovascular risk factors. Hypertension 1994; 23: 195–199.
32. Pedrinelli R, Giampietro O, Carmassi F, et al. Microalbuminuria and endothelial dysfunction in essential hypertension. Lancet 1994; 344: 14–18.
33. Scaglione R, Ganguzza A, Corrao S, et al. Central obesity and hypertension: pathophysiologic role of renal haemodynamics and function. Int J Obesity 1995; 19: 403–409.
34. Gibbons GH, Dzau, VJ. Mechanisms of disease: emerging concept of vascular remodeling. N Eng J Med 1994; 330, 1431.
35. Bennett, MR, Evan GT, Schwartz SM. Apoptosis of human vascular smooth muscle cells derived from normal vessels and coronary atherosclerotic plaques. J Clin Invest 1995; 95, 2266.
36. Brooks PC, Clark RAF, Cheresh DA, et al. Requirement of vascular integrin avb3 for angiogenesis. (1994); Science 264, 569.
37. Isner, J. M., Kerney, M., Bortman, S., Passeri, J. Apoptosis in human atherosclerosis and restenosis. (1995); Circulation 91, 2703.
38. Pignoli P, Tremoli E, Poli A, Oreste P, Paoletti R. Intima plus media thickness of the arterial wall: a direct measurement with ultrasound imaging. Circulation 1986; 74: 1399–1406.
39. Delcker A, Diener HC. Quantification of atherosclerosis plaques in carotid arteries by three dimensional ultrasound. Br J Radiol 1994; 67: 672–678.
40. Suurküla M, Agewall S, Fagerberg B, et al. Ultrasound evaluation of atherosclerosis manifestations in the carotid artery in high-risk hypertensive patients. Arterioscler Thromb 1994; 14: 1297–1304.
41. Pinto A, Scaglione R, Galati D, et al. Evaluation of regional haemodynamics and alterations of vascular wall of the lower limbs in hypertensive subjects. Eur Heart J 1995; 1692–1697.
42. Di Silvestre G, Cecala M, Amato P, et al. Ultrasonographic assessment of common carotid artery wall in hypertensives with familial hypercholesterolaemia. (Abs). Am J Hypertens 1996; 9: 62A.
43. Craven TE, Ryu JE, Espeland MA, et al. Evaluation of the associations between carotid artery atherosclerosis and coronary artery stenosis: a case-control study. Circulation 1990; 82: 1230–1242.
44. Howard G, Ryu JE, Evans GW, et al. Extracranial carotid atherosclerosis in patients with and without transient ischaemic attacks and coronary artery disease. Arteriosclerosis 1990; 10: 714–719.
45. Emeri RV, Cohn LH, Witimore AD. Coexistent carotid and coronary artery disease. Arch Surg 1983; 118: 1035–1039.
46. Mathur KS, Kashyap SK, Kumar U. Correlation of the extent and severity of atherosclerosis in the coronary and cerebral arteries. Circulation 1963; 27: 929–934.
47. Gai V, Forneris M, Colussi A. Pluridistrettualità arteriosclerotica in un gruppò di coronaropatici. In : Angiologia 86. Monduzzi Ed., Bologna 1986; 159–163.

48. Avellone G, Di Garbo V, Cordova R, et al. Sindrome trombofilica in pazienti affetti da pregresso infarto del miocardio con o senza lesioni aterosclerotiche carotidee. Cardiologia 1995; 40 (11): 845–850.
49. Lüscher TF. Imbalance of endothelium-derived relaxing and contracting factors: a new concept in hypertension? Am J Hypertens 1990; 3: 317.
50. Taddei S, Virdis A, Mattei P, Salvetti A. Vasodilation to acetylcholine in primary and secondary forms of human hypertension. Hypertension 1993; 21: 929–933.
51. Treasure CB, Klein JL, Vita JA, et al. Hypertension and left ventricular hypertrophy are associated with impaired endothelium-mediated relaxation in human coronary resistance vessels. Circulation 1993; 87: 86–93.
52. Taddei S, Virdis A, Mattei P, et al. Response to acetylcholine in offspring of essential hypertensive patients. Hypertension 1996, in press.
53. Levin ER, Endothelius. N Engl J Med 1995; 333 (6): 356–363.
54. Lüscher TF, Seo B-G, Bühler FR. Potential role of endothelin in hypertension. Hypertension 1993; 21: 752–757.
55. Brunner F, Du Toit EF, Opie LH. Endothelin release during ischaemia and reperfusion of isolated perfused rat hearts. J Mol Cell Cardiol 1992; 24: 1291–1305.
56. Omland T, Lie RT, Aakvaag A, et al. Plasma endothelin determination as a prognostic indicator of 1-year mortality after acute myocardial infarction. Circulation 1994; 89: 1573–1579.
57. Douglas SA, Louden C, Vickery-Clark LM, et al. A role for endogenous endothelin-1 in neointimal formation after rat carotid artery balloon angioplasty: protective effects of the novel non-peptide endothelin receptor antagonist SB 209670. Circ Res 1994; 75: 190–197.
58. Parrinello G, Scaglione R, Pinto A, et al. Central obesity and hypertension: role of plasma endothelin. Am J Hypertens 1996;9:1186–1191.
59. HaaK T, Jungmann E, Felber A, et al. Increased plasma levels of endothelin in diabetic patients with hypertension. Am J Hypertens 1992; 5: 161–166.
60. Kurihara Y, Kurihara H, Suzuki H, et al. Elevated blood pressure and craniofacial abnormalities in mice deficient in endothelin-1. Nature 1994; 368: 703–710.
61. Davenport AP, Ashby MJ, Easton P, et al. A sensitive immunoassay measuring endothelin-like immunoreactivity in human plasma: comparison of levels in patients with essential hypertension and normotensive control subjects. Clin Sci 1990; 78: 261–264.
62. Haynes WG, Hand MF, Johnstone HA, et al. Direct and sympathetically mediated venoconstriction in essential hypertension. Enhanced response to endothelin-1. J Clin Invest 1994; 94: 1359–1364.
63. Lerman A, Hildebrand FL, Aarthus LL, Burnett JC. Endothelin has biological actions at pathophysiological concentrations. Circulation 1991; 83: 1808–1814.
64. Vanhoutte PM. Is endothelin involved in the pathogenesis of hypertension? Hypertension 1993; 21: 747–751.
65. Omboni S, Frattola A, Parati G, Mancia G. Clinical value of blood pressure measurements: Focus on ambulatory blood pressures. Am J Cardiol 1992; 70: 4D-8D.
66. Licata G. Epidemiologia dell'ipertensione arteriosa e danno d'organo. Ann Ital Med Int 1994; 9(Suppl): 44–49.
67. Licata G, Scaglione R, Ganguzza A, et al. Central obesity and hypertension. Relationship between fasting serum insulin, plasma renin activity and diastolic blood pressure in young obese subjects. Am J Hypertens 1994; 7: 314–320.
68. Licata G, Corrao S, Ganguzza A, et al. Microalbuminuria in obese subjects: relationship between body fat distribution, blood pressure and left ventricular structure and function. Submitted to Am J Cardiol.
69. O'Brien E, Sheridan J, O'Malley K. Dippers and non-dippers. Lancet 1988; ii: 397.
70. Staessen JA, Fagard RH, Lijnen PJ, et al. Mean and range of the ambulatory pressure in normotensive subjects from a meta-analysis of 23 studies. Am J Cardiol 1991; 67: 723–727.
71. Verdecchia P, Porcellati C, Schillaci G et al. Ambulatory blood pressure. An independent predictor of prognosis in essential hypertension. Hypertension 1994; 24: 793–801.
72. Grosse P, Ansoborlo P, Lemetayer P, Clementy J. Daytime and nighttime ambulatory blood pressures should be calculated over the true sleep/waking cycle and not over arbitrary periods. Am J Hypertens 1996; 9: 269–272.
73. Gatzka CD, Schmieder RE. Improved classification of dippers by individualized analysis of ambulatory blood pressure profiles. Am J Hypertens 1995; 8: 666–671.
74. Corrao S, Scaglione R, Arnone S, et al. Analysis of 24-h non-invasive ambulatory blood pressure profiles by a third degree polynomial approach. J Cardiovasc Diagn Proc 1996; 13 (4):237–242.
75. Brunner HR, Laragh JH, Baer L. Essential hypertension: renin and aldosterone heart attack and stroke. N Engl J Med 1972: 286: 441–449.

76. Brunner HR, Sealey JE, Laragh JH. Renin as a risk factor in essential hypertension: more evidence. Am J Med 1973; 55: 295–302.
77. Gavras H, Kremer D, Brown JJ, et al. Angiotensin and norepinephrine induced myocardial lesions: experimental and clinical studies in rabbits and man. Am Heart J 1975; 89: 321–332.
78. Camargo MJ, Campbell WG, Volpe M, et al. Abnormal renin secretory response to high sodium diet in stroke prone spontaneously hypertensive rats. Kidney Int 1990; 37: 383A.
79. Volpe M, Rubattu S, Mirante A, et al. Early impairment of sodium handling in stroke-prone spontaneously hypertensive rats. Am J Hypertens 1992; 5: 48A.
80. Kurtz TW, Morris RC, Pershadsingh HA. The Zucker fatty rat as a genetic model of obesity and hypertension. Hypertension 1989; 13: 896–901.
81. Licata G, Volpe M, Scaglione R, Rubattu S. Salt regulating hormones in young normotensive obese subjects. Effects of saline load. Hypertension 1994; 23 (suppl 1): 20–24.
82. Volpe M, Lembo G, De Luca N, et al. Abnormal hormonal and renal responses to saline load in hypertensive patients with parental history of cardiovascular accidents. Circulation 1991; 84: 92–100.
83. Stier CT, Benter IF, Ahmad S. Enalapril prevents stroke and kidney dysfunction in salt-loaded stroke-prone spontaneously hypertensive rats. Hypertension 1989; 13: 115–121.
84. Alderman MH, Madhavan S, Ooi WL, et al. Association of the renin-sodium profile with the risk of myocardial infarction in patients with hypertension. N Engl J Med 1991; 324, 16: 1098–1104.
85. Rigat B, Hubert C, Corvol P, Soubrier F. PCR detection of the insertion/deletion polymorphism of the human angiotensin converting enzyme (DCPI). Nucleic Acids Res 1992; 20: 1433.
86. Cambien F, Poirier O, Lecerf L, et al. Deletion polymorphism in the gene for angiotensin-converting enzyme is a potent risk factor for myocardial infarction. Nature 1992; 359: 641–644.
87. Tiret L, Poirier O, Lecerf L, et al. Deletion polymorphism in angiotensin-converting enzyme gene associated with parental history of myocardial infarction. Lancet 1993; 341: 991–992.
88. Schunkert H, Hense HW, Holmer SR, et al. Association between a deletion polymorphism of the angiotensin-converting enzyme gene and left ventricular hypertrophy. N Engl J Med 1994; 330: 1634–1638.
89. Lindpaintner K, Pfeffer MA, Kreutz R, et al. A prospective evaluation of an angiotensin-converting enzyme gene polymorphism and the risk of ischaemic heart disease. N Engl J Med 1995; 332: 706–711.
90. Eschwege E, Richard JL, Thibault N, et al. Coronary heart disease plasma insulin levels: the Paris prospective study, ten years later. Horm Metab Res 1985; 15 (Suppl): 41–46.
91. Pyorala K. Relationship of glucose tolerance and plasma insulin to the incidence of coronary heart disease: results from two population studies in Finland. Diabetes Care 1989; 2: 131–141.
92. Ducimetiere P, Eschwege R, Papoz L, et al. Relationship of plasma insulin levels to the incidence of myocardial infarction and coronary heart disease mortality in a middle-aged population. Diabetologia 1980; 19: 205–210.
93. Zavaroni I, Bonora E, Pagliara M, et al. Risk factors for coronary artery disease in healthy persons with hyperinsulinemia and normal glucose tolerance. N Engl J Med 1989; 320: 702–706.
94. Bigazzi R, Bianchi S, Baldari G, Campese VM. Clustering of cardiovascular risk factors in salt-sensitive patients with essential hypertension: role of insulin. Am J Hypertens 1996; 9: 24–32.
95. Cigolini M, Seidell JC, Targher G, et al. Fasting serum insulin in relation to components of the metabolic syndrome in european healthy men: the european fat distribution study. Metabolism 1995; 44: 35–40.
96. Stout RW. The impact of insulin upon atherosclerosis. Horm Metab Res 1994; 26: 125–128.
97. King GL, Goodman DA, Buzney S, et al. Receptors and growth-promoting effects of insulin and insulin like growth factors in cells from bovine retinal capillaries and aorta. J Clin Invest 1985; 75: 1028–1036.
98. Anderson EA, Balon TW, Hoffman RP, et al. Insulin increases sympathetic activity but not blood pressure in borderline hypertensive humans. Hypertension 1992; 19: 621–627.
99. Jeng JR, Sheu WHH, Jeng CY, et al. Impaired fibrinolysis and insulin resistance in patients with hypertension. Am. J. Hypertens 1996; 9: 484–490.
100. Connel JMC, Mc Lellan AR. Hypertension, insulin and atherogenesis. J Cardiovasc Pharmacol 1991; 18 (Suppl 2): 45–50.
101. Rocchini AP, Katch V, Kveselis D, et al. Insulin and renal sodium retention in obese adolescents. Hypertension 1989; 14: 367–374.
102. Landsberg L, Young JB. Insulin mediated glucose metabolism in the relationship between dietary intake and sympathetic nervous systemic activity. Int J Obesity 1985; 9 (Suppl 2): 63–68.
103. Rocchini AP, Moorehead C, De Runer S, et al. Hyperinsulinemia and the aldosterone and pressor response to angiotensin II. Hypertension 1990; 15: 861–866.
104. Trevisan R, Fioretto P, Semplicini A. Role of insulin and atrial natriuretic peptide in sodium ritention in insulin-treated IDDM patients during isotonic volume expansion. Diabetes 1990; 39: 289–298.
105. Berg K. New serum type system in man: the Lp system. Acta Pathol Scand 1963; 69: 369–382.

106. Rosengren A, Wilhelmsem L, Eriksson E, Risberg B, Wedel H. Lipoprotein(a) and coronary heart disease: a prospective case-control study in a general population sample of middle aged men. BMJ 1990; 301: 1248–1251.
107. Schaefer EJ, Lamon-Fava S, Jenner JL . Lipoprotein levels and risk of coronary heart disease in men: the lipid research clinics coronary primary prevention trial. JAMA 1994; 271: 999–1003;
108. Genest J, Jenner JL, McNamara JR et al. Prevalence of lipoprotein (a) [Lp(a)] excess in coronary artery disease. Am J Cardiol 1991; 67: 1039–1045.
109. Bailleul S, Conderc R, Rossignol C, et al. Lipoprotein (a) in childhood: relation with other atherosclerosis risk factor and family history of atherosclerosis. Clin Chem 1995; 41 (2): 241–245.
110. Watts GF, Mazurkiewicz JC, Tonge K, et al. Lipoprotein (a) as a determinant of the severity of angiographically defined carotid atherosclerosis. Q J Med 1995; 88: 321–326.
111. Brown G, Albers JJ, Fisher SM, Schaefer SM, Lin JT, Kaplan C, et al. Regression of coronary artery disease as a result of intensive lipid-lowering therapy in men with high levels of apolipoprotein B. N Engl J Med 1990; 323: 1289–1298.
112. Seed M, Hoppichler F, Reaveley D, et al. Relation of serum lipoprotein (a) phenotype to coronary heart disease in patients with familiar hypercholesterolemia. N Engl J Med 1990; 322: 1494–1499.
113. Gaubatz JW, Ghanem KI, Guevara J, et al. Polymorphic forms of human apolipoprotein (a): inheritance and relationship of their molecular weights to plasma levels of lipoprotein (a). J Lipid Res 1990; 31: 603–613.
114. Parlavecchia M, Pancaldi A, Taramelli R, et al. Evidence that Apolipoprotein (a) phenotype is a risk factor for coronary artery disease in men <55 years of age. Am J Cardiol 1994; 74: 346–351.
115. Scaglione R, Corrao S, Ganguzza A, et al. Lipoprotein (a) in obese subjects with central fat distribution: relationship with ambulatory blood pressure monitoring and left ventricular structure and function. Submitted to NMCD.
116. Mudd SH, Skovby F, Levy HL. The natural history of homocystinuria due to cystathionine ß-synthase deficiency. Am J Hum Genet 1985; 37: 1–31.
117. Mayer EL, Jacobsen DW, Robinson K. Homocysteine and coronary atherosclerosis. JACC 1996; 27(3): 517–527.
118. Wilcken DEL, Wilcken B. The pathogenesis of coronary artery disease. A possible role for methionine metabolism. J Clin Invest 1976; 57: 1079–1082.
119. Dudman NPB, Hicks C, Lynch JF, et al. Homocysteine thiolactone disposal by human arterial endothelial cells and serum in vitro. Arterioscler Thromb 1991; 11: 663–670.
120. Di Minno G, Davì G, Margaglione M, et al. Abnormally high thromboxane biosynthesis in homozygous homocystinuria. Evidence for platelet involvement and probucol-sensitive mechanism. J Clin Invest 1993; 92: 1400–1406.
121. Hilden M, Brandt NJ, Nilsson IM, et al. Investigation of coagulation and fibrinolysis in homocystinuria. Acta Med Scand 1974; 195: 533–535.
122. Ubink JB, Vermaak WJH, Becker PJ, et al. The prevalence of homocysteinemia and hypercholesterolemia in angiographically defined coronary heart disease. Klin Wochenschr 1991; 69: 527–534.
123. Glueck CJ, Shaw P, Lang J, et al. Evidence that homocysteine is an independent risk factor for atherosclerosis in hyperlipidemic patients. Am J Cardiol 1995; 75: 132–136.
124. Valleisen L, Bailey J, Epping Ph, et al. Epidemiological study on factor VII, factor VIII and fibrinogen in an industrial population. I. Baseline data on the relation to age, gender, body weight, smoking, alchool, pill-using and menopause. Thromb Haemost 1985; 54: 475–479.
125. ECAT Angina Pectoris Study Group. Baseline associations of haemostatic factors with extent of coronary arteriosclerosis and other coronary risk factors in 3000 patients with angina pectoris undergoing coronary angiography. Eur Heart J 1993; 14: 8–17.
126. Masuda T, Yasue H, Ogawa H, et al. Plasma plasminogen activator inhibitor activity and tissue plasminogen activator levels in patients with unstable angina and those with coronary spastic angina. Am Heart J 1992; 124: 314–319.
127. Licata G, Scaglione R, Avellone G, et al. Haemostatic function in young obese subjects with central obesity: relationship with left ventricular function. Metabolism 1995; 44, 11: 1417–1421.
128. Licata G, Corrao S, Parrinello G, et al. Obesità e malattie cardiovascolari. Relazione al 93° Congresso Nazionale della società Italiana di Medicina Interna, Firenze 17–21 Ottobre 1992.
129. Hollister AS, Inagami T. Atrial natriuretic factor and hypertension. A review and metaanalysis. Am J Hypertens 1991; 4: 850–865.
130. Volpe M, Tritto C, De Luca N, et al. Failure of atrial natriuretic factor to increase with saline load in patients with dilated cardiomyopathy and mild heart failure. J Clin Invest 1991; 88: 1481–1489.
131. Fricker J. Brain natriuretic peptide indicates post-MI outlook. Editorial the Lancet 1996; 347: 1753.

132. Yasue H, Morita E, Yoshimura M, et al. Increased plasma levels of brain natriuretic peptide in acute myocardial infarction [abstract]. Circulation 1991; 84 (Suppl II): 29.
133. Liuzzo G, Biasucci L, Gallimore R, et al. The prognostic value of C-reactive protein and serum amyloid A protein in severe unstable angina. N Engl J Med 1994;331:417–424.
134. Neri Serneri GG, Abbate R, Gori AM, et al. Transient intermittent lymphocyte activation is responsible for the instability of angina. Circulation 1992;86:790–797.
135. Muscari A, Bozzoli C, Puddu GM, et al. Association of serum C3 levels with the risk of myocardial infarction. Am J Med 1995;98:357–364.

15

CONGESTIVE HEART FAILURE IN THE ELDERLY

Franco Rengo,[1,2] Domenico Acanfora,[2] Luigi Trojano,[2] Giuseppe Furgi,[2] Costantino Picone,[2] S. Pollice,[1] and Gian Luca Iannuzzi[1]

[1]Institute of Internal Medicine
Cardiology and Cardiovascular Surgery
Department of Geriatry
"Federico II" University, School of Medicine
Naples, Italy
[2]"Salvatore Maugeri" Foundation
Institute of Care and Scientific Research
Rehabilitation Institute of Campoli del Monte Taburno
(BN) Italy

Congestive heart failure is the common end-point of several heart diseases and is a relevant issue in world health sanitary policy. Its incidence and mortality rate increases rapidly in the elderly (1,2). However, it is still unknown whether high incidence and mortality rate of congestive heart failure are due to the severity of heart diseases in the elderly or if they can be ascribed to the frequent association of several cardiac and extracardiac chronic diseases with age-associated changes in cardiovascular system and other systems.

Neither it is known which role aging processes exert upon prognosis of congestive heart failure. Some authors suggest that age is the main factor of reduced survival in patients with congestive heart failure (3,4), while others do not agree with this hypothesis (5).

EPIDEMIOLOGY

The main sources about epidemiology of congestive heart failure are Gibson et al. (6) and Framingham studies (7). According to both of them incidence and prevalence of congestive heart failure increase as age increases (6,7).

Since early observations by McKee and Kannel (7), incidence of congestive heart failure is only slightly decreased during the following 40 years (8), notwithstanding the development of new therapeutic agents in last decades. This observation is consistent with Yusuf's theory (9) according to which medical therapy, particularly antihypertensive drugs, cannot prevent congestive heart failure but can only delay its clinical manifestations. It is thus clear the relevance of congestive heart failure in the elderly: its annual incidence is 13 to 50/1000 in subjects aged 75–90 years, while it is 1.6/1000 in subjects aged 45–54 years (7).

Recent Advances in Geriatrics, edited by Barbagallo, Licata, and Sowers.
Plenum Press, New York, 1998.

Also the prevalence of congestive heart failure increases with age: it is reported to be about 3% in subjects aged 45–64 years, 6% in subjects aged 65–74 years, and 10% in subjects aged ≥75 years (10). However, a great variability exists in prevalence esteems: Klainer et al. (11) claim that diagnostic criteria may critically influence prevalence rates in different studies. If the diagnosis is based on first diagnosis in death certificates the prevalence of congestive heart failure appears to be low; if death certificates are examined by experienced cardiologists, or if the prevalence is calculated on diagnosis at the time of hospitalization, or if the diagnosis is made on the basis of autopsy reports, then prevalence of congestive heart failure is much higher. More accurate esteems can be obtained by examining medical prescriptions or by means of specific questionnaires compiled by physicians. However, the best methodology is the population-based survey: such studies report that the prevalence of congestive heart failure can be found between 0.5 and 13/1000. Even with this methodological approach, some variability is found. It may be attributed to width of population samples, to different demographic conditions, to different sources of information, but above all, to different diagnostic tools. For instance, Schocken et al. (10) made diagnosis of congestive heart failure on the basis of use of cardioactive glucosides, while Sutton (2) and Gibson et al. (6) considered the use of diuretics and digitalis. On the other hand, McKee et al. (7) (in the Framingham study), and, more recently, Schocken et al. (10) used a set of clinical criteria not yet validated. Harlan et al in Duke study (11) utilized for the diagnosis of congestive heart failure the presence of third tone and of a cardiothoracic ratio >0.48, and validated their criterion against left ventricular end-diastolic pressure in patients affected by coronary heart disease. More recently Carlson et al. (12) identified a clinical-radiographic score for the diagnosis of congestive heart failure and validated their criterion by measurement of wedge pulmonary pressure. Marantz et al. (13) verified the criteria of Framingham, Duke and Boston studies in relation to left ventricular ejection fraction at rest, evaluated by a radionuclide technique: sensitivity and specificity of the three sets of criteria appeared to be similar, but diagnosis of congestive heart failure was not correlated to left ventricular ejection fraction at rest, in agreement with other studies (14,15).

It appears clear that the most common diagnostic criteria have different drawbacks: some have not been validated, others have been validated only in superselected samples, others need very sophisticated instrumental tools. A new set of criteria, that is adequately validated on patients with different heart diseases and does not require instrumental techniques, has been recently proposed by our group. These criteria are purposes based only on clinical examination, medical history and current drug use. They have been developed and validated on a sample of 520 consecutive patients with heart disease of different etiology, aged 45 years or more. We selected 37 items from literature about clinical examination, medical history and drug use information. On the basis of the lack of empirical correlations with the criterion standard [clinical and radiological criteria - Battler's criteria (16)], 15 items were removed from the scale. Of the 22 remaining items, 15 showed higher intercorrelations and were included in the final form of the score.

The clinical-history form achieved adequate reliability: the score was significantly higher in patients with CHF according to Battler's criteria (Cronbach's alpha: no CHF=0.72; CHF=0.82) and progressively increased as NYHA class increased (Cronbach's alpha: class I-II NYHA=0.71; class III-IV NYHA=0.80). Sensitivity of clinical-history form for detecting CHF was 88.6%, the specificity 86.8% and the predictive accuracy 87%. The clinical-history form was significantly correlated with left ventricular ejection fraction (r=.42; p<0.0005) and peak oxygen consuption (r=.69; p<0.0001). Test-retest examination on 250 patients showed no statistical difference.

The clinical-history form may represent a useful instrument for the diagnosis of CHF, suitable for clinical and epidemiological purposes (17).

Recently we have applied this clinical-history form in an Italian Cooperative Study on Congestive Heart Failure in elderly hospitalized patients with heart disease (CHF Italian Study). The prevalence of CHF in our 1.320 study sample was 49.3% in patients aged 65 to 74 years and 66.3% in patients aged 75 years or more. CHF was most frequent in the males patients aged 65 to 74 years (male=50.4%; female=47.7%), while in the older patients the prevalence of CHF was similar in both sex (male=67.4%; female=65.3%) (18). The age-related increases of prevalence of CHF, evaluated via clinical-history form, was also confirmed in our population based study on 1.339 non-istituzionalized subjects (Osservatorio Geriatrico della Campania) (19).

ETIOLOGY

Hypertension and coronary heart disease are reported to be the most frequent causes of heart failure in the Framingham Study (7,20). Seventy-five percent of patients affected by hypertension develop congestive heart failure, while ischemic cardiopathy not associated with hypertension precedes congestive heart failure only in 10% of patients. In the same study, valvulopathies increase risk for congestive heart failure only when associated to hypertension (7). However, these data showing a critical role of hypertension, might not be still valid because in recent years new preventive and therapeutic measures have dramatically modified natural history of heart diseases, particularly in elderly patients.

In the Italian CHF Study I (18) hypertensive cardiopathy (40.1%) and ischemic heart disease (37.8%) were the most frequent heart diseases, but they appear to have different roles in the development of congestive heart failure: the risk associated to hypertensive cardiopathy is very low (+2%; RR=1.02, CI 95%: 0.92–1.12; P=NS). In this study, 19.6% of patients presented an association of two or more heart diseases, which are closely correlated with age and congestive heart failure. This observation suggests that multiple etiology of heart diseases increases the risk for the development of congestive heart failure in elderly patients. It is worth mentioning that the association of other chronic extra-cardiac diseases may influence the mechanisms of compensation in the elderly (18).

PATHOPHYSIOLOGY

Congestive heart failure, defined as that condition in which abnormal heart function does not assure sufficient blood delivery to satisfy metabolic requirements of organs and systems, is frequently due to a defect in myocardial contraction. The inability to keep an optimal perfusion of body tissues induces a series of peripheric changes which represent possible mechanisms of compensation but which can also hamper blood circulation.

The possible mechanisms of compensation include some hemodynamic changes (e.g. heart rate variations, changes in ventricular volumes), but also complex biochemical and hormonal modulations.

Changes of Cardiovascular Structures and Function during Congestive Heart Failure and Aging

The study of pathophysiology of congestive heart failure has to take into account the relationships between congestive heart failure and aging. Generally, congestive heart failure is considered to depend on loss of myocardial tissue, reduction of myocardial contractility, pressure and volume overload or restrictive myocardial diseases. The most frequent cause of congestive heart failure secondary to loss of myocardial tissue is coronary heart disease; acute myocardial infarction provokes brisk loss of contractile tissue. On the other hand, a chronic progressive loss of myocites (about 25 million per year) has been demonstrated in the aging heart (21).

Several factors affect myocardial contractility: loss of muscular fibers, intrinsic depression, circulating catecholamines, autonomic nervous function, anoxia, hypercapnia, acidosis. An impairment of contractility determines a reduction of left ventricular ejection fraction; for instance, in primitive dilatative cardiomyopathy the left ventricular ejection fraction is reduced even at rest.

In aging, left ventricular ejection fraction at rest is not reduced, while it decreases during physical activity, because of the inability of aged myocardium in modulating its contractility (22).

During pathological conditions the reduction of left ventricular ejection fraction is associated with volume overload. This change has the aim of keeping sufficient the cardiac output. Telediastolic and telesystolic volumes at rest are similar in young and elderly individuals. However, relevant differences between young and elderly subjects are found during physical activity. In the elderly, physical stress induces smaller changes in heart beat than in young people, while telesystolic volume does not reduce (22); cardiac output is kept adequate mainly by an increased telediastolic volume via Frank-Starling mechanism. These adaptive changes in aged heart are probably related to: i) an intrinsic impairment of the excitation-contraction mechanism, but also to a reduction of beta-adrenergic modulation of this mechanism itself; ii) an age-dependent increase of aortic impedance (and consequently of after-load), due to a reduced beta-adrenergic modulation of vascular smooth musculature and to stuctural changes of aorta and large vessel (23).

The increase of left ventricular volumes and the reduction of aortic compliance generally determines an increase of systemic arterial pressure (Table 1). This pressure overload is a mechanical signal of activation for myocardial cells (membrane stretch), which

Table 1. Age-related changes of hemodynamic parameters in patients with congestive heart failure (III-IV NYHA class)

	<65 years n=25	≥65 years n=18	p
Age (years)	44 ± 9	69 ± 3	<.001
Left ventricular ejection fraction (%)	21.5 ± 5.6	31 ± 6.1	<.001
Heart rate (bpm)	78 ± 14	74 ± 15	NS
Systolic blood pressure (mmHg)	131 ± 17	147 ± 16	<.005
Diastolic blood pressure (mmHg)	80 ± 12	81 ± 13	NS
Mean blood pressure (mmHg)	97 ± 13	102 ± 12	NS
Mean right atrial pressure (mmHg)	5.3 ± 2.8	9.6 ± 3.3	<.001
Mean pulmonary pressure (mmHg)	28 ± 11	29 ± 9	NS
Mean wedge pressure (mmHg)	20.4 ± 4.7	25.2 ± 4.5	<.005
Cardiac index (L/min/m2)	2.8 ± 0.7	2.1 ± 0.6	<.005
Total pulmonary resistances (dyne · cm · sec^{-2})	427 ± 260	465 ± 256	NS
Vascular pulmonary resistances (dyne · cm · sec^{-2})	213 ± 140	236 ± 178	NS
Systemic vascular resistances (dyne · cm · sec^{-2})	3209 ± 781	3699 ± 784	<.05

may induce cellular hypertrophy, through activation of cationic channels and the consequent activation of phosphorilating mechanisms. In left ventricular hypertrophy the number of nuclei per myocite is reduced while their volume increases. In elderly people Olivetti et al (24) have demonstrated that the number of myocites is reduced and their volume increases in the physiological aging process. Loss of cells and enlargement of the remaining myocites may represent the structural basis for the reduced compensatory capacity in the aging heart and at the same time may contribute to the development of myocardial dysfunction and failure in the elderly (24).

Hypertrophy provokes continous re-modeling of myocardium and a consequent diastolic stiffness which, together with relaxation alterations caused by reduced calcium reuptake, determine diastolic dysfunction.

During congestive heart failure, left ventricular compliance decreases and it is possible to observe both ventricular asinergy and stiffness. Age-dependent alterations of diastolic features of left ventricle have been demonstrated (25,26). Moreover, a high percentage of elderly patients with congestive heart failure shows a preserved systolic function.

Age- and Congestive Heart Failure-Related Changes of Autonomic Nervous System

Congestive heart failure is associated with complex neuro-humoral and autonomic modifications. The increase in sympathetic activity appears the most important compensatory mechanism to maintain cardiac output. From the standpoint of the regulation of receptor-mediated contractility, human ventricular myocardium is a "β-adrenergic organ". Ventricular myocardium relies on β-adrenergic stimulation to augment contractility. Human ventricular myocardium contains β_1 and β_2-adrenergic receptors with a relatively high proportion of subtype β_2-receptors that are coupled to adenylate cyclase and muscle contraction. These heterogeneity in β receptor subtypes is not entirely clear, the presence of two structurally and genetically distinct subtypes provides the human heart with two β-adrenergic receptors that exhibit differences in pharmacological specificity and regulatory behavior.

In human ventricular myocardium, α_1-receptor density is extremely low, α_1-stimulation of the second-messenger inosytol triphosphate is only marginal, and α_1-mediated positive inotropic effects are inconsistently obtained in isolated tissue preparations. In heart failure, α_1-receptor density is unchanged or slightly increased, suggesting that the α_1-adrenergic pathway has no compensatory role in supporting cardiac function in the failing human heart. The unchanged α_1-receptor population seems to play a role in the stimulation of cardiac hypertrophy.

Congestive heart failure exerts major effects on β-receptor-G protein-adenylate cyclase complex. Ventricular myocardial β_1-receptors downregulate in direct relation to the severity of ventricular dysfunction, while β_2-receptor density in myocitic membrane does not change. The selective loss of subtype of β_1-receptor leads to a marked decrease in the contractility. On the other hand, the still normal density of β_2-receptors does not ensure their normal function: selective stimulation of β_2-receptor obtained from failing hearts determines a lower adenylate cyclase stimulation, likely due to G-protein alterations (uncoupling of β_2-receptors).

The adrenergic activation increases with severity of ventricular dysfunction. Coronary sinus plasma concentration of norepinephrine increases in patients with severe left ventricular failure, notwithstanding the reduction of β_1-receptor density. Chronic high levels of cathecolamines may have a toxic effect and loose any compensatory activity.

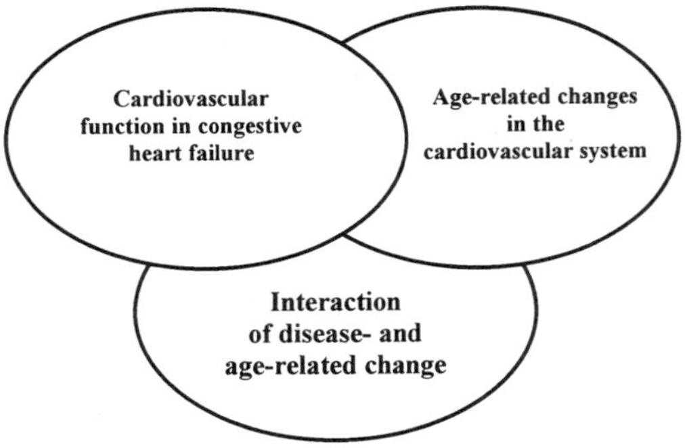

Figure 1. Age-dependent and disease-related changes in the cardiovascular system.

Age-dependent changes in the cardiovascular system are difficult to delineate because of the confounding effects of disease-related changes (Figure 1). The autonomic nervous system changes in the elderly are very difficult to interpret because most of the available data have been derived from animal studies. However, some well-established effects of age and congestive heart failure on autonomic nervous system changes are summarized in Table 2.

The parasympatethic activity is reduced during both physiological aging and congestive heart failure. This change has been demonstrated by baroreflex sensitivity assays and by heart rate variability studies in the time and the frequency domains. Further light on this matter has been shed by a recently-developed visual approach to the study of heart rate variability (Poincarè Plots) (27). By quantifying the Poincarè Plots, we have obtained several objective measures of heart rate variability based on non-linear analysis of RR intervals (28). Such parameters, together with data about heart rate variability in the time and the frequency domains, have been evaluated in a study on a population of 100 patients with heart disease, with or without congestive heart failure. These data show that both congestive heart failure and aging affect heart rate variability. However, further studies are needed to better characterize the autonomic nervous system changes during congestive heart failure and aging.

Role of Neurohormonal Mechanisms during Congestive Heart Failure and Aging

Adrenergic stimulation during congestive heart failure modulates activation of other neurohormonal mechanisms, which in turn determine haemodynamic variations. It is well

Table 2. Effects of age and congestive heart failure (CHF) on autonomic nervous system changes

	CHF changes		Age-related changes
↑	Plasma norepinephryne concentration at rest	↑	Plasma norepinephryne concentration at rest
↓	Plasma norepinephryne concentration at peak exercise	↑	Plasma norepinephryne concentration at peak exercise
↓	Cardiac norepinephryne stores	↓	Cardiac norepinephryne stores
↓	Regulation of β_1-receptors	↓	Affinity of β_1-receptors
	Uncoupling of β_2-receptors		
↓	Inotropic and chronotropic response to β-agonists	↓	Inotropic and chronotropic response to β-agonists
↓	Baroreflex sensitivity	↓	Baroreflex sensitivity

known that plasma renin activity is increased in patients with congestive heart failure; the kidney is the likely source of most of this proteolytic enzyme, but the blood vessels may also contribute to its plasma levels. The β-adrenergic stimulation is among major mechanisms responsible for renin release; the final product of the renin-angiotensin system is angiotensin II, a potent direct arteriolar constrictor which may further facilitate the release of norepinephrine from terminal sympathetic nerve endings. Additionally, angiotensin II acts on the adrenal cortex to release aldosterone, a potent salt- and water-retaining hormone. Aldosterone also has a potent kaliuretic effect, thereby contributing to hypokaliemia and setting the stage for ventricular arrhythmias.

Plasma renin activity declines with age in normal subjects; this phenomenon is associated with a fall in aldosterone plasma concentration. Cleland et al. (29) demonstrated that in middle-aged and elderly patients with congestive heart failure resting renin and angiotensin II were similar and rose on standing with a further increase during exercise. However, aldosterone rose during exercise only in younger patients, while increments in plasma noradrenaline were greater in the elderly. These observations suggest that the angiotensin converting enzyme inhibitors may be useful also in elderly patients with congestive heart failure. Although plasma renin activity reduces with age, Duggan et al. (30) demonstrated that platelet angiotensin II receptors density increases with age and receptor affinity does not change.

The antidiuretic hormone is an important and powerful endogenous vasoconstrictor and increases during heart failure. Angiotensin II is known to increase concentration of antidiuretic hormone, but the stimuli that raise antidiuretic hormone levels during heart failure are not well known. In general, levels of antidiuretic hormone increase about twice in patients with congestive heart failure, but there are many patients with normal levels. Mild increases in vasopressin levels do increase vascular resistance and lower cardiac output in patients with congestive heart failure; actually, antidiuretic hormone vascular antagonists can improve cardiac output when given to patients with increased basal level of antidiuretic hormone. Nonpressor increments of antidiuretic hormone may potentiate the vasoconstriction due to angiotensin II and norepinephrine.

Some factors can inhibit plasma renin activity in congestive heart failure. Digoxin administration in never treated patients with congestive heart failure reduces plasma renin activity and aldosterone concentration of about 50%.

The most important suppressor of renin and aldosterone release is the atrial natriuretic factor; this is a hormone produced by mammalian atria in response to atrial distension, increased extracellular sodium or tachycardia. The atrial natriuretic factor has a wide range of potent biological effects including natriuresis, vasodilatation, and inhibition of renin and aldosterone secretion, and plays an important role in the homeostasis of body fluids and blood pressure. Burnett et al. (31) demonstrated that plasma concentration of the atrial natriuretic factor increases during congestive heart failure when right atrial pressure is elevated. Recent investigations have shown the existence of a family of structurally related peptides, atrial (ANP), brain (BNP) and C-type (CNP) natriuretic peptides. All of them reduce cardiac preload, but only ANP and BNP have a natriuretic effect. ANP and BNP have been localized to the heart, while recent studies failed to detect CNP messenger RNA in the human myocardium; small CNP concentrations have been found in endothelial cells, consistent with a paracrine role for CNP in the control of the vascular tone.

During congestive heart failure plasma concentration of ANP are significantly increased secondary to enhanced atrial and ventricular synthesis and decreased ANP clearance in liver and kidneys; circulating BNP is also increased as a result of enhanced cardiac production. Several studies support a functional role for these hormones in cardio-renal regulation in congestive heart failure. The circulating and cardiac tissue concentration of CNP remains undefined.

Naruse et al. (32) demonstrated a significant age-dependent increase of plasma concentration of ANP and BNP in healthy subjects, while CNP plasma levels were similar in young and elderly normal controls and in patients with congestive heart failure but raise in patients with cor pulmonale compared with age-matched controls (33).

Increased ANP plasma levels in elderly patients without congestive heart failure is a very strong marker for subsequent development of this syndrome (34). Recently, we have confirmed high ANP plasma levels in healthy elderly subjects but we have also demonstrated reduced natriuresis after ANP administration. This finding suggested an ANP-resistance in elderly subjects (35), a phenomenon detected also in middle-aged patients with primitive cardiomyopathy (36).

CLINICAL MANIFESTATIONS OF CONGESTIVE HEART FAILURE

Diagnosis of congestive heart failure is made upon clinical history, physical examination and chest X-ray findings. In many elderly patients, clinical manifestations of congestive heart failure are often altered, distorted or overshadowed by other symptoms. The presenting symptoms may not be clearly expressed by patients with confusional states, uremia, or pre-existing dementia. Pulmonary rales and peripheral edema are not specific for congestive heart failure in the elderly, while elevated jugular venous pressure and positive hepatojugular reflux are excellent confirming signs of congestive heart failure. Left ventricular fourth sound is a normal finding in the elderly, but third heart sound correlates well with elevated left ventricular diastolic pressure.

As stated above, congestive heart failure may be associated with a relatively spared left systolic function in the elderly (15,37). Actually, data from CHF Italian study I showed that an increased cardio-thoracic ratio on chest X-ray (>0.50) is present in 40.8% of the total study sample and only in 69% of patients with congestive heart failure; however, this finding is significantly associated with congestive heart failure [OR=1.72 (1.47–2.00); χ^2=48.2; p<0.0001].

On the other hand, it is worth remembering that a number of precipitants can contribute to development and to dramatic evolution of congestive heart failure, particularly in elderly patients (Table 3).

SPECIFIC FEATURES OF ELDERLY PATIENTS

Many cardiovascular changes during chronic congestive heart failure in middle-aged patients are similar to those observed in physiological aging. This observation implies that the development of congestive heart failure in advanced age has a "multiplicative", and not only additional, effect on clinical manifestations. The congestive heart failure is indeed a very dangerous syndrome in the elderly.

Moreover, it must be remembered that the aging process involves not only the cardiovascular system but also many other systems and organs; for this reason, the elderly patient often presents comorbidity, atypical clinical presentations, higher risks for loss of autonomy and iatrogenic diseases.

Recently, Hughes et al. (38) compiled an aging-related meta-analysis of V-HeFT I and II studies. Hughes et al. (38) found that congestive heart failure is associated with more severe functional impairment in elderly patients (VO_2 max 13.6 mL · min^{-1} · Kg^{-1} in

Table 3. Common precipitants of heart failure in the elderly

Cardiovascular factors	Extra-cardiac factors
• Myocardial ischemia or infarction	• Dietary sodium excess
• Uncontrolled hypertension	• Excess fluid intake
• Atrial fibrillation or flutter	• Nonadherence to medications
• Ventricular arrhythmias	• Fever
• Bradiarrhythmias	• Infections
Drugs	• Hyperthyroidism
• Alcohol	• Anemia
• β-blockers	• Renal failure
• Calcium antagonists	• Acute or chronic lung diseases
• Anti-arrhythmic agents	
• Nonsteroidal anti-inflammatory agents	
• Corticosteroids	

patients aged ≥65 years versus 14.3 mL · min^{-1} · Kg^{-1} in patients aged <65 years), longer disease duration (3.8 years versus 3.1 years), and more frequent edema (19% versus 13%), although left ventricular ejection fraction was better in elderly patients (31% versus 29%). We observed similar findings in 142 consecutive patients with mild to moderate congestive heart failure (Table 4). Hughes et al. and our data suggested that although elderly patients seem to be "sicker" (i.e. they show longer disease duration and more frequent edema), the more severe clinical manifestations of congestive heart failure can be likely ascribed to different pathophysiological mechanisms. Actually, in elderly patients left ventricular systolic function is relatively preserved; this observation is in agreement also with epidemiological data showing an age-dependent diastolic dysfunction (4,15,125). On the other hand, it is well known that the physiological aging process determines an alteration of left ventricular diastolic function which can precipitate functional impairment in presence of heart disease.

We have recently completed a multi-centric cooperative study in elderly hospitalized patients with heart disease. We evaluated the prevalence and the ethiology of heart failure

Table 4. Ergometric findings in 142 patients with congestive heart failure classified according to the NYHA class and age

	II NYHA			III NYHA		
	<65 years n=37	≥65 years n=45	p	<65 years n=40	≥65 years n=20	p
Age (years)	46 ± 12	68 ± 3	<.001	51 ± 7	66 ± 1	<.001
Weight (Kg)	75.8 ± 13.4	69.2 ± 17.5	NS	77.5 ± 10	72.6 ± 2.4	NS
LVEF (%)	23.5 ± 6.6	31.7 ± 7.2	<.001	18.3 ± 5.4	28.4 ± 5	<.001
MWL (Watts)	103 ± 31	89 ± 20	NS	83 ± 22	76 ± 8	NS
Rest HR (bpm)	85 ± 17	74 ± 10	<.001	86 ± 22	76 ± 8	<.001
Peak HR (bpm)	146 ± 20	119 ± 21	<.001	134 ± 26	111 ± 12	<.001
Rest SBP (mmHg)	114 ± 16	121 ± 12	<.05	110 ± 12	122 ± 21	<.05
Peak SBP (mmHg)	154 ± 27	164 ± 15	NS	139 ± 20	168 ± 12	<.001
Rest VO_2 (ml/min)	394 ± 95	367 ± 96	<.001	350 ± 100	396 ± 76	NS
Peak VO_2 (ml/min)	1434 ± 547	1198 ± 306	<.05	1046 ± 239	730 ± 49	<.001
Peak VO_2 (ml/min/Kg)	19.1 ± 5.5	16.6 ± 4.2	<.05	13.5 ± 3	10.1 ± 1	<.001
Peak VE (L/min)	55.9 ± 16.4	45.8 ± 12.1	<.005	50.7 ± 14	41.6 ± 5.4	<.01

LVEF=Left ventricular ejection fraction; MWL=Maximal work-load; HR=Heart rate; SBP=Systolic blood pressure; VO_2=O_2 consumption; VE=Ventilation.

in a sample of consecutive elderly patients enrolled from April 4, 1992 to June 30, 1992 and from November 8, 1992 to February 28, 1993. We studied 1319 patients (643 male, 676 female; mean age 77±7 yrs), 581 of whom aged 65 to 74 yrs. (322 male, 259 female), 738 aged more than 75 yrs. (321 male, 417 female). In our sample, 25.6% patients were classified in Class I NYHA, 40.5% in Class II, 24.4% in Class III, and 9.6% in Class IV. Diagnosis of congestive heart failure was made by means of a clinical-history score, when patients' score was ≥4 (17). Congestive heart failure has been identified in 633 patients (58.6%) (312 male, 321 female). The prevalence of congestive heart failure increased significantly with age (65–74 yrs.: 37.9%; ≥75 yrs.: 62.1%; χ^2=33.4; p<0.0001), while it was not affected by sex. Table 5 shows the ethiology and risk ratios adjusted by age-group for congestive heart failure.

Valvular heart disease, cor pulmonare and primary cardiomiopathy increase significantly the risk for congestive heart failure in elderly patients, while hypertensive cardiomiopathy and coronary heart disease do not.

Comorbidity and Congestive Heart Failure. Data from CHF Italian Study I show a direct relationship between age and number of chronic conditions associated with heart disease. Furthermore, the presence and the number of extra-cardiac chronic diseases modify risk profile of congestive heart failure in elderly patients. The risk-ratios for congestive heart failure demostrated that any not-reversible condition (diabetes; hepatic, respiratory and artero-venous diseases) exerts a detrimental effect on clinical picture. Cerebrovascular diseases do not emerge as a strong risk factor, likely because they most often determine severe loss of autonomy, and limitation of physical activity, preserving residual cardiac reserve, and thus avoiding manifestation of clinical signs and symptoms of congestive heart failure.

Quality of Life and Congestive Heart Failure. Comorbidity and congestive heart failure accelerate loss of autonomy in elderly patients. The Italian Cooperative Study Group on heart failure in elderly patients analyzed some psycho-social variables to better characterize patients' sample. The case report-form collected information about educational level, type of job, marital status, familiar environment and free-time activities of patients. Moreover, the study included some standardized scales to evaluate autonomy, mood, and general cognitive abilities. In our patients illiteracy and prevalence of residence in an institution increased significantly with age. Furthermore, standardized scales showed a significant reduction of personal autonomy: at ADL the percentage of dependent subjects increased from 31.6% to 62.7% (χ^2=119; p<.0001); at IADL it reduced from 10.5±4 to 7±4.5 (F=196; p<.0001). In the oldest group of patients higher percentages of cognitive

Table 5. Age-adjusted risk ratios (OR_{MH}) and confidence intervals at 95% (CI 95%) for congestive heart failure in 1320 consecutive elderly patients in relation to the etiology of heart disease (CHF Italian study)

	Prevalence (%)	OR_{MH}	CI 95%	χ^2	p
Hypertensive heart disease	34.9	1.08	0.80–1.47	0.21	NS
Coronary heart disease	32.3	0.75	0.55–1.02	3.29	NS
Valvular heart disease	10.9	2.78	1.61–4.71	15.2	<.0001
Cor pulmonare	6.40	15.4	4.69–64.4	34.1	<.0001
Primitive cardiomyopathy	2.60	6.52	1.69–26.0	9.25	<.005

Table 6. Age-adjusted risk ratios (OR_{MH}) and confidence intervals at 95% (CI 95%) for congestive heart failure in 1320 consecutive elderly patients in relation to some psychosocial variables (CHF Italian study)

	OR_{MH}	CI 95%	χ^2	p
Illiteracy	2.13	1.46–2.94	23.65	<.0001
Social dependence (IADL)	2.03	1.46–2.82	18.96	<.0001
Physical dependence (ADL)	2.10	1.59–2.77	29.42	<.0001
Depression (GDS)	2.02	1.33–3.05	14.42	<.001
Cognitive impairment (MMS)	1.66	1.22–2.25	10.76	<.005

impairment (low scores at MMSE) and depression (measured by GDS) were detected. The risk ratio of developing heart failure associated to each of these psycho-social variables was calculated stratifying by age-group and sex. Our analysis showed that some conditions determine a significant increase of risk for heart failure, so that their presence deserves special attention in elderly patients affected by CHF (Table 6).

PROGNOSIS

Congestive heart failure is a clinical condition associated with a poor prognosis. Many studies report that mortality-rate becomes higher when surgically-correctable mechanical alterations are not present [male=82%, (RR=4.0); female=67%, (RR=5.8)]. Mortality is 4 to 8 times greater of age-matched based population. Many patients with CHF died suddenly (8,20).

To determine which of the many clinical parameters routinely collected influence mortality in patients with low left ventricular ejection fraction (less than 45% at radionuclide ventriculography), 128 elderly patients (mean age 79±3 years) with various heart diseases were followed-up for 3 years. Twenty-eight percent had coronary heart disease, 16% hypertensive heart disease, 7% valvular heart disease. The remaining 62 patients (48%) made up a group comprising patients with primitive cardiomyopathy, cor pulmonare with no evidence of coronary heart disease, valvular disease or hypertensive heart disease. Thirty-four percent of all patients were classified as having congestive heart failure. Thirty-seven clinical variables were analyzed using a Cox proportional model. Forty-four patients died, 36 (82%) of sudden cardiac death. Ten characteristics at study entry predicted an increased mortality risk: S_3 gallop [Hazard Ratio=1.80 (1.33–2.46); p<.0001], number of clinical signs ≥3 [Hazard Ratio=1.44 (1.18–1.76); p<.0001], left ventricular ejection fraction ≤25% [Hazard Ratio=1.34 (1.14–1.58); p<.0001], New York Heart Association functional class ≥III [Hazard Ratio=1.32 (1.12–1.57); p<.0001], dyspnea [Hazard Ratio=1.32 (1.16–1.50); p<.0001], digoxin treatment [Hazard Ratio=1.32 (1.08–1.46); p<.0001], rales [Hazard Ratio=1.31 (1.11–1.54); p<.002], number of symptoms ≥4 [Hazard Ratio=1.27 (1.09–1.47); p<.002], asthenia [Hazard Ratio=1.27 (1.09–1.47); p<.002], associated pulmonary disease [Hazard Ratio=1.22 (1.06–1.40); p<.01]. Long-term survival of very elderly patients with low ejection fraction is related to the functional capacity, the severity of symptoms and the number of clinical signs. Moreover a LVEF ≤25% selects a subgroup of patients at higher risk. Our results suggest that these variables may influence the long-term survival of elderly patients with heart disease. Further studies with a greater number of patients are necessary to better delineate the prognostic value of the clinical and instrumental variables routinely collected in these patients (39).

Also in-hospital mortality is higher in elderly patients with CHF. Data from CHF Italian Study demonstrated a 22.7% total mortality rate without any diffecences between age-groups (65–74 years=23.8%, ≥75 years=21.9%; χ^2=0.68, p=NS). The most frequent clinical condition associated with death is the CHF (26.4%) with an age-related increment (65–74 years=14.5%, ≥75 years=36.4%; χ^2=15.85, p<0.0001).

THERAPEUTIC CONSIDERATIONS AND CONCLUSIONS

No specific drugs exist for the pharmacologic treatment of heart failure in the elderly, so that the geriatric specificity in the treatment of heart failure can be recognized in the art of drug choice and dosage, to obtain the best results with the least side effects.

Association of multiple heart diseases, comorbidity, loss of autonomy, and cognitive impairment call for a multidimensional approach to elderly patients with heart disease and in particular with congestive heart failure. The multidimensional approach and the continuative intervention have indeed been proved to be effective in improving survival and quality of life in elderly patients with chronic illnesses (40,41).

The increased prevalence, incidence and mortality rate of congestive heart failure in the elderly suggest that age-related changes in the cardiovascular system are important determinants of congestive heart failure. However, other major factors, such as comorbidity, loss of autonomy, and cognitive impairment, can contribute to development and to dramatic evolution of the syndrome.

Further studies on disease- and age-related changes are necessary to develop new and more potent strategies to secure "*successful aging*".

REFERENCES

1. Ghali, J.K., Cooper, R., Ford, E. (1990): Trends in hospitalization rates for heart failure in United States, 1973–1986: Evidence for increasing population evidence. Arch Int Med, 150, 769–773.
2. Sutton, G.C. (1990): Epidemiologic aspects of heart failure. Am Heart J, 120, 1538–1540.
3. Willens, H.J., Blevins, R.D., Wrisley, D., Antionishen, D., Reinstein, D., Rubenfire, M. (1987): The prognostic value of functional capacity in patients with mild to moderate heart failure. Am Heart J, 114, 377–382.
4. Judge, K., Pawitan, Y., Caldwell, J., Gersh, B.J., Kennedy, J.W. (1991): Congestive heart failure in patients with preserved left ventricular systolic function. Analysis of the CASS registry. J Am Coll Cardiol, 18, 377–382.
5. Likoff, M., Chandler, S., Kay, H. (1987): Clinical determinants of mortality in chronic congestive heart failure secondary to idiopathic or to ischemic cardiomiopathy. Am J Cardiol, 59, 634–638.
6. Gibson, T.C., White, K.L., Klainer, L.M. (1966): The prevalence of congestive heart failure in two rural comunities. J Chronic Dis, 19, 141–152.
7. McKee, P.A., Castelli, W.P., McNamara, P.M., Kannel, W.B. (1971): The natural history of congestive heart failure: The Framingham Study. N Engl J Med, 285, 1441–1446.
8. Ho, K.K.L., Pinsky, J.L., Kannel, W., Levy, D. (1993): The epidemiology of heart failure: The Framingham Study. J Am Coll Cardiol, 22(Supplement A), 6–13.
9. Yusuf, S., Thom, T., Abbott, R.D. (1989): Changes in hypertension treatment and in congestive heart failure mortality in the United States. Hypertension, 13, 174–179.
10. Schocken, D.D., Arrieta, M.I., Leaverton, P.E., Ross, E.A. (1992): Prevalence and mortality rate of congestive heart failure in the United States. J Am Coll Cardiol, 20, 301–306.
11. Harlan, W.R., Oberman, A., Grimm, R., Rosati, R.A. (1977): Chronic congestive heart failure in coronary artery disease: Clinical criteria. Ann Inter Med, 86, 133–138.
12. Carlson, K.J., Lee, D.C.S., Goroll, A.H., Leahy, M., Johnson, R.A. (1985): An analysis of physicians' reasons for prescribing long-term digitalis therapy in outpatients. J Chron Dis, 38, 733–739.

13. Marantz, P.R., Tobin, J.N., Wassertheil-Smoller, S., Steingart, R.M., Wexler, J.P., Budner, N., Lense, L., Wachpress, J. (1988): The relationship between left ventricular systolic function and congestive heart failure diagnosed by clinical criteria. Circulation, 77, 607–612.
14. Franciosa, J.A., Park, M., Levine, T.B. (1981): Lack of correlation between exercise capacity and indexes of resting left ventriucular performance in heart failure. Am J Cardiol, 47, 33–39.
15. Dougherty, A.H., Naccarelli, G.V., Gray, E.L., Hicks, C.H., Goldstein, R.A. (1984): Congestive heart failure with normal systolic function. Am J Cardiol, 54, 778–782.
16. Battler, A., Karliner, J.S., Higgins, C.B., Slutsky, R., Gilpin, E.A., Froelicher, V.F., Ross, J. Jr. (1980): The initial chest X-ray in acute myocardial infarction. Prediction of early and late mortality and survival. Circulation, 61, 1004–1009.
17. Acanfora, D., Trojano, L., Maggi, S., Harris T., Furgi, G., Rossi, M., Papa, A., Iannuzzi, G.L., Picone C., Regno C., Rengo, F. (1996). Development and Validation of a Clinical-History Form for the Diagnosis of Congestive Heart Failure. J Heart Failure, 3,18.
18. Rengo, F., Acanfora, D. (1994): Lo scompenso cardiaco nell'anziano. G Ital Cardiol, 24, 1423–1434.
19. Cacciatore F., Abete P., Paolisso G., Amato L., Canonico S., Maggi S., Varricchio M., Franco R., for the Osservatorio Geriatrico Campano Group. (1997): The role of blood pressure in cognitive impairment in an elderly population. J Hyperten, 15, 135–142.
20. Ho, K.K.L., Anderson, K.M., Kannel, W.B., Grossman, W.B., Levy, D. (1993): Survival after the onset of congestive heart failure in Framingham heart study subjects. Circulation, 88, 107–115.
21. Olivetti, G., Melissari, M., Capasso, J.M., Anversa, P. (1991): Myocite loss and reactive cellular hypertrophy. Circulation Research, 68, 1560–1568.
22. Rodeheffer, R.J., Gerstenblith, G., Becker, L.C., Fleg, J.L., Weisfeldt, M.L., Lakatta, E.G. (1984): Exercise cardiac output is maintained with advancing age in healthy human subjects: cardiac dilatation and increased stroke volume compensate for a diminished heart rate. Circulation, 69(No 2), 203–213.
23. Katz, A.M. (1990): Cardiomiopathy of overload. N Engl J Med 0, 322(No2), 100–110.
24. Olivetti, G., Melissari, M., Balbi, T., Quaini, F., Sonnelblick, E.H., Anversa, P. (1994): Myocyte nuclear and possible cellular hyperplasia contribute to ventricular remodeling to the hypertrophic senescent heart in humans. J Am Coll Cardiol, 24, 140–149.
25. Nicolino, A., Ferrara, N., Longobardi, G., Acanfora, D., Rengo, C., Rengo, F. (1993): Left ventricular diastolic filling in elderly hypertensive patients. J Am Geriatr Soc, 41, 217–222.
26. Bonow, R.O., Vitale, D.F., Bacharach, S.L., Maron, B.J., Green, M.V. (1988): Effects of aging on asyncronous left ventricular regional function and global ventricular filling in normal human subjects. J Am Coll Cardiol, 11, 50–58.
27. Woo, M.A., Stevenson, W.G., Moser, D.K., Trelase, R.B., Harper, R.M. (1992): Patterns of beat-to-beat heart rate variability in advanced heart failure. Am Heart J, 123, 704–710.
28. Marciano, F., Migaux, M.L., Acanfora, D., Furgi, G., Rengo, F. (1994): Quantification of Poincarè maps for the evaluation of heart rate variability. Computers in Cardiology, 577–580.
29. Clealand, J.G.F., Dargie, H.J., Robertson, J.I.S., Ball, S.G., Hodsman, G.P. (1984): Renin and angiotensin responses to posture and exercise in elderly patients with heart failure. Eur Heart J, 5(Suppl E), 9–11.
30. Duggan, J., Kilfeather, S., O'Brien, E., O'Malley, K., Nussberger, J. (1992): Effects of aging and hypertension on plasma angiotensin II and platelet angiotensin II receptor density. Am J Hypertens, 5, 687–693.
31. Burnett, J.C. Jr., Granger, J.P., Opgenorth, T.J. (1984): Effects of synthetic atrial natriuretic factor on renal function and renin release. Am J Physiol, 247, 863–866.
32. Naruse, M., Takeyama, Y., Tanabe, A., Hiroshige, J., Naruse, K., Yoshimoto, T., Tanaka, M., Katagiri, T., Demura, H. (1994): Atrial and brain natriuretic peptides in cardiovascular diesases. Hypertension, 23(Suppl. I), 231–234.
33. Cargill, R.I., Barr, C.S., Coutie, W.J., Struthers, A.D., Lipworth, B.J. (1994): C-type natriuretic peptide levels in cor pulmonare and in congestive heart failure. Thorax, 49, 1247–1249.
34. Davis, K.M., Fish, L.C., Elahi, D., Clark, B.A., Minaker, K.L. (1992): Atrial natriuretic peptide levels in the prediction of congestive heart failure rish in frail elderly. JAMA, 267, 2625–2629.
35. Leosco, D., Ferrara, N., Landino, P., Romano, G., Cacciatore, F., Longobardi, G., Dal Canton, A., Rengo, F. (1996): Effects of age on the role of atrial natriuretic factor in renal adaptation to physiologic variations of dietary salt intake. J Am Soc Nephrol, 7, 1045–1051.
36. Iervasi, G., Clerico, A., Berti, S., Pilo, A., Biagini, A., Bianchi, R., Donato, L. (1995): Circulation, 91, 2018–2027.
37. Rengo, F., Ferrara, N., Leosco, D. (1991): Ventricular function in the elderly. Aging, 3, 9–17.
38. Hughes, C.V., Wong, M., Johnson, G., Cohn, J.N. (1993): Influence of age on mechanisms and prognosis of heart failure. Circulation, 87(Suppl VI), 111–117.

39. Acanfora, D., Crisci, C., Rengo, C., Vitale, D.F., Picone, C., Papa, A., Rengo, F. (1995): Clinical determinants of long-term mortality in elderly patients with heart disease. Arch of Gerontology, 21, 233–240.
40. Rubenstein, L.Z., Josephson, K.R., Wieland, G.D., English, P.A., Sayre, J.A., Kane, R.L. (1984): Effectiveness of geriatric evaluation unit (GEU): a randomized clinical trial. N Engl J Med, 311, 1664–1170.
41. Rubenstein, L.Z., Wieland, G.D., Josephson, K.R., Rosbrook, B., Sayre, J.A., Kane, R.L. (1988): Improve survival for frail elderly inpatients on a geriatric evaluation unit (GEU): who benefits? J Clin Epidemiol, 41, 441–449.

16

THE ROLE OF THE AUTONOMIC NERVOUS SYSTEM IN CONGESTIVE HEART FAILURE

Gianfranco Piccirillo, Carmela Bucca, Sabrina Tarantini, Elvira Santagada, Michele Durante, Silvia Remediani, Maria Luce Nocco, and Vincenzo Marigliano

Istituto di I Clinica Medica
Cattedra di Geriatria
Policlinico Umberto I
Viale del Policlinico 155, 00161 Roma, Italy

1. ABSTRACT

Altered sympathovagal balance could be a substrate for malignant ventricular arrhythmias in congestive heart failure. The aim of this study is to assess neuroautonomic function by power spectral analysis in patients with congestive heart failure and the effects of treatment with carvedilol in these patients. We compared the LF/HF ratio of all patients at baseline and after sympathetic stress (tilt). In group I, we considered 10 patients with congestive heart failure and 10 controls mean aged 60 years, while in group II were 10 patients with heart failure 70 years old and normal subjects age-matched. In group I, at rest the subjects with congestive heart failure had a significantly greater LF/HF ($p<0.001$) than controls. In contrast, it increased significantly after tilt in control subjects. In group II, at rest LF/HF did not differ between patients with congestive heart failure and normal subjects, while after tilt it resulted higher in controls ($p<0.05$). After a month of 25 mg daily of carvedilol administration in patients with heart failure in group I, both at rest and after tilt, LF/HF was significantly greater in patients in wash-out than treated ($p<0.001$). In group II there weren't significant differences both at rest and after tilt. This study showed increase of sympathetic activity in patients with congestive heart failure mean aged 60 years, less evident in patients aged 70 years. Carvedilol can exert beneficial myocardial effects in these patients, because reduces morbidity and mortality and can favorably influence the course of disease and prolong survival.

2. INTRODUCTION

Congestive heart failure is a serious medical condition manifested by signs and symptoms of abnormal cardiac ventricular performance. It is becoming a very important

Recent Advances in Geriatrics, edited by Barbagallo, Licata, and Sowers.
Plenum Press, New York, 1998.

problem due to the increasing geriatric population. The Framingham Heart Study estimated the prevalence of congestive heart failure to be between 3 and 10/1000. The dominant etiologic precursor is hypertension, which preceded failure in 75% of the cases; coronary heart disease is noted in 39%, but in 29% it is accompanied by hypertension; precursive rheumatic heart disease is in 21% of patients with congestive heart failure, and it is accompanied by hypertension in 11%. Despite modern management, congestive heart failure proved to be extremely lethal. The probability of dying within five years from onset of congestive heart failure is 62% for men and 42% for women. (1,2). According to data derived from the NHANES-I Epidemiologic Follow-up Study (1982–1986), mortality at 10 and 15 years increases in graded fashion with advancing age, with men more likely to die than women. In patients over 55 years old, the 15-year total mortality rate is 39.1% for women and 71.8% for men (3).

Activation of the sympathetic nervous system is one of the cardinal pathophysiologic abnormalities in patients with chronic heart failure and plays an important part in the progression of heart failure. Levels of circulating catecholamines increase in patients with heart failure in proportion to the severity of disease (4) and those with the highest plasma levels of norepinephrine have the most unfavorable prognosis (5). In Sweden in the 1970s, controlled clinical trials have shown that beta blockers, previously considered to be contraindicated, can produce hemodynamic and symptomatic improvement in chronic heart failure (6). These drugs can reduce symptoms, improve left ventricular function, and increase functional capacity.

Carvedilol is a non selective beta-receptor antagonist that also blocks alfa-1-receptors and, unlike beta blockers, exerts antioxidant effects, which may contribute to its actions in heart failure. It reduces the risk of death as well as the risk of hospitalization for cardiovascular causes in patients with heart failure who are receiving treatment with digoxin, diuretics, and an angiotensin-convertining-enzyme inhibitor. Moreover, as compared with placebo, carvedilol therapy is accompanied by a reduction in the risk of hospitalization for cardiovascular causes and in the combined risk of hospitalization or death (7).

One of the preferred methods that offers notable advantages for assessing sympathovagal balance is spectrum analysis. This technique is simple to perform and permits to evaluate overall autonomic modulation non invasively and repeatedly so that it could be utilized in follow up of these patients. By applying an autoregressive algorithmo a computerized ECG trace of 512 consecutive RR intervals spectrum analysis yelds two spectral bands, a high-frequency band (HF: 0.25Hz) influenced mainly by vagal activity and a low-frequency band (LF: 0.1Hz) predominantly under the control of sympathetic activity. The ratio of LF to HF (LF:HF) is usually indicated as a marker of sympathovagal interaction. Spectrum analysis also detects a very-low frequency component (VLF: 0.04Hz) probably influenced by the renin-angiotensin system (8,9).

Our aim in this study is to evaluate sympathetic function in elderly subjects with congestive heart failure and the effects of treatment with carvedilol in these patients.

3. MATERIALS AND METHODS

3.1. Study Subjects and Protocol

For this randomized study, subjects enrolled from our outpatients clinic underwent an initial screening consisting of a complete history and physical examination. None were undergoing pharmacological therapy at the time of the study. Subdividing the sample into

Table 1. Basal characteristics of the study subjects

	Group 1 (~60 ys)		Group 2 (~70 ys)	
Variable	Subjects with CHF (n=10)	Controls (n=10)	Subjects with CHF (n=10)	Controls (n=10)
Age (years)	60.4 ± 3	60.2 ± 1.2	70.4 ± 3.3	70.2 ± 1.3
Sex (M/F)	6/4	8/2	8/2	7/3
BMI (Kg/m^2)	23.4 ± 1.2	22.4 ± 1.2	22.6 ± 1.3	21.2 ± 1.4
EF (%)	30.9 ± 1.4	65.4 ± 1.2	29.9 ± 6.4	63.4 ± 1.3
Functional classification (NYHA)	II	II	II	II

Comparison between the two groups of subjects with congestive heart failure (CHF) and two age-matched control groups: composition of the subgroups, age, EF (ejection fraction), class NYHA (New York Heart Association), BMI (body mass index). Data are expressed as mean ±SEM.

two groups according to onset of symptoms of heart failure with slight limitation of physical activity, (II class NHYA: patients were confortable at rest; ordinary physical activity resulted in fatigue, palpitation, dyspnea or palpitation) for at least three months and ejection fraction < 0.35%(despite at least two months of treatment with diuretics and an angiotensin-converting-enzyme inhibitor) provided group of subjects with heart failure and a normal control group (Table 1).

Criteria for exclusion included a body mass index (BMI) higher than 26 Kg/m^2, smoking (> 5 cigarettes/day), systolic blood pressure of more than 160 or less than 85 mmHg or diastolic blood pressure of more than 100 mmHg, conditions likely to affect neuroautonomic function (neuropathies, diabetes, heart disease, renal failure, cardiac arrhythmia and liver disease) and a story of acute myocardial infarction, acute cerebrovascular events or systemic disease.

All subjects underwent echocardiography and power spectrum analysis of R-R interval variability. Power spectra were evaluated at baseline (rest) and after head-up tilt, a manoeuvre causing sympathetic stress (tilt).

In the second part of study in the subjects with congestive heart failure we evaluated spectral data after a month of 25 mg daily of carvedilol administration. During this time, the patients' other drug therapies for heart failure were kept constant, unless side effects occurred that were thought to be related either to these other medications or to the study drug itself.

3.2. Power Spectrum Analysis of R-R Interval Variability

All subjects were studied at 8.00 a.m., in a quiet and confortable environment; they rested supine for at least 30 min before undergoing a 15-min baseline electrocardiographic (ECG) recording. After resting, all subjects underwent head-upright tilt testing, a passive manoeuvre obtained with a motorized tilt table (10,11). After 15 min upright (90°) the subjects were returned to the supine position (0°) for the second 15-min ECG recording. If hypotension (a > 20 mmHg fall in SBP) or if symptoms indicating the onset of syncope or nausea, or gastric pyrosis developed during tilt, testing was stopped and the subject was excluded from the study. The ECG signal was immediately digitized and sampled at 500 Hz, with 12 precision bits. Tracings were transferred and directly stored in hard-disk memory on an IBM compatible personal computer with a 486 microprocessor. An autoregressive algorithm was then used to compute power spectral densities from the electrocardiografic data (12,13). The QRS (II lead) was automatically recognized by a classic derivative/threshold algorithm (14). Statistical data on the R-R intervals, including the mean R-R duration obtained after eliminating anomalous beats, the maximum and minimum duration, the variance and the normalized R-R series after subtracting the mean. Spectral power was calculated as follows, from a series of 512 consecutive R-R intervals. The autocorrelation functions were applied to the complete R-R series; the Yule-Walker matrix (autocorrelation values matrix) was calculated with the method of Levinson-Durbin (15) and the matrix order was determined with the Anderson test and Akaike Information Criteria (16). The spectral decomposition method was then applied to estimate the power and center frequency of each spectral component (17). Spectral power was expressed in ms^2. The frequency of the oscillations was calculated in cycles/beat and divided by the mean R-R interval expressed in seconds, for conversion into Hertz equivalents (Hz Eq).

To evaluate autonomic nervous system function we analyzed three power spectral components: a high-frequency component (from 0.16 to 0.40 Hz Eq), a low-frequency component (from 0.04 to 0.15 Hz Eq) and a very low- frequency component (from 0.0033 to 0.04 Hz Eq) (18–21). We considered total power (TP) as the spectral density from 0.0033 to 0.04 Hz Eq (22,23). Because of the skewness of power spectral data these were also transformed into the natural logarithm of the variable (ln) and into normalized units (NUs) (24). Transforming data into NUs also helped to accentuate sympathovagal balance activity. NUs were calculated as follows: LF NUs = LF power / TP-VLF power × 100; HF NUs = HF power / TP-VLF power × 100.

The last calculation was the ratio between LF and HF powers (LF/HF).

3.3. Statistical Analysis

Data were analyzed with the statistical package SPSS. An analysis of variance was used to compare the general characteristics (including age, BMI, heart rate, EF) and LF/HF ratio. Mann Whitney analysis was applied for comparing the two groups. Wilcoxon's test was used to compare the results in the same subgroup before and after tilt. All data are expressed as mean ± standard error (SE). A p value < 0.05 was considered to indicate statistical significance.

4. RESULTS

Twenty subjects with congestive heart failure (ten with mean age 60.4 ± 3.3 years, EF: 30.9 ± 1.4 and ten with 70.4 ± 3.3 years, EF: 29.9 ± 6.4) and twenty normal subjects (ten with mean age 60.2 ± 1.2 years, EF: 65.4 ± 1.2 and ten with 70.2 ± 1.3 years, EF: 63.4 ± 1.3) were selected and completed the study. We distinguished these patients in two groups: group I, including patients with heart failure and controls mean aged 60 years and group II, comprehending patients with heart failure 70 years old and normal subjects age-matched (Tab. 1).

In group I, at rest the subjects with congestive heart failure had a significantly greater LF/HF ($p < 0.001$) than controls. In contrast, it increased significantly after tilt in control subjects.

In group II, at rest LF/HF did not differ significantly between patients with congestive heart failure and normal subjects, while after tilt it resulted higher in controls ($p < 0.05$) (Tab. 2).

After a month of 25 mg daily of carvedilol in patients with heart failure in group I, both at rest and after tilt, LF/HF was significantly greater in patients in wash-out than

Table 2. Ratio of low frequency power to high frequency power in subjects with congestive heart failure and age-matched control group

	Group 1		Group 2	
	Subjects with CHF	Controls	Subjects with CHF	Controls
Rest LF/HF	2.3 ± 0.3*	1.5 ± 0.2	1.0 ± 0.3	0.9 ± 0.2
Tilt LF/HF	3.2 ± 0.2*	4.2 ± 0.1	1.0 ± 0.2**	2.2 ± 0.1

Change in ratio of low frequency power to high frequency power in subjects with congestive heart failure and age-matched control group at baseline (Rest) and after a passive orthostatic manoeuvre (Tilt).
LF/HF = ratio of low frequency power to high frequency power.
*p< 0.001 subjects with CHF vs controls; **p< 0.05 subjects with CHF vs controls.

treated (p<0.001). In Group II there weren't significant differences both at rest and after tilt (Tab. 3).

5. DISCUSSION

Although neurohormonal responses are thought to have a role in the preservation of circulatory homeostasis, it is now obvious that the progressive activation of the renin-angiotensin and adrenergic systems that occurs during the natural history of heart failure has a role in the development of progressive cardiac disfunction (25,26). The compensatory stimulation of heart rate and myocardial contractility is initially favorable, but prolonged adrenergic activation may be unable to prevent progression of heart failure past a critical point (27). In chronic heart failure desensitization phenomena involving myocardial beta receptors and G proteins occur, as well as direct and indirect toxic myocardial effects mediated by intracellular Ca^{++} overload and effects on macromolecular synthesis.

This study showed increase of sympathetic activity at rest in patients with congestive heart failure 60 years old, less evident in subjects 70 years old because of desensitization of myocardial beta receptors with increasing age.

Although the precise mechanisms stimulating the sympathetic nervous system in congestive heart failure are not fully understood, the magnitude of increase in LF/HF ratio may be a more sensitive indicator of cardiac functional status than the more traditional measurements of cardiac performance. Furthermore, since simpathetic stimulation may precipitate ventricular fibrillation (28) and sudden death is common among patients with severe heart failure, activation of sympathetic nervous system could be a causative factor of the high mortality rate in this syndrome.

Table 3. Ratio of low frequency power to high frequency power after a month of 25 mg daily of carvedilol administration

	Group 1		Group 2	
	Subjects with CHF before carvedilol	Subjects with CHF after carvedilol	Subjects with CHF before carvedilol	Subjects with CHF after carvedilol
Rest LF/HF	2.3 ± 0.3*	0.9 ± 0.2	1.0 ± 0.3	1.0 ± 0.1
Tilt LF/HF	3.2 ± 0.2*	2.0 ± 0.2	1.0 ± 0.2	2.5 ± 0.1

Change in ratio of low frequency power to high frequency power after a month of 25 mg daily carvedilol in subjects with congestive heart failure at baseline (Rest) and after a passive orthostatic manoeuvre (Tilt).
LF/HF = ratio of low frequency power to high frequency power.
*p<0.001 LF/HF before of carvedilol administration vs after of carvedilol administration.

Bristow demonstrated that direct inhibition of the biologic effects of catecholamine neurotransmitter (norepinephrine) or hormones (epinephrine and norepinephrine) may produce beneficial myocardial effects (29). These findings have led investigators to propose that sympathetic antagonists (beta-blockers) might be useful in the management of heart failure.

Controlled trials of several different beta-blockers have shown that these drugs can reduce symptoms, improve left ventricular function, and increase functional capacity (30). Particularly third-generation beta blocking agents exert alpha-1-adrenergic blockade, peripheral vascular beta-agonist activity and a direct action that cause vasodilatation (29).

In this study we evaluated spectral data after a month of 25 mg daily of carvedilol administration and we found a decrease of LF/HF ratio, index of inhibition of sympathetic activity.

Carvedilol has vasodilatatory activity due to alpha-1-receptor antagonism (31) that results in moderate arteriolar dilation and reduced total peripheral resistance in subjects with heart failure (32). In heart failure from idiopathic dilated cardiomyopathy carvedilol has been well tolerated (33) and has substantially improved resting left ventricular function as assessed by left ventricular ejection fraction in both idiopathic and ischemic dilated cardiomyopathy (34). Packer et al. demonstrated in a double-blind, placebo-controlled, stratified study the safety of carvedilol on mortality in patients with congestive heart failure: the reduction in risk attributable to carvedilol was 65%. In addition, carvedilol therapy was accompanied by a 27% reduction in the risk of hospitalization for cardiovascular causes, as well as a 38% reduction in the combined risk of hospitalization or death (7).

6. CONCLUSION

Increased systemic and cardiac adrenergic drive is associated with heart failure and is directly related to an adverse outcome. Initially these events may be protective, but the long-term effects are deleterious. Circulating catecholamines increase in proportion to the severity of congestive heart failure and indicate unfavorable prognosis. The activation of simpathetic nervous system can precipitate ventricular fibrillation (28) and sudden death and it is responsable of the high mortality rate in heart failure.

Power spectral analysis permits to evaluate overall autonomic modulation non invasively and repeatedly so that it could be utilized in follow up of these patients.This study showed increase of sympathetic activity in patients with congestive heart failure mean aged 60 years, less evident in patients aged 70 years. Third-generation beta blocking agents exert beneficial myocardial effects in congestive heart failure. Carvedilol reduces morbidity and mortality and can favorably influence the course of disease and prolong survival (7).

The question of whether other beta-blockers prolong survival in heart failure is being addressed in ongoing trials.

REFERENCES

1. McKee PA, Castelli WP, McNamara PM, Kannel WB. The natural hystory of congestive heart failure. The Framingham Study. N.Engl.J.Med.1971;285: 1442–6.
2. Kannel WB, Plehn JF, Cupples LA. Cardiac failure and sudden death in the Framingham Study. Am.Heart J.1988;115: 869–75.
3. Douglas D. Schocken, Martha I Arrieta, PE Leaverton, EA Ross. Prevalence and mortality rate of Congestive heart failure in the United States. J Am Coll Cardiol 1992; 20: 301–6.

4. Thomas JA, Marks BH. Plasma norepinfrine in congestive heart failure. Am.J.Cardiol 1978;41:233–43.
5. Cohn JN, Levine TB, Olivari MT et al. Plasma norepinefrine as a guide to prognosis in patients with chronic congestive heart failure. N.Engl J Med 1984;311:819–823.
6. Swedberg K, Hjalmarson A, Waagstein F, Wallentin I. Prolongation of survival in congestive cardiomyopathy by beta-receptor blockade.Lancet 1979;1:1374–6
7. M.Packer, MR Bristow, JN Cohn, WS Colucci, MB Fowler, EM Gilbert, NH Shusterman. The effect of carvedilolon morbidity and mortality in patients with chronic heart failure. N Engl J Med 1996;334:1349–55.
8. Akselrod S, Gordon D, Ubel FA, Shannon DC, Barger AC, Cohen RJ. Power spectral analysis of heart rate fluctuation: a quantitative probe of heart rate fluctuation: a quantative probe of beat-to-beat cardiovascular control. Science 1981;213:220–222.
9. Bonaduce D,Marciano F, Petretta M, Migaux ML, Morgano G, Bianchi V, Salemme L, Valva G, Condorelli M. Effects of converting enzyme inibition on heart period variability in patients with acute myocardial infarction. Circulation 1994; 90:108–113.
10. Pomeranz B, Macaulay RJB, Caudill MA, Gordon D, Kilborn KM, Barger AC, Shannon DC, Cohen RJ, Benson H. Assessment of autonomic function in humans by heart rate spectral analysis. Am J Phisiol 1985; 248: H151-H153.
11. Yo Y, Nagano N, Iiyama K, Higaki J, Mikami H, Ogihara T. Effects of age and hypertension on autonomic nervous regulation during passive head-up tilt. Hypertension 1994; 23 (supp I): I-82-I-86.
12. Pagani M, Lombardi F, Guzzetti S, Rimoldi O, Furlan R, Pizzinelli P, Sandrone G, Malfatto G, DellOrto G, Piccaluga E, Tureil M, Baselli G, Cerutti S, Malliani A. Power spectral analysis of heart rate and arterial pressure variability as a marker of sympathovagal interaction in man and conscious dog. Circ. Res. 1986; 59: 178–193.
13. Ripley KL, Murray A. Introduction to automated arrhythmia detection. New York TEEE Comp. Society Press, 1980.
14. Kay SM, Marple SL Jr. Spectrum analysis. A modern prospective. Proc. IEEE 1981; 69 (11): 1380–1419.
15. Akaike H. Statistical predictor identification. Ann. Int. Stat. Math. 1970; 22: 203–217.
16. Zetterberg LH. Estimation of parameters for a linear difference equation with application to EEG analysis. Math Biosci 1969; 5: 227–275.
17. O'Brien IAD, O'Hare P, Corral RJM. Heart rate variability in healthy subjects: effect of age and the derivation of normal ranges for tests of autonomic function. Br. Heart J. 1986; 55: 348–35?
18. Weise F, Heydeinreich F, Runge U. Contribution of sympathetic and vagal mechanisms to genesis of heart rate fluctuation during orthostatic load: a spectral analysis. J. Aut. Nerv. Syst. 1987; 21: 127–134.
19. Rottmann JN, Steinman RC, Albrecht P, Bigger JT, Jr, Rolnitzky LM, Fleiss JL. Efficient estimation of the heart period power spectrum suitable for physiologic or pharmacologic studies. Am. J. Cardiol. 1990; 66: 1522–1524.
20. Malliani A, Pagani M, Lombardi F, Cerutti S. Cardiovascular neural regulation explored in the frequency domain. Circulation 1991; 84: 482–492.
21. Saul JP, Albrecht P, Berger RD, Cohen RJ. Analysis of long term heart rate variability: methods, scaling and implications. IEEE 1988; 88: 409–412.
22. Bigger JT, Fleiss JL, Rolnitzky LM, Steinman RC. The ability of several short-term measures of R-R variability to predict mortality after myocardial infarction. Circulation 1993; 88: 927–934.
23. Gottdiener JS, Reda DJ, Matterson BJ, Massie BM, Notargiacomo A, Hamburger RJ, Williams DW, Henderson WG. Importance of obesity, race and age to the cardiac structural and functional effects of hypertension. J Am Coll Cardiol 1994; 24: 1992–1498.
24. Brovelli M, Baselli, Cerutti S. Computerized analysis for an experimental validation of neurophysiological models of heart rate control. In Computers in Cardiology. Silver Spring Md, IEEE Computer Society Press 1983: 205–208.
25. Bristow MR, Kantrowitz NE, Ginsburg R, Fowler MB. Beta-adrenergic function in heart muscle disease and heart failure. J Mol Cell Cardiol 1985; 17: 41–52.
26. Packer M Neurohormonal interactions and adaptations in congestive heart failure. Circulation 1988; 77: 721–730.
27. Feldman AM, Bristow MR. Adrenergic neuroeffector mechanisms in the failing human heart. In: Braunwald E, ed. Clinical Update, 3rd ed. Heart disease. Philadelphia: W.B. Saunders, 1990: 206–216.
28. Lown B, Verrier RL. Neural activity and ventricular fibrillation. N Engl J Med 1976; 294 : 1165–70.
29. Bristow MR. Pathophysiologic and pharmacologic rationales for clinical management of chronic heart failure with beta-blocking agents. Am J Cardiol 1993; 71: 12C-22C.
30. Krum H, Sackner-Bernstein JD, Goldsmith RL. Double-blind placebo-controlled study of the long-term efficacy of carvedilol in patients with severe chronic heart failure. Circulation 1995; 92: 1499–506.

31. Wendt TH, van der Does R. Schrader R, Landgraf H, Kober G. Acute hemodinamic effects of the vasodilating and beta-blocking agent carvedilol in comparison to propranolol. J Cardiovasc Pharmacol 1987; 10 (suppl 11): S147-S150.
32. Das Gupta P, Broadhurst P, Lahiri A.The effects of intravenous carvedilol, a new multiple action vasodilating beta-blocker, in congestive heart failure. J Cardiovascul Pharmacol 1991; 18 (suppl.4): S12-S16.
33. Olsen SL, Gilbert EM, Renlund DG, Mealey PC, Volkman K, O'Connel JB, Yanowitz FD, Bristow MR. Carvedilol improves left ventricular function in idiopathic dilated cardiomyopathy. Circulation 1991; 84: II-564.
34. Olsen SL, Gilbert EM, Renlund DG, Mealey PC, Taylor DO, Volkman AK, Bristow MR Carvedilol improves symptoms and left ventricular function in patients with congestive heart failure due to ischemic or idiopathic dilated cardiomyopathy. J Am Coll Cardiol 1993; 21: 11A.

17

TREATMENT OF CONGESTIVE HEART FAILURE IN THE ELDERLY

Gaspare Parrinello, Pietra Amato, Anna Licata, Salvatore Paterna, Antonio Pinto, Ligia J. Dominguez, Mario Barbagallo, and Giuseppe Licata*

Istituto di Medicina Interna
University of Palermo

1. INTRODUCTION

Congestive heart failure (CHF) is a complex clinical syndrome which constitutes the epilogue of the natural history of virtually all heart diseases and in its advanced stages, has a poor prognosis. In the elderly, heart failure exhibits particular characteristics linked to the age-related alterations of cardiovascular system, to the association with other pathologies, to the atypical clinical presentation and to the increased iatrogenic risk. Heart failure now afflicts over 1% of the general population with nearly 1 in 10 elderly subjects affected, and the frequency of CHF is progressively increasing in most industrialized societies[1,2]. Further, CHF remains a significant cause of death and hospitalization especially among elderly populations. As such, 37,927 deaths and 722,000 hospital discharges were attributed to heart failure in 1990 (Fig. 1).[3] Therefore, continued efforts are needed for the primary and secondary prevention of this syndrome.

The aim of therapy in CHF should be not only to improve symptoms and signs of CHF but also to prevent major morbid events such as hospitalization, recurrent myocardial infarction, and to improve quality of life, and prolong survival. The proportion of patients reported to die suddenly or from progressive circulatory failure is not consistent among similar studies of CHF. Lack of an adequate or consistent classification of how patients die may contribute to the current confusion about the mode of death in heart failure. Defining how patients with heart failure die could be important in developing strategies to reduce the continuing high mortality associated with this condition.[4]

2. SELECTION AND TARGETS OF THERAPY IN THE ELDERLY

Selection of anti-heart failure drugs should be based on knowledge of the impact of specific therapies on the pathophysiological events of CHF and on the morbidity and mor-

* Correspondence to: Giuseppe Licata, MD, Pizza delle Cliniche N.2, 90127 Palermo, Italy. Tel: 39-91-6552152/1; fax: 39-91-6552153.

Recent Advances in Geriatrics, edited by Barbagallo, Licata, and Sowers.
Plenum Press, New York, 1998.

tality risks. The target for therapeutic intervention may be categorized and directed to the hemodynamic, neuro-endocrine and metabolic components of CHF, to the symptoms and quality of life, and to the morbidity and mortality risks[5].

Among neurohumoral mechanism contributing to CHF development, increased activation of the sympathetic nervous system, increased activity of renin-angiotensin-aldosterone system (RAS-A) and increased levels of vasopresin are included[6].

Diuretics, vasodilators and ACE-inhibitors are now accepted as standard treatment, particularly when used in combination. Controversy continues to surround the efficacy of digitalis glycosides; they improve symptoms in some patients but their impact on morbidity and mortality is still uncertain. Despite available treatment with diuretics, digitalis, vasodilators and ACE-inhibitors, the morbidity and mortality risks of congestive heart failure remain high. It is important to mention that none of these drug groups directly modulate the excessive excitation of the sympathetic-adrenal system, one of the major neuro-endocrine hazards of CHF.

The sympathetic activation in CHF, although initially useful to maintain cardiac output, is deleterious to cardiac function and survival in the long term. Levels of circulating catecholamines increase in patients with heart failure in proportion to the severity of the disease and those with the highest plasma levels of norepinephrine have the most unfavorable prognosis. As such, Cohn et al. reported that plasma norepinephrine concentration is an independent predictor of mortality for patients with heart failure[7]. This has led clinicians to consider the possibility of using therapies that reduce sympathetic activity or its consequences.

Indeed, sustained neurohormonal activation may be one of the factors responsible for the transition from asymptomatic left ventricular dysfunction to established CHF. Patients whose neurohormonal systems are ponderously activated have the highest mortality independently of other clinical variables such as symptoms and left ventricular ejection fraction[8].

3. TREATMENT OPTIONS IN THE ELDERLY

3.1. Diuretics

Diuretics have long been accepted as the traditional first-line treatment for patient with symptomatic heart failure whatever its etiology or dysfunctional stage. This is probably due to the rapid improvement of congestive symptoms experienced by most patients after diuretic administration. The effects of diuretic treatment are to reduce cardiac dilatation and ventricular wall stress and to counteract peripheral vascular stiffness by inhibiting renal retention of salt and water. Four classes of diuretics are available, including drugs acting on the proximal tubule, the distal tubule, the loop of Henle or the convoluted tubule. The "high-ceiling" loop diuretics are those most commonly used in clinical practice for the treatment of acute CHF. These loop diuretics, which include furosemide, ethacrinic acid, bumetamide, piretamide and torasemide, increase the fractional excretion of sodium to a maximum of 25% of the filtered load, and their efficacy is largely independent of the glomerular filtration rate.

In severe CHF, large doses of diuretics in isolation become ineffective, and additional strategies may be useful: i) constant infusion of loop-active diuretics providing large doses at relatively low infusion rates may increase efficacy and reduce side effects; ii) combination of diuretics acting at different sites may provide synergism; this is especially true with the addition of loop-active diuretics to thiazides, which appears to increase thiazide-sensitive NaCl transport in the distal convoluted tubule; and iii) the use of diuretics may be potentiated by the infusion of renal doses of dopamine to increase renal blood

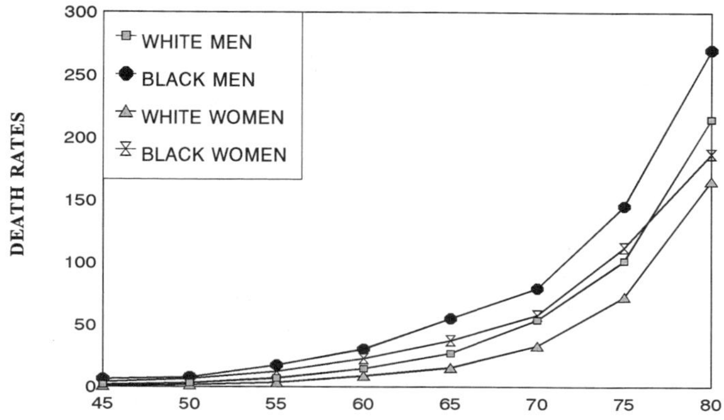

Figure 1. Death rates per 100,000 subjects, for congestive heart failure in the United States in 1990. Modified from Gillum RF (3).

flow[9]. In fact, in a study by Dormans et al, the addition of hydrochlorothiazide to high dose furosemide in patients with severe heart failure was effective even in patients with a significantly reduced renal function[10].

Preliminary data from our laboratory have demonstrated that the association of hypertonic saline solution infusion with concomitant intravenous (iv) diuretic administration, is able to improve refractory CHF. We have evaluated 30 hospitalized patients (11 females and 19 males) with refractory CHF, not responsive to usual treatment (digitalis, oral diuretic, ACE-inhibitors and other vasodilators), in NYHA functional class IV, aged 65 to 85 years (mean age 76.2±8.86). All the patients were treated with hypertonic saline solution (150 ml of NaCl 0.9% plus NaCl 10 mEq/ml 20–40 ml and KCl 10 mEq/ml 10–20 ml) and furosemide (250–500 mg qd, iv) for 6–12 days. We observed a prominent improvement in clinical parameters such as dyspnea, lower limbs edema or anasarca and weakness, as well as reduction in body weight, NYHA functional class (IV to II) and hospitalization period (Table 1) in all 30 patients. Twenty patients in frank anasarca (ascitis, pleural and pericardial efusion) experienced complete resolution of this state after treatment. After administration of this combined therapy, there was a significant increase in serum sodium and a decrease in serum potasium, but the values remained between normal ranges. Both systolic and diastolic blood pressure were decreased without clinical manifestations and heart rate was corrected to normal values (Table 1). Patients did not complain of any major discomfort during treatment and tolerated well the i.v. infusion. Our findings suggest that this new therapeutic approach to refractory CHF is able to improve the symptoms (dispnea, lower limbs edema, weakness) and to reduce body weight, functional class and hospitalization period. The long-term effects are ongoing.

3.2. Digitalis

For many physicians, digitalis glycosides together with diuretics, continue to be a mainstay of the treatment of symptomatic heart failure. The symptomatic benefits conferred by digitalis may be less clear-cut than those induced by diuretics but this may be due to their nearly universal combined prescription. Several studies (RADIANCE, PROVED, DIG trials) have shown that chronic digoxin therapy in heart failure has favor-

Table 1. Clinical and laboratory parameters of 30 patients with refractory CHF before and after treatment with IV furosemide and hypertonic solution[a]

Parameter	Before	After	p<
Weight (Kg)	73.5 ± 12.6	63.8 ± 11.4	0.001
Diuresis/24 h	350 ± 175	2100 ± 626.9	0.001
Na (mEq/l)	138.1 ± 7.4	142.2 ± 3.8	0.01
K (mEq/l)	4.4 ± 0.6	3.9 ± 0.6	0.01
Creat (mg%)	1.4 ± 0.9	1.5 ± 0.9	NS
BUN (mg%)	62.1 ± 4.1	90.5 ± 6.5	0.001
Uric acid (mg%)	8.1 ± 2.7	9.1 ± 2.7	NS
SBP (mmHg)	142 ± 23.8	121.7 ± 22.7	0.001
DBP (mmHg)	80.7 ± 13.8	73.2 ± 12.4	0.01
HR (beats/min)	82.7 ± 13.7	77.1 ± 10.2	0.01
EF (%)	35.3 ± 7.3	36.8 ± 5.4	NS

[a]Data are expressed as mean±SD

able effects on symptoms, exercise capacity and rate of hospitalization[11–14]. The recent DIG trial (7788 patients with CHF in sinus rhythm) has also shown that digoxin has little effect on mortality in CHF[13]. There is general agreement in the notion that digoxin is indicated for most patients with CHF and systolic dysfunction. However, the question of whether chronic digoxin therapy is indicated in diastolic dysfunction heart failure has not been rigorously tested. It is noteworthy that the heart failure patients of the DIG trial who had normal or near normal systolic function (EF > 45%) also experience a reduction in hospitalization rate during long-term digoxin administration compared to placebo[14]. In fact over the years, digoxin has been proved to be a complex agent and it is probable that most of its beneficial effects are probably rendered by non-inotropic properties[15–17]. We know that digoxin blunts the high sympathetic nervous system tone and RAS-A activity and normalizes the disordered baroreceptor function and responsiveness associated with CHF[14,15]. Some studies have also indicated that the addition or withdrawal of digitalis has led to clinical deterioration or improvement, respectively.[13,18]

3.3. ACE Inhibitors

In the last years, ACE inhibitors represent a step forward in the treatment of CHF. Numerous trials have convincely demonstrated the efficacy of ACE inhibitors to improve the clinical signs and symptoms of patients with CHF, to reduce mortality and to slow the progression of myocardial dysfunction, as well as to favorably modify the natural history of the disease. The main rationale for ACE inhibition in chronic CHF, in left ventricular dysfunction, and after myocardial infarction is the modulation of prolonged neurohormonal activation. In particular, the beneficial effects of ACE-inhibition on survival in heart failure appear to depend largely on the degree to which neurohormonal systems are activated in this condition[8]. Results of some of the survival trials with ACE inhibitor treatment will be commented below.

3.4. Other Vasodilators

The vasodilators comprise an heterogeneous group of drugs with the only common property being dilatation of the vessels of the systemic vascular system. All vasodilators have the universal property of reducing cardiac afterload and/or preload, and some, such as the nitrates, have dose-dependent activity: at low doses nitrates dilate the systemic venous capacitance system and in high doses also dilate the arterial resistance vessels. Small studies have shown that nitrates may have a role in heart failure management[19,20]. They remain an important approach in patients with concomitant angina pectoris and myocardial ischemia. From the standpoint of large trials, the best studied vasodilators are the calcium channel blockers.

The newer dihydropiridines underwent randomized controlled investigation in the PRAISE and VHeFT III trials. Amlodipine did not affect overall survival in heart failure, but appeared to reduce mortality in the subset of non-ischemic dilated cardiomyopathy in the PRAISE trial. On the other hand, felodipine did not affect mortality in the V-HeFT III trial, but most of the patients in V-HeFT III had ischemic cardiomyopathy and failure. Perhaps the most reliable statement to make about the new dihydropyridines is that they do not appear to increase mortality when used as vasodilators in symptomatic heart failure[21,22].

3.5. β-Blockers

β-blockers, especially metoprolol, appear to be beneficial in some patients with CHF, possibly related to their reduction in sympathetic nervous activity and restoration of β-receptor population, with resultant improved contractile performance, enhanced myocardial relaxation, and overall increase in cardiac efficiency.[23]

Clinical trials have shown that β-adrenergic blocking agents are effective and well tolerated in patients with mild to moderate CHF, but the utility and safety of these agents in patients with advanced disease have not been evaluated[24].

For this reason, amongst the many newer drugs in development, the β-adrenoceptor antagonists hold considerable promise as the next step towards a more comprehensive treatment of CHF. In fact, recent studies have demonstrated that β-blockers therapy in CHF may be beneficial. This is in contrast with the earlier belief that the negative inotropic action of β-blocking agents leads to deterioration of the failing heart. Controlled clinical trials have shown that the long-term administration of metoprolol, bucindolol, nebivolol, bisoprolol and carvedilol can improve ventricular function and clinical status in selected patients with an idiopathic dilated cardiomyopathy[25–30]. In addition, long-term therapy with propanolol can reduce mortality in patients with left ventricular dysfunction after myocardial infarction.[31]

Pathophysiological targets for β-blocker therapy in CHF are myocardial protection or stabilization towards incidental ventricular fibrillation. This may explain the observation of a reduction in cardiac death after β-blockade. Moreover, β-blockers may improve cardiac function by reducing heart rate, resulting in lower myocardial energy expenditure, prolonged diastolic filling and increased effective myocardial blood flow due to the prolonged coronary vascular diastolic perfusion time. The restoration of physiological reflex, e.g. a normalization of the regularly abnormal baroreceptor reflex in heart failure, may be important. Thus, the normalization of down-regulated sympathetic receptors in the myocardium with a return to normal responsiveness to sympathetic stimulation has been proposed as a possible mechanism of action of β-blockers in CHF.[32,33]

The new agent carvedilol combines a non-selective β-receptor antagonistic action with α-1 receptor blockade. Additionally, it has antioxidant properties *in vitro*, which may protect against the continuing loss of cardiac myocytes and inhibit vascular smooth muscle cell proliferation.[34,35] These actions seem to be independent of β-receptor blockade. Inhibition of vascular smooth muscle cell proliferation could retard the progression of coronary atheroma and alter the vascular remodeling that occurs in CHF. In the United

States, Carvedilol HF Study Group reported that the addition of carvedilol to conventional therapy is associated with a decrease in mortality among patients with CHF.

Therapy with β-blockers though, is not included currently in the guidelines for treatment of CHF and there are no trials directed to elderly populations at the moment. However, these agents appear a promising option that merit further study.

4. SURVIVAL TRIALS

Studies of CHF reported over the last 60 years have emphasized the poor prognosis of the condition, particularly when LV systolic dysfunction is the cause. Recent clinical trials have demonstrated that ACE inhibitors, and possibly some others vasodilators, can improve prognosis.

The Cooperative New Scandinavian Enalapril Survival Study (CONSENSUS) was the first trial to show that treatment with the ACE-inhibitor enalapril may improve survival in patients with severe heart failure (NYHA Functional Class IV).[36] Subsequent data from SOLVD have demonstrated that the chronic therapy with enalapril is able to reduce mortality and incidence of cardiovascular events, also in patients with low grade CHF (II-III class NYHA).[37] In VHeFT II, in which the effects on mortality of treatment with enalapril and the association nitrates + hydralazine were compared in patients with CHF, it was concluded that not only mortality was significantly lower in the enalapril-treated group respect to the group treated with the combination of nitrates and hydralazine, but also enalapril treatment was associated with a lower incidence of sudden death.[38] Further, the benefit of enalapril on survival compared with hydralazine-isosorbide dinitrate was more evident in patients with higher plasma noradrenaline values and those with higher plasma renin activity. Another ACE inhibitor, captopril, has also proved to reduce mortality after myocardial infarction when compared to placebo in the Survival and Ventricular Enlargement (SAVE) trial.[39] A recent large trial, the AIRE Study, demonstrated that ramipril reduces mortality and progression to heart failure resistant to non-ACE inhibitor treatment, among patients with evidence of CHF early after myocardial infarction.[40]

Hughes et al. have reported a meta-analysis of VHeFT I and II data, with particular reference to geriatric parameters. In addition to the efficacy of the different therapies used in these trials, it is interesting to remark on the peculiar characteristics of the adult and aged populations studied. In fact, patients over 65 years of age present a significantly increased duration of CHF (3.8 vs 3.1 years), of edema (19 vs 13%), a higher ejection fraction (31 vs 29%), and a lower VO_2. These data suggest that, although CHF seems to be more complex in the elderly patients (because of the longer duration and the particular clinical signs), this may be due to a different physiopathogenic mechanism of this syndrome in the elderly. These data are in accordance with epidemiological reports of an increased incidence of diastolic dysfunction in elderly patients, who have a lesser involvement of left ventricular systolic function even in the presence of a decreased VO_2.[41]

Although, there is no dispute about the overall effects of ACE inhibitors therapy on prognosis, there is considerable disagreement among different studies when considering the proportion of patients who die suddenly and the effects of treatment on the relative likelihood of sudden death or death due to circulatory failure. In view of this disagreement, Poole Wilson and coworkers proposed a framework for the classification of the mode of death in which clear separation of the activity and place at the time of death, cause of death, mode of death and events prior to death is made (ACME: Activity, Cause, Mode and Event). Classifying mortality in this way may help identify the mechanisms leading to death and hence may help develop therapies and strategies to reduce mortality in patients with CHF, a group of patients whose prognosis remains poor.[4]

5. CONCLUSIONS

The drug treatment of congestive heart failure has undergone substantial evolution during the past few years but when considered in the overall contest of the high mortality risk of the syndrome, despite such treatment, there is much further to go. Respect to the treatment of this condition in the elderly, the particular characteristics and common associated conditions in these patients should be considered. At the present time, many relevant questions of practical importance remain to be answered before new proposed drugs can be safely recommended for general use in the treatment of CHF. Among these questions, it is important to consider the age of patients to be treated, the etiology of heart failure, the degree of functional disability, and the different mechanisms of action and individual dose-responses of the therapeutical options currently available or to be used in the future. Extensive clinical research programs and large scale survival trials should be directed towards the goal of comprehensive treatment of the patients with CHF, considering the possibility of pharmacological modulation of neurohormonal activation.

REFERENCES

1. Kannel WB, Ho K, Thom T. Changing epidemiological features of cardiac failure. Br Heart J 1994;72:(Suppl):S3–9.
2. Licata G. Moderni orientamenti terapeutici nello scompenso cardiaco congestizio. G Clin Med 1991;LXXII:489–506.
3. Gillum RF. Epidemiology of heart failure in the United States. Am Heart J 1993;126:1042–1047.
4. Narang R, Cleland JGF, Erhardt L, et al. Mode of death in chronic heart failure .A request and proposition for more accurate classification. Eur Heart J 1996;17:1390–1403.
5. Taylor SH. Congestive heart failure. Towards a comprehensive treatment. Eur Heart J 1996;17 (suppl. B):43–56.
6. Cohn JN. Current therapy of the failing heart. Circulation 1988; 78:1099–1107.
7. Cohn JN, Levine TB, Olivari M.T. et al. Plasma norepinephrine as a guide to prognosis in patients with chronic congestive heart failure. N Engl J Med 1984;311:819–823
8. Sigurdsson A, Swedberg K. Neurohormonal activation and congestive heart failure: today's experience with ACE inhibitors and rationale for their use. Eur Heart J, 1995;16(suppl.N): 65–72.
9. Ellison DH. The physiologic basis of diuretic synergism: its role in treating diuretic resistance. Ann Int Med 1991;114:886–894.
10. Dormans TPJ, Gerlag PGG. Combination of high-dose furosemide and hydrochlorothiazide in the treatment of refractory congestive heart failure. Eur Heart J 1996;17:1867–1874.
11. The Captopril-Digoxin Multicenter Research Group: Comparative effects of therapy with captopril and Digoxin in patients with mild to moderate heart failure. JAMA 1988; 259:539–544.
12. Packer M., Gheorghiade M, Young JB, for the RADIANCE Investigators. Withdrawal of digoxin from patients with chronic heart failure treated with angiotensin-converting enzyme inhibitors. N Engl J Med 1993;329:1–7.
13. Uretsky BF, Young JB, Shahidi FE, et al. Randomized study assessing the effect of digoxin withdrawal in patients with mild to moderate chronic heart failure: results of the PROVED trial. J Am Coll Cardiol 1993;22:955–962.
14. The Digitalis Investigation Group. The effect of digoxin on mortality and morbidity in patients with heart failure. N Engl J Med 1997;336:525–534.
15. Covit AB, Schaer GL, Sealey JE, Cody RJ, Laragh J. Suppression of the renin-angiotensin system by intravenous digoxin in congestive heart failure. Am J Med 1983;75:445–447.
16. Ferguson DW, Abboud FM, Mark AL. Selective impairment of baroreceptor mediated vasoconstrictor responses in patients with ventricular dysfunction. Circulation 1984;69:451–460.

17. Strickler JC, Kessler RH. Direct renal action of some digitalis steroids. J Clin Invest 1961;40:311–319.
18. Aronow WS, Starling I, Etienne F. Lack of efficacy of digoxin in treatment of compensated congestive heart failure with third heart sound and sinus rhythm in elderly patients receiving diuretic therapy. Am J Cardiol 1986;58:168–169.
19. Leier CV, Huss P, Magorien RD, Unverferth DV. Improved exercise capacity and differing arterial and venous tolerance during chronic isosorbide dinitrate therapy for congetive heart failure. Circulation 1983; 67:817–822.
20. Franciosa JA, Goldsmith SR, Cohn JN. Contrasting immediate and long-term effects of isosorbide dinitrate on exercise capacity in congestive heart failure. Am J Med 1980;69:559–566.
21. Packer M, for the prospective Randomized Amlodipine Survival Evaluation Study Group. Effect of amlodipine on morbidity and mortality in severe chronic heart failure N Engl J Med 1996;335:1107–1114.
22. Boden WE, Ziesche S., Carson PE et al. Rationale and design of the third vasodilator-heart failure trial (V-HeFTIII): felodipine as adjunctive therapy to enalapril and loop diuretics with or without digoxin in chronic heart failure. V-HeFT III investigators. Am J Cardiol 1996;77:1078–82.
23. Fisher ML, Gottlieb SS, Plotnik G, et al.Beneficial effects of metoprolol in heart failure associated with coronary artery disease: a randomized trial. J Am Coll Cardiol 1994;23:943–50.
24. Krum H, Sackner-Bernstein JD, Goldsmith RL, et al. Double-blind, placebo-controlled study of the long-term efficacy of carvedilol in patients with severe chronic heart failure. Circulation 1995;92:1499–1506.
25. Gilbert EM, Anderson JL, Deitchman D, et al. Chronic β-blocker-vasodilator therapy improves cardiac function in idiopathic dilated cardiomyopathy: a double-blind, randomized study of bucindolol versus placebo. Am J Med 1990;88:223–229.
26. Wisenbaugh T, Katz I, Davis J, et al. Long term (3 month) effects of a new beta-blocker (nebivolol) on cardiac perfomance in dilated cardiomyopathy. J Am Coll Cardiol 1993;21:1094–1100.
27. Bristow MR, O' Connell JB, Gilbert EM, et al. For the bucindolol Investigators. Dose response of chronic β-blocker treatment in heart failure from either idiopathic dilated cardiomyopathy or ischemic cardiomyopathy. Circulation 1994;89:1632–1642.
28. Metra M, Nardi M, Giubbini R, Dei Cas L. Effects of short- and long-term carvedilol administration on rest and exercise capacity and clinical conditions in patients with idiopathic dilated cardiomyopathy. J Am Coll Cardiol 1994;24:1678–1687.
29. Waagstein F, Bristow M.R., Swedberg K, et al. Beneficial effects of metoprolol in idiopathic dilated cardiomyopathy. Lancet 1993;342:1441–1446.
30. CIBIS Investigators and Committees. A randomized trial of β-blockade in heart failure: the Cardiac Insufficiency Bisoprolol Study (CIBIS). Circulation 1994;90:1765–1773.
31. Chadda K, Goldstein S, Byington R, Curd JD. Effect of propanolol after myocardial infarction in patients with congestive heart failure Circulation 1986;73:503–510.
32. Merlino G, Scaglione R, Corrao S, et al. Association between reduced lymphocyte β-adrenergic receptors and left ventricular dysfunction in young obese subjects. Int J Obesity 1994;18:699–703.
33. Merlino G, Scaglione R, Paterna S, et al. Lymphocyte β-adrenergic receptors in young subjects with peripheral or central obesity: relationship with central hemodynamics and left ventricular function. Eur Heart J 1994;15:786–794.
34. Yue T-L, Cheng HY, Lysko PG, et al. Carvedilol, a new vasodilator and β-adrenoceptor antagonist, is an antioxidant and free radical scavenger. J Pharmacol Exp Ther 1992;263:92–98.
35. Ohlstein EH, Douglas SA, Sung C-P, et al. Carvedilol, a cardiovascular drug, prevents vascular smooth muscle cell proliferation, migration and neointimal formation following vascular injury. Proc Natl Acad Sci USA 1993;90:6189–6193.
36. Consensus Trial Study Group. Effect of Enalapril on mortality in severe congestive heart failure: results of Cooperative North Scandinavian Enalapril Survival Study. N Engl J Med 1987;316:1429.
37. The SOLVD Investigators. Effect of Enalapril on survival in patients with reduced left ventricular ejection fractions and congestive heart failure. N Engl J Med 1991;325:293–302
38. Cohn JN Johnson G., Ziesche S, et al. A comparison of enalapril with hydralazine-isosorbide dinitrate in the treatment of chronic congestive heart failure. N Engl J Med 1991;325:303–10
39. Pfeffer MA et al. ACM and SAVE Investigators: Effect of captopril on mortality and morbidity in patients with left ventricular disfunction after myocardial infarction: Result of the Survival and Ventricular Enlargement Trial. New Engl J Med 1992:327:669–77.
40. Cleland JGF, Erhardt L, Murray G, Halls AS, Balls SG. Effect of ramipril on morbidity and mode of death among survivors of acute myocardial infarction with clinical evidence of heart failure. A report from the AIRE study Investigators. Eur Heart J 1997;18:41–51.
41. Hughes CV, Wong M, Jonhson G, et al. Influence of age on mechanisms and prognosis of heart failure. Circulation 1993;87(Suppl VI):111–117.

18

APOLIPOPROTEIN E GENOTYPE IN VASCULAR DEMENTIA

Carlo Vergani,* Ludovica Caputo, Anthony Ryan, Jacopo Tagliabue, and Giorgio Annoni

Istituto di Medicina Interna
Cattedra di Gerontologia e Geriatria
Università di Milano and Ospedale Maggiore
IRCCS, Milano
Via Pace 9, 20122 Milano, Italy

1. INTRODUCTION

The ε4 allele of apolipoprotein E (ApoE) has been associated with Alzheimer's disease (AD): the frequency of the ε4 allele is elevated in samples of AD patients[1,2] and individuals with a single or double dose of the ε4 allele have earlier onset of AD symptoms[1]. Furthermore, subjects with one or two ε4 alleles have been shown to have increased amounts of the neurofibrillary tangles and amyloid plaques associated with AD[3].

The ε4 allele can therefore be regarded as a risk factor for AD, while there is some evidence that the ε2 allele may offer some protection[4] or at least delay the appearance of symptoms in early onset familiar AD[5,6].

It has been suggested that the main utility of the ApoE genotype test, from a clinical point of view, is in the differential diagnosis of dementia[7]. However, Italian[2,8] and Japanese[9] studies have also shown an association of the ε4 allele with vascular dementia (VaD), enlighten a possible broader role of the Apo E in the pathogenesis of the cognitive impairment.

Since Down's syndrome (DS) exhibits many of the histological hallmarks of AD, an understanding of the importance of ApoE in this condition is of considerable interest. Chromosome 21 encodes the amyloid precursor protein (APP) and DS individuals who exceed the age of 40 years develop increased amyloid deposition. Moreover, a heavier "amyloid burden" has been associated with the ε4 allele in DS patients[10]. An increase in the occurrence of the ε2 allele has been reported in a DS population[11] but other authors have concluded that the frequencies of the ApoE alleles in DS do not greatly differ from those of the general population[12–14]. Finally, the influence of the ε4 allele on the risk of dementia

* Corresponding author: Fax: 0039-2-55017492; phone: 0039-2-5503 5412; e-mail: vergani@imiucca.csi.uni.

Recent Advances in Geriatrics, edited by Barbagallo, Licata, and Sowers.
Plenum Press, New York, 1998.

in 82 DS patients was found important and similar to that of non trisomic subjects[24]. This report strenghten the hypothesis coming from one postmortem series[10], who suggested that inheritance of the ε4 is an indipendent risk factor, along with age, for developing higher amounts of amyloid in the brain, which are directly correlated with dementia.

Here we present ApoE genotype data of 116 Italian people: elderly controls, demented elderly and DS subjects; other results were based on phenotypic analysis[8] or on genotyping of early onset sporadic and familiar AD patients[6,5,15].

2. MATERIALS AND METHODS

2.1. Subjects

Elderly subjects were out-patients of the Geriatrics Department, Ospedale Maggiore, IRCSS of Milano. A number of samples were provided by two nursing homes for the elderly. For ApoE genotyping 116 subjects were recruited, of whom 30 were assigned to the control group on the basis of absence of cognitive decline (MMSE > 24). For all demented patients (n = 55) extensive neurological testing and brain CT scans were performed. 42 were diagnosed as AD using NINCDS-ADRDA criteria[16] and 13 as VaD using NINDS-AIRDEN criteria[17]. Finally, blood samples were collected from 31 DS subjects, all of whom had been karyotypically confirmed. The mean ages (±SD) of the subjects in the different groups are shown in Table 1.

2.2. Apo E Genotype Characterization

Nuclear DNA was prepared by standard methods. A 244 base pair portion of the apoE gene was PCR amplified using the F4 and F6 primers[18] at 96°C for 5 minutes, 30 cycles of 95°C for 1 minute, 60°C for 1 minute 10 seconds and 70°C for 2 minutes, and a final 10 minutes at 70°C. Ten units of *Hha* I restriction enzyme were added directly to the PCR reaction mix and the mixture incubated for three hours at 37°C. The resulting DNA fragments were electrophoresed on 8% polyacrylamide gels for three hours at 35 mA constant current. Gels were stained using ethidium bromide and fragments visualized under UV light. Figure 1 is a paradigmatic example of the obtained polymorphism.

2.3. Statistical Analysis

Data were analysed statistically using the χ^2 and Fisher's exact tests. Age at onset of AD symptoms was analysed using Kaplan Mayer product limit distributions.

Table 1. Genotype and allele frequencies in the different groups[a]

			Genotypes+						Alleles		
	N	Age	ε2/ε2	ε2/ε3	ε3/ε3	ε2/ε4	ε3/ε4	ε4/ε4	ε2	ε3	ε4
C	30	73.3 ± 7.1	ND	1 (3)	23 (77)	ND	6 (20)	ND	1 (2)	53 (88)	6 (10)
AD	42	78.9 ± 5.8	ND	3 (7)	20 (48)	ND	17 (40)	2* (5)	3 (4)	60 (71)	21 (24)
VaD	13	77.7 ± 6.7	ND	1 (8)	3 (23)	1 (8)	8 (60)	ND**	2 (7)	15 (58)	9 (35)
DS	31	30.3 ± 11.6	ND	2 (7)	25 (80)	ND	4 (13)	ND	2 (3.5)	56 (90)	4 (0.65)

[a]N=number of subjects. Age is given as the mean years ± SD. Genotype and allele frequencies are shown in brackets. C=Controls; AD=Alzheimer's disease; VaD=Vascular dementia; ND=Not detected.

*χ^2 = 4.918, $p < 0.05$ for comparison of the frequency of ε4 heterozygotes plus homozygotes in AD vs controls.

**$p < 0.01$ (Fisher's exact test) for comparison of the frequency of ε4 carriers in VaD vs controls.

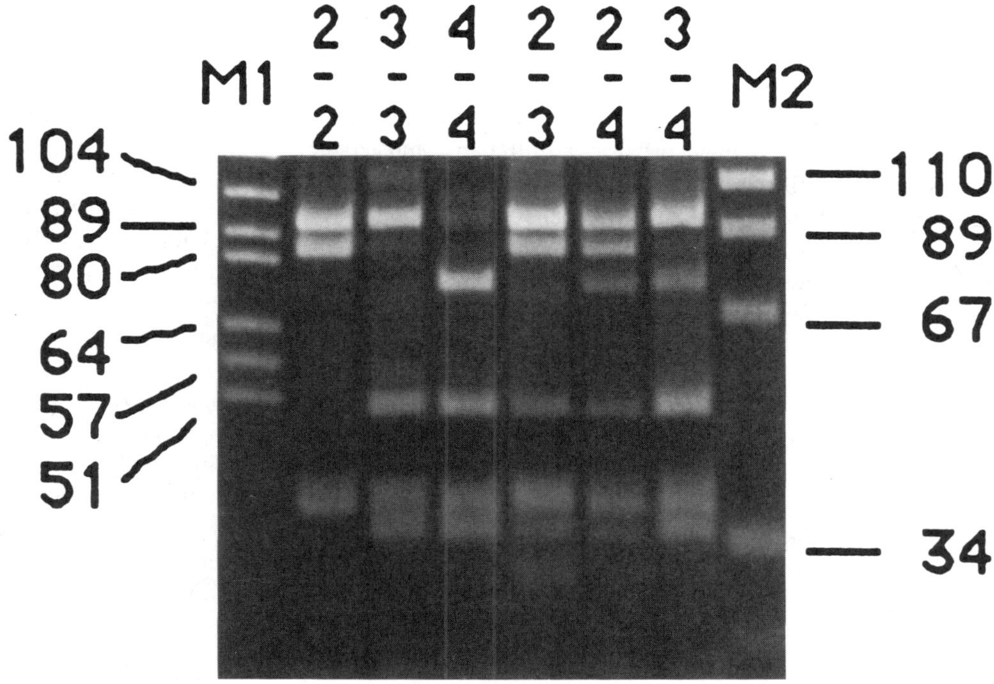

Figure 1. Apo E restriction patterns.

3. RESULTS

The data are summarised in Table 1. Within the AD group the number of individuals with a single or double dose of the ε4 allele was significantly increased with respect to the control group ($\chi^2 = 4.918$, $p < 0.05$).

The same increase in ε4 carriers can also be seen in VaD ($p < 0.01$, Fisher's exact test). There were no statistically significant differences between the control and DS groups.

Figure 2 relates ApoE genotype to the age at onset of AD symptoms. While in general the age of onset of AD symptoms is slightly lower for patients with one or two ε4 alleles, this difference is not statistically significant (log rank test, $p > 0.55$).

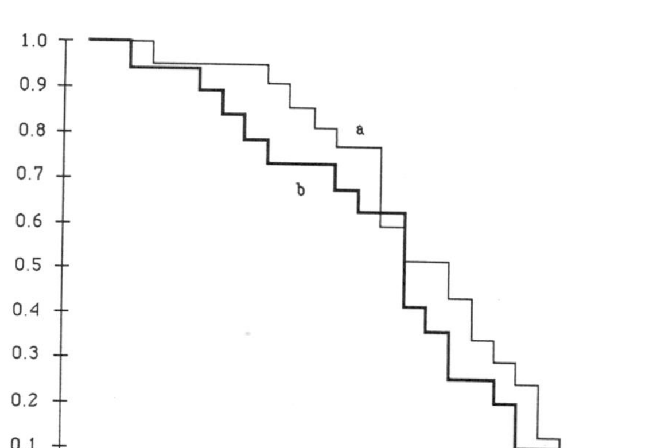

Figure 2. Onset curve showing the proportion of patients unaffected by AD symptoms after the age of 60 years. The bold curve (b) represents patients carrying one or two copies of the ε4 allele. Two patients were homozygotes for ε4 and had onset at ages 65 and 75. The remainder of the ε4 carriers had the ε3/ε4 genotype. The lighter curve (a) represents patients without an ε4 allele.

4. DISCUSSION

The results of this study agree with the previously reported association between the ε4 and AD[1,8]. However, at least in this group of patients, this can be seen also in the VaD group. Our findings are in accordance with Italian[2,8] and Japanese[9] reports.

We can confirm a general trend in the relationship between ApoE genotype and the age at onset of AD, but this lacked statistical significance. The discrepancy may be related to sample size. However, the same analysis has been used with similar numbers[19]. Since the diagnostic criteria used in other studies have been reproduced exactly by us, it is unlikely that the difference seen here could be abscribed to variance in the diagnosis of dementia or in the dimention of the sample. The reported elevated frequency of ε4 carriers in VaD[2,8,9] and recently in motor neuron disease[20] points to a much broader role for ApoE in neurological disorders. In particular Apo E alleles may confer a different vascular risk in that ε4 elevates plasma LDL cholesterol and accelerates the development of atherosclerosis whereas ε3 and ε2 yield lower risk. Moreover, since ApoE is involved in growth and repair processes in the nervous system[21], it is possible that this function may offer an explanation for the part played by the protein in neurological disorders[9]. In addition, the connection between the ε4 allele and other amyloid-forming conditions, such as Creutzfeldt-Jakob disease and DS, is still under question. Amouyel *et al.*[19] reported a strong link between ε4 and Creutzfeldt-Jakob disease, but other reports are not in keeping with this.[13,22,23]

Moreover, despite the fact that ε4 has been related to increased amyloid deposition also in DS[10], the lowest ever ε4 frequency for an AD population was recorded in a sample of DS patients with AD[14]. In our group of DS subjects, which was not characterized by neuro-psychological analysis, there were no statistically significant differences in genotype frequencies compared with controls.

On the basis of the data presented here it seems that the ApoE test is of limited utility in the differential diagnosis of dementia. Nonetheless, it appears that ε4 is a risk factor for the development of dementia and that ApoE genotype is useful in the identification of high-risk subjects.

ACKNOWLEDGMENTS

The authors wish to thank ViviDown, Milano, Dr G. Guerrini at the Istituto Arici Sega, Brescia, and Dr B. Bernardini at the Istituto Redaelli, Milano, for the provision of some blood samples. Statistical analysis was performed by Dr C. Zocchetti, Università di Milano. Dr A. Ryan is the holder of a research grant from AGER, The Association for Geriatric Research and the Study of Longevity, Milano. This project was partly funded by Ricerca Corrente Ospedale Maggiore, IRCCS, Milano.

REFERENCES

1. Corder EH, Saunders AM, Strittmatter WJ, Schmechel DE, Gaskell PC, Small GW, Roses AD, Haines JL and Pericak-Vance MA. Gene dose of Apolipoprotein E type 4 allele and the risk of Alzheimer's disease in late onset families. Science 1993; 261: 921–923.
2. Frisoni GB, Calabresi L, Geroldi C, Bianchetti A, D'Acquarica AL, Govoni S, Sirtori CR, Trabucchi M and Franceschini G. Apolipoprotein E ε4 allele in Alzheimer's disease and Vascular dementia. Dementia 1994; 5: 240–242.

3. Polvikoski T, Sulkava R, Haltia M, Kainulainen K, Vuorio A, Verkkoniemi A, Niinisto L, Halonen P and Kontula K. Apolipoprotein E, dementia and cortical deposition of β-amyloid protein. N Engl J Med 1995; 333: 1242–1247.
4. Talbot C, Lendon C, Craddock N. Protection against Alzheimer's disease with apoE ε2. Lancet 1994; 343: 1432–1433.
5. Nacmias B, Latorraca S, Piersanti P, Forleo P, Piacentini S, Bracco L, Amaducci L and Sorbi S. ApoE genotype and familial Alzheimer's disease: a possible influence on age of onset in APP717 Val->Ile mutated families. Neurosci Lett 1995; 183: 1–3.
6. Sorbi S, Nacmias B, Forleo P, Piacentini S, Latorraca S, Amaducci L. Epistatic effect of APP717 and Apolipoprotein E genotype in familial Alzheimer's disease. Ann Neurol 1995; 38: 124–127.
7. Roses AD. Apolipoprotein E genotyping in the differential diagnosis, not prediction, of Alzheimer's disease. (Point of View) Ann Neurol 1995; 38: 6–14.
8. Frisoni GB, Bianchetti A, Govoni S, Trabucchi M, Calabresi L, Franceschini G. Association of Apolipoprotein E e4 with vascular dementia. (Letter) JAMA 1994; 271(17): 1317.
9. Noguchi S, Murakami K, Yamada N. Apolipoprotein E genotype and Alzheimer's disease. Lancet 1993; 342:737–738.
10. Hyman BT, West HL, Rebeck GW, Lai F, Mann DM. Neuropathological changes in Down's syndrome hippocampal formation. Effect of age and apolipoprotein E genotype. Arch. Neurol 1995; 52: 373–378.
11. Pickering-Brown S, Mann DM, Bourke JP, Roberts DA, Balderson D, Burns A, Byrne J and Owen F. Apolipoprotein E4 and Alzheimer's disease pathology in Lewy body disease and in other b-amyloid-forming diseases. Lancet 1994; 343: 1155.
12. Hardy J, Crook R, Perry R, Raghaven R, Roberts G. ApoE genotype and Down's syndrome. Lancet 1994; 343: 979–980.
13. Saunders AM, Schmader K, Breitner JCS, Benson MD, Brown WT, Goldfarb L, Goldgaber D, Manwaring MG, Szymanski MH, McCown N, Dole KC, Schmechel DE, Strittmatter WJ, Pericak-Vance MA and R-oses AD. Apolipoprotein E ε4 allele distributions in late-onset Alzheimer's disease and in other amyloid forming diseases.Lancet 1993; 342: 710–711.
14. Van Gool WA, Evenhuis HM, Van Duijn CM. A case control study of Apolipoprotein E genotypes in Alzheimer's disease associated with Down's syndrome. Ann Neurol 1995; 38: 225–230.
15. Sorbi S, Nacmias B, Forleo P, Piacentini S, Amaducci L. Alzheimer's disease and apolipoprotein E in Italy. Ann N Y Acad Sci 1996; 777: 260–265.
16. McKahn G, Drachman D, Folstein M, Katzmann R, Price D, Stadlan EM. Clinical diagnosis of Alzheimer's disease: Report of the NINCDS-ADRDA work group under the auspices of Department of Health and Human Services task force on Alzheimer's disease. Neurology 1994; 34: 939–944.
17. Roman GC, Tatemichi TK, Erkinjuntti T, Cummings JL, Masdeu JC, Garcia JH, Amaducci L, Orgogozo JM, Brun A, Hofman A, Moody DM, O'Brien MD, Yamaguchi T, Grafman J, Drayer BP, Bennet DA, Fisher M, Ogata J, Kokmen E, Bermejo F, Wolf PA, Gorelick PB, Bick KL, Pajeau AK, Bell MA, De Carli C, Culebras A, Korczyn AD, Bogousslavski J, Hartmann A and Scheinberg P. Vascular dementia: diagnostic criteria for research studies. Report of the NINDS-AIRDEN International workshop. Neurology 1993; 43: 250–260.
18. Hixon JE, Vernier DT. Restriction isotyping of human apolipoprotien E by gene amplification and cleavage with HhaI. J. Lip. Res 1990; 31: 545- 548.
19. Amouyel P, Vidal O, Launay JM, Laplanche JL. The Apolipoprotein E alleles as a major susceptibility factors of Creutzfeldt-Jakob disease. Lancet 1995; 344: 1315–1318.
20. Al-Chalabi A, Enayat ZE, Bakker MC, Sham PC, Ball DB, Shaw CE, Lloyd CM, Powell JF and Leigh PN. Association of Apolipoprotein E ε4 allele with bulbar-onset motor neuron disease. Lancet 1996; 347: 159–160.
21. Mahley RW. Apolipoprotein E: Cholesterol transport protein with expanding role in cell biology. Science 1988: 240; 622–630.
22. Nakagawa Y, Kitamoto T, Furukawa H, Ogomori K, Tateishi J. Apolipoprotein E in Creutzfeldt-Jakob disease. Lancet 1995; 345: 68.
23. Salvatore M, Seeber AC, Nacmias B, Petraroli R, D'Alessandro M, Sorbi S, Pocchiari M. Apolipoprotein E in sporadic and familial Creutzfeldt-Jakob disease. Neurosci Lett 1995; 199 (2): 95–98.
24. Schupf N, Kapell D, Lee JH, Zigman W, Canto B, Tycko B, Mayeux R. Onset of dementia is associated with Apolipoprotein E ε4 in Down's syndrome. Ann Neurol 1996; 40: 799–781.

19

RISK FACTORS FOR DELIRIUM IN THE ELDERLY

Gianfranco Salvioli* and Chiara Mussi

University of Modena
Department of Internal Medicine
Geriatric and Gerontology Section
Modena, Italy

1. INTRODUCTION

Delirium is defined as an organic brain syndrome with global cognitive impairment of abrupt onset and relatively short duration (usually less than 1 month) and with concurrent disturbance of attention, sleep-wake cycle and psychomotor behaviour (1). No formal guidelines exist to recognize this syndrome, which remains a clinical diagnosis: the current criteria are chiefly characterized by changes in consciousness and cognition during a brief period (Table 1) (2); advanced age is a crucial variable in delirium: DSM IV has made great progress in including age-related conditions that were not present in previous DSMs.

Although the prevalence of delirium in older inpatients is 10 to 25% and it is associated with a mortality up to 40%, significantly increased hospital length of stay, istitutionalization and functional disability, little is known about its pathophysiology (3). Unfortunately this common picture is frequently unrecognized expecially in old patients (4): in a study, 32% of cases went unrecognized by physicians (5). This is important since the mean length of hospitalization for patients with delirium is longer than for nondelirious controls (about 10 days) (6).

Sometimes delirium shows a non-specific presentation, above all in the elderly; it is often misdiagnosed as depression or psychosis, or misattributed to dementia or senescence. The problems are many: the essential features of delirium are not directly rated and often incomplete or difficult to identify. Many efforts have been done to increase the recognition of delirium in the elderly to improve the outcomes: DSM criteria remain the gold standard to make the precise diagnosis, but screening for its presence and the quantifica-

* Correspondence address: Prof. Gianfranco Salvioli, Ospedale Estense, Viale Vittorio Veneto 9, 41100 Modeno, Italy. Tel: 39 59 436082.

Recent Advances in Geriatrics, edited by Barbagallo, Licata, and Sowers.
Plenum Press, New York, 1998.

Table 1. Diagnostic criteria for delirium

1. Disturbance of consciousness (that is, reduced clarity of awareness of the environment) in conjunction with reduced ability to focus, sustain, or shift attention
2. A change in cognition (such as memory deficit, disorientation, or language disturbance) or the development of a perceptual disturbance that is no better accounted for by a preexisting, established, or evolving dementia
3. Development of the disturbance during a brief period (usually hours to days) and a tendency for fluctuation during the course of the day
4. Evidence from the history, physical examination, or laboratory findings that the disturbance is caused by
   a. A general medical condition
   b. A substance intoxication or side effects
   c. A substance withdrawal
   d. Multiple factors

From *Diagnostic and Statistical Manual of Mental Disorders*, Fourth Edition (2).

tion of its symptoms is best accomplished using other assessment instruments (7). The Confusion Assessment Method (table 2) has been developed to be used in the elderly by nonpsychiatric clinicians, but its sensitivity, though a high specificity, is poor (6).

Other instruments are available: the Saskatoon Delirium Checklist was assessed to rate symptoms derived from DSM III-R according to how often the single feature (e.g. altered attention, hallucinations, modified sleep-wake cycle etc.) was present; though not validated, this scale permits to weight delirious symptoms one by one, even if the patient doesn't develope the complete picture of delirium (8). The Delirium Symptom Interview has been created by an interdisciplinary group and has been proposed as a reliable method for identifying hospitalized patients having key symptoms of delirium (9): it offers independent evaluation of delirium features, but it has not been validated for it doesn't distinguish delirium from dementia. The Delirium Symptom Rating Scale distinguishes patients whose delirium improved within 1 week from patients who didn't show changes during the same period: the former had a significantly lower score than the latter (10).

Table 2. The Confusion Assessment Method (CAM) diagnostic algorithm

Feature 1. Acute onset and fluctuating course

This feature is usually obtained from a family member or nurse and is shown by positive responses to the following questions: Is there evidence of an acute change in mental status from the patient's baseline? Did the (abnormal) behaviour fluctuate during the day, that is, tend to come and go, or increase and decrease in severity?

Feature 2. Inattention

This feature is shown by a positive response to the following question: Did the patient have difficulty focusing attention, for example, being easily distractable, or having difficulty keeping track of what was being said?

Feature 3. Disorganized thinking

This feature is shown by a positive response to the following question: Was the patient's thinking disorganized or incoherent, such as rambling or irrelevant conversation, unclear or illogical flow of ideas, or unpredictable switching from subject to subject?

Feature 4. Altered level of consciousness

This feature is shown by any answer other than "alert" to the following question: Overall, how would you rate this patient's level of consciousness? (alert [normal], vigilant [hyperalert], lethargic [drowsy, easily aroused], stupor [difficult to arouse], or coma [unarousable])

The diagnosis of delirium by CAM requires the presence of feature 1 and 2 and either 3 or 4 (6).

2. RISK FACTORS FOR DELIRIUM IN THE ELDERLY

The development of a strategy to prevent the appearance of delirium requires the identification of risk factors, which can be predisposing or precipitating factors. The formers represent the vulnerability of the patient at hospital admission: advanced age, cognitive impairment, chronic and severe illness and disability are well identifiable conditions. On the other hand, it is difficult to define the independent contribution of predisposing and precipitating conditions; there are many situations in which a predisposing factor becomes a precipitating one and viceversa. It is important to keep in mind that delirium developed during hospitalization must be conceptually separated from delirium at admission (11). The comprehensive history and the physical examination are cornerstones of both the diagnosis and the evaluation of delirious patients; in particular, a detailed review of taken medication has great importance. Drugs, metabolic disturbances, dehydration, acute urinary retention, fever, environmental features, use of restraint, etc, have been proposed as principal precipitating factors; many others are listed in table 3 (11,12).

Few studies have been carried out to find a predictive model for the occurrence of delirium in hospitalized elderly medical patients based on the clinical features present at the admission. A strong univariate unadjusted association has been found between incident inhospital delirium and functional decline: delirious subjects lost a mean of one ADL as measured 3 months after hospital discharge (13). In a prospective study Inouye et al (14) identified four independent baseline risk factors using proportional hazards analysis: vision impairment, severe illness, cognitive impairment and a high urea nitrogen/creatinine ratio (Relative Risks: 3.5, 3.5, 2.8, 2.0, respectively); the four risk factors were tested in a separated cohort of patients to validate the model.

Many Authors have proposed other protocols to identify risk factors for delirium, but the outcomes are different one to another (table 4).

This is the principal reason why the National Institute of Health is organizing a complex study to obtain a better concordance in the evaluation of this scarcely known syndrome (22).

2.1. Postoperative Delirium

In 1955 Bedford reported on 120 elderly patients who developed postoperative "dementia" (23): the diagnosis of delirium was not already defined and probably those persons were affected by delirium more than true dementia. Many studies conducted in surgical

Table 3. Predisposing factors for delirium

Neurologic:	Dementia, stroke, seizure, head injury
Genitourinary:	Uremia, urosepsis, urinary retention
Cardiopulmonary:	Myocardial infarction, congestive heart failure, pulmonary embolism, pneumonia, hypoxia (from any cardiopulmonary disease), hypertensive encephalopathy
Gastrointestinal:	Hepatic encephalopathy, severe fecal impaction
Infections:	Potentially every kind of infection, sepsis
Metabolic:	Electrolyte abnormalities, fluid imbalance, hyper/hypoglycemia, hyper/hypothyroidism, hyper/hypothermia, vitamin deficiency (thiamin, folate), malnutrition
Drugs	(See chapter)
Miscellanea:	Advanced age, sensory deprivation and sensory overload, visual and auditory impairment, alcohol use/dependence, trauma (hip fractures, falls), recent surgical procedures, physical restraints

Table 4. Clinical studies regarding the appearance of delirium, its evaluation and associated conditions

Author	Study and cohort	Methods	Risk factors	Conclusions
Jitapunkul (15)	184 patients with acute illness (60–97 yrs)	DSM III at admission; serial use of AMT	Infections, stroke	D was present in 22% of patients; its presence suggested a poor prognosis; AMT, if repeated helps in the detection of D.
Inouye (14)	Two prospective cohort studies; 107 hospitalized elderly (>70 yrs) and a validation cohort of 174 comparable patients	CAM daily; APACHE II score; biochemical parameters	Vision impairment, severe illness, cognitive impairment, high urea/creatinine ratio	D developed in 25% of patients and 17% in the validation cohort; the predictive on 4 risk factors can be used at the admission to identify elderly at greatest risk.
Murray (13)	Predictive study on 325 hospitalized community and nursing home elderly; 3-6 months	DSM III criteria; monitored with DSI; daily ADL and PDS	Delirium is the only factor significantly associated with loss of function over time	Delirious subjects lost a mean of almost one ADL as measured 3 month after hospital discharge.
Rockwood (16)	12-month prospective descriptive study of 168 consecutively admitted patients	DSM IV and DSM iII criteria; Barthel index; MMSE		Prevalence of D: 18%; incidence of D: 7%; mean duration: 8 days. Complete symptoms recovery: only 52%.
Pompei (17)	432 patients (age>65 yrs, derivation cohort) and 323 (>70 yrs, test cohort)	DSM III R; CAM; MMSE	Cognitive impairment, burden of comorbidity, depression and alchoholism	D was present in 15% of derivation cohort population. In test cohort the predictive model was validated (26% developed D).
Fisher (18)	80 older patients undergoing elective orthopedic surgery	CAM; clock-drawing; MMSE	Male gender, clock-drawing score <6 (normal=10)	17.5% had postoperative D.
Inouye (19)	196 patients aged >70 yrs with no delirium (development cohort) and 312 comparable delirious patients (validation cohort)	CAM to define the onset of delirium at day 9	Physical restraint, malnutrition, more than 3 medications, use of bladder catheter and any iatrogenic event	Respectively 18 and 15% in development and validation cohorts developed D. The predictive model identifies elderly patients at risk for D.
Lerner (20)	199 community dwelling patients with dementia (retrospective study)	MMSE; ADL; Clinical Dementia Rating scores; Brief Psychiatric Rating Scale	Urinary tract infections, stressful events, surgery, medical illness, medications	22% of dementing patients had D; these had worse ADL scores and higher incidence of hallucination and paranoid delusions.
O'Keeffe (21)	225 patients admitted to an acute geriatric unit	DSM III criteria every 48 hours	Dementia, severe acute illness, multiple comorbid conditions, disability	D is an independent predictor of adverse outcomes in older hospital patients (as prolonged hospital stay and increased admission to long term care).

Abbreviations: ADL: Activity Daily Living; AMT: Abbreviated Mental Test; CAM: Confusion Assessment Method; D: delirium; DSI: Delirium Symptom Interview; MMSE: Mini Mental State Examination; PDS: Performance Daily Score; yrs: years.

populations had revealed the potential of a geriatric anesthesiologic program in preventing the onset of postsurgical confusion, the correlation of postoperative delirium with perioperative hypoxemia and the predictive value of quantitative electroencephalographic monitoring. Its incidence ranges from 10 to 60%; differences in diagnostic criteria, population under study and methods of surveillance account for the wide range of the results (24).

A key factor for explaining the pathogenesis of postoperative delirium seems to be either cerebral hypoxia which reduces the levels of neurotransmitters within the brain or the use of drugs with anticholinergic activity (8), but also the increased levels of serum cortisol due to the surgery stress could play a role (25). It is recommended to use anesthetics with shorter elimination half-lives; no difference in the effects of general, epidural, or spinal anesthesia has been found in postoperative confusion (24).

Postoperative delirium has a greater incidence in orthopedic than in general surgery (44–55% vs 10–14%). Two potential preoperative risk factors are male gender and a clock-drawing score of less than 6. An abnormal clock-drawing test seems to reflect alterations of the nondominant parietal lobe, which is associated not only with visuospatial activity, but also with maintenance of attention and integration of sensory informations — functions that are impaired in delirium (18).

2.2. Delirium and Drugs

Drug consumption is particularly high in older people and, as a result, side effects are often prevalent. Delirium is a dangerous side effect of many drugs frequently prescribed in the elderly: medications contribute to the onset of 22 to 39% of delirium cases. Diminished function of the central cholinergic neurotransmitter system is the most preminent proposed mechanism of delirium. Numerous medications with significant antimuscarinic action inhibiting brain postsynaptic receptors can cause drug-induced delirium, above all in older people. Changes in cholinergic brain receptors may increase the sensitivity to anticholinergic drugs (26). Alzheimer patients have been reported to be more sensitive to anticholinergic drugs because of severe depletion of cholinergic system: Sunderland et al. reported that central nervous system functions such as recognition and certain elements of behaviour were more compromized by temporary cholinergic blockade with scopolamine in patients with Alzheimer dementia than in normal-matched controls (27).

It is well established that many functions of the blood brain barrier change with age: as consequence, the passage of many drugs into cerebrospinal fluid of old patients is facilitated, as the contact of the molecules with muscarinic receptors. Moreover, the reduced metabolic activity of hepatic enzymes, as well as diminished liver blood flow, may decrease drug clearance. Impaired renal function may result in accumulation of active metabolites. Serum albumin is often decreased in the elderly because of malnutrition, severe illnesses and pressure sores; so, a high free fraction of drugs due to reduced albumin binding increases toxicity in old patients. The relative increase in body fat occurring in the elderly may cause accumulation and lower clearance of lipid-soluble compounds (28).

Older people are also at risk of receiving more than one medication with anticholinergic effect. The anticholinergic activity of many drugs and their metabolites is often unknown. So it is possible that a high serum anticholinergic activity and related symptoms could result from complicated medication regimens in which several drugs, some or all of which have modest anticholinergic effect, are prescribed.

Tune et al. (29) investigated the anticholinergic effects of the 24 drugs most frequently prescribed for the elderly; some of them are tipically associated with anticholinergic side effects, some others (e.g. warfarin) are not. Table 5 presents the anticholinergic

Table 5. Anticholinergic drug levels in 24 medications ranked by the frequency of their prescription for elderly patients

Medication[a]	Anticholinergic drug level (ng/ml of atropine equivalents)
Furosemide	0.22
Digoxin	0.25
Dyazide	0.08
Hydrochlorothiazide	0.00
Propranolol	0.00
Salicylic acid	0.00
Dipyridamole	0.11
Theophylline anydrous	0.44
Nitroglycerin	0.00
Insulin	0.00
Warfarin	0.12
Prednisolone	0.55
Alpha-methyldopa	0.00
Nifedipine	0.22
Isosorbide dinitrate	0.15
Ibuprofen	0.00
Codeine	0.11
Cimetidine	0.86
Diltiazem hydrochloride	0.00
Captopril	0.02
Atenolol	0.00
Metoprolol	0.00
Timolol	0.00
Ranitidine	0.22

[a]at a 10^{-8} M concentration (very close to common blood concentration) (29).

activity of commonly used medications: of the enounced drugs, 13 produced detectable anticholinergic effects and 9 of these (ranitidine, codeine, dipyridamole, warfarin, isosorbide, theophylline, nifedipine, digoxin and prednisolone) produced anticholinergic levels that are been shown to cause significant impairment in tests of recent memory and attention in normal elderly control subjects (8).

Physostigmine challenge test (1–2 mg) has been proposed to diagnose delirium due to central anticholinergic toxicity, but it has not been evaluated in elderly patients (30).

3. CAN DELIRIUM BE PREVENTED?

Delirium in the elderly is a multifactorial syndrome in which predisposing associated factors (table 4) can amplify the effects of many precipitating risk factors (19).

Inouye and Charpentier identified five risk factors (use of psychoactive medications, dehydration, immobility, sensory impairment, indwelling catheters) and proposed a model to predict the developement of delirium during the first 9 days of hospitalization; even though baseline factors play an important role in determining delirium; the five precipitating factors are modifiable with intervention strategies that could prevent the onset of delirium (19). This is particularly relevant since delirium, as mentioned before, is associated with increased morbidity and mortality with a great impact on health care costs. Early recognition of the syndrome is essential; the possibility to prevent delirium should be proved in clinical trials. The prognosis of the elderly with delirium could be influenced by concomitant severe physical illness or dementia; nevertheless, the outcomes in studies that exclude subjects with dementia are similar to those including them (22).

4. CONCLUSIONS

These findings emphasize the need to prevent delirium in the hospitalized elderly. A correct assessment at the admission and during hospital stay for the presence of known risk factors for delirium should be carried out to improve the prevention of this clinical feature so strongly associated to functional decline, prolonged hospital stay and increased admission to long term care. A validated method for the early diagnosis of delirium has not jet been defined (11,31). The correct evaluation of predisposing factors seems a key point to identify the elderly at risk of delirium during hospitalization. Many risk factors such as polipharmacy, immobility, dehydration, physical restraints, bladder catheter and others, must be revised with appropriate protocol: the importance of these conditions is that they are modifiable by appropriate interventions; the outcomes could be not only the reduced incidence of confusion but also the prevention of functional decline (21,22). Therefore the correction of reversible underlying causes and the limitated use of the above mentioned drugs and restraints (where it is possible) represent the basis for the prevention of delirium; on the other hand it is of great importance for the delirious patient to avoid unfamiliar surrounding and to help him with constant orientation, intervention that must be recommended in every geriatric ward.

REFERENCES

1. Lipowsky ZJ (1983). Transient cognitive disorders (delirium, acute confusional state) in the elderly. Am J Psychiatry, 140, 1426–1436.
2. American Psychiatric Association (1994). Diagnostic and Statistical Manual of Mental Disorders. 4th ed. Washington (DC): American Psychiatric Association, 123–133.
3. Mach JR jr, Dysken MW, Kuskowski M, Richelson E, Holden L, & Jilk KM (1995). Serum anticholinergic activity in hospitalized older persons with delirium: a preliminary study. J Am Geriatr Soc, 43, 491–495.
4. Levkoff SE, Evans DA, Liptzin B, Cleary PD, Lipsitz LA, Wetle TT, Reilly CH, Pilgrim DM, Schor J, & Rowe J (1992). Delirium. The occurrence and persistence of symptoms among elderly hospitalized patients. Arch Intern Med, 152, 334–340.
5. Inouye SK, Van Dick CH, Alessi CA, Balkin S, Siegal AP, & Horwitz RI (1990). Clarifying confusion: the Confusion Assessment Method. A new method for detection of delirium. Ann Intern Med, 113, 941–948.
6. Thomas RI, Cameron DJ, & Fahs MC (1988). A prospective study of delirium and prolonged hospital stay. Exploratory study. Arch Gen Psychiatry, 45, 937–949.
7. Trzepac PT, Baker RW, & Greenhouse J (1988). A symptom rating scale for delirium. J Psychiatr Res, 23, 89–97.
8. Miller PS, Richardson JS, Jyu CA, Lemay JS, Hiscock M, & Keegan DL (1988). Association of low serum anticholinergic levels and cognitive impairment in elderly presurgical patients. Am J Psychiatry, 145, 342–345.
9. Albert MS, Levkoff SE, Reilly CH, Liptzin B, Pilgrim DM, Cleary PD, Evans DA, & Rowe J (1992). The Delirium Symptom Interview: an interview for the detection of delirium symptoms in hospitalized patients. J Geriatr Psychiatr Neurol, 5, 14–21.
10. Wada Y, & Yamaguchi N (1993). Delirium in the elderly: relationship of clinical symptoms to outcome. Dementia, 4, 113–116.
11. Inouye S (1994). The dilemma of delirium: clinical and research controversies regarding diagnosis and evaluation of delirium in hospitalized elderly medical patients. Am J Med, 97, 278–288.
12. Seymour DG, Henschke PJ, Cape RDT, & Campbell AC (1980). Acute confusional states and dementia in the elderly: the role of dehydration, volume depletion, physical illness and age. Age Aging, 9, 137–146.

13. Murray AM, Levkoff SE, Wetle TT, Beckett L, Cleary PD, Schor JD, Lipsitz LA, Rowe JW, & Evans DA (1993). Acute delirium and functional decline in the hospitalized elderly patients. J Gerontol, 48, M181-M186.
14. Inouye SK, Viscoli CM, Horwitz RI, Hurst LD, & Tinetti ME (1993). A predictive model for delirium in hospitalized elderly medical patients based on admission characteristics. Ann Intern Med, 119, 474–481.
15. Jitapunkul S, Pillay I, & Ebrahim S (1992). Delirium in newly admitted elderly patients: a prospective study. Quart J Med, 300, 307–314.
16. Rockwood K (1993). The occurence and duration of symptoms in elderly patients with delirium. J Gerontol, 48, M162-M166.
17. Pompei P, Foreman M, Rudberg MA, Inouye SK, Braund V, & Cassel CK (1994). Delirium in hospitalized older persons: outcomes and predictors. J Am Geriatr Soc, 42, 809–815.
18. Fisher BW,& Flowerdew G (1995). A simple model for predicting postoperative delirium in older patients undergoing elective orthopedic surgery. J Am Geriatr Soc, 43, 175–178.
19. Inouye SK,& Charpentier PA (1996). Precipitating factors for delirium in hospitalized elderly persons. Predictive model and interrelationship with baseline vulnerability. JAMA, 275, 852–857.
20. Lerner AJ, Hedera P, Koss E, Stukey J, & Friedland RP (1997). Delirium in Alzheimer Disease. Alzh Dis Assoc Disord, 11, 16–20.
21. O'Keeffee S, & Lavan J (1997). The prognostic significance of delirium in older hospital patients. J Am Geriatr Soc, 45, 174–178.
22. Francis J (1997). Outcomes of delirium: can systems of care make a difference? J Am Geriatr Soc, 45, 247–248.
23. Bedford PD (1955). Adverse cerebral effects of anaesthesia on old people. Lancet, II, 259–263.
24. Parikh SS, & Chung F (1995). Postoperative delirium in the elderly. Anaesth Analg, 80, 1223–1232.
25. Gustafson Y, Brannstrom B, Berggren D, Ragnarsson JI, Sigaard J, Bucht G, Reitz S, Norberg A, & Winblad B (1991). A geriatric-anaesthesiologic program to reduce acute confusional states in the elderly patients treated for femoral neck fractures. J Am Geriatr Soc, 39, 655–662.
26. Fastbom J, Claesson CB, Cornelius C, Thorslund M, & Winblad B (1995). The use of medicines with anticholinergic effects in older people: a population study in urban area of Sweden. J Am Geriatr Soc, 43, 1135–1140.
27. Sunderland T, Tariot PN, Cohen RM, Wiengartner H, Mueller EA, & Murphy DL (1987). Anticholinergic sensitivity in patients with dementia of the Alzheimer type and age-matched controls. A dose-response study. Arch Gen Psychiatry, 44, 418–426.
28. Mooradian AD (1994). Potential mechanisms of the age-related changes in the blood-brain barrier. Neurobiol Aging, 15, 751–755.
29. Tune L, Carr S, Hoag E, & Cooper T (1992). Anticholinergic effects of drugs commonly prescribed for the elderly: potential means for assessing risk of delirium. Am J Psychiatry, 149, 1393–1394.
30. Mogelnicki SR, Waller JL, & Finlayson DC (1979). Physostigmine reversal of cimetidine-induced mental confusion. JAMA, 241, 826–827.
31. Rockwood K, Cosway S, Stolee P, Kydd D, Carver D, Jarrett P, & O'Brien B (1994). Increasing the recognition of delirium in elderly patients. J Am Geriatr Soc, 42, 252–256.

20

DEFINITION OF OUTCOMES IN A DEMENTIA EVALUATION AND REHABILITATION UNIT

Cristina Geroldi, Angelo Bianchetti, and Marco Trabucchi

Geriatric Research Group
Brescia, Italy
IRCCS S. Giovanni di Dio
Sacro Cuore Fatebenefratelli Hospital
Brescia, Italy

SUMMARY

In geriatric medicine, outcome as measure of the quality of care has made up of importance only in the last decade. In the care of irreversible dementia, the recovery is not a reachable goal, but a number of outcomes can be identified. The improvement of clinical picture (daily function, cognition, and behavioral disturbances), of the somatic symptoms and of the quality of life in the demented patients can be reached and easily assessed during a relatively brief stay in a Dementia Evaluation and Rehabilitation Unit.

INTRODUCTION

The quality of care and services in medicine can be defined according to different domains (structures, processes, output, and outcome). In several medical fields (e.g., surgery, cardiology) measures of outcome are considered of primary importance in determining quality of treatment. In geriatric medicine, and even more so in the care of dementia patients, only recently outcomes acquired attention and a major role in measuring quality of care.

Impairment of cognitive function represent one of the more prevalent cause of disability in the elderly, affecting about 10–15% of people older than 65, and 25–50% of those aged 85 and over, in the general population, and 50–80% of the subjects living in nursing homes (1,2). Several clinical entities are associated with cognitive impairment in the elderly, such as delirium, dementia syndrome, depressive pseudodementia, paranoid states and other psychoses. Dementia has a number of causes: Alzheimer's disease is the most frequent (50–60%), multi-infarct dementia and mixed forms account for 20–30% of cases, and 5–10% of patients have potentially reversible causes (3). Imprecise definition and incomplete differential diagnoses have led to the underdiagnosis, misdiagnosis, or

Recent Advances in Geriatrics, edited by Barbagallo, Licata, and Sowers.
Plenum Press, New York, 1998.

overdiagnosis of dementia syndrome in many clinical settings. Inappropriate management of patients affected by dementia can increase mortality and morbidity, determine worse quality of life of patients and caregivers, and increase health care expenditures. Are reduction of morbidity and mortality -the historically basic goals in the care of demented patients- the only possible outcomes in non-reversible dementia? Is it possible to characterize "positive outcomes", and to aim at sensible and clinically relevant treatment-induced improvements in the course of a fatally progressive disease? What is the appropriate clinical setting to reach "positive outcomes"?

In the last 20 years different health services were designed to diagnose dementia more accurately and to improve the care of patients. Aims of these services (diagnostic evaluation, treatment/referral, case management, research, training and continuing education, rehabilitation programs, special programs of care), their target subjects (outpatients, inpatients, nursing home residents), organization, and costs are specific.

In June 1991, the first Italian Dementia Evaluation and Rehabilitation Unit, a hospital ward for demented patients, started in Brescia. It is devoted to the diagnosis and treatment of complex cases of dementia syndromes, to the formation of physicians and nurses, to establish protocols and the control of the cost-benefit ratio of dementia services.

Aim of the paper is to define possible clinical outcome in the care of demented patients admitted in our Dementia Evaluation and Rehabilitation Unit.

METHODS

The Dementia Evaluation and Rehabilitation Unit is a multidisciplinary center designed to provide comprehensive assessment of medical, psychological and social problems of the demented elderly, to provide them with therapy, rehabilitation, counseling, and social, legal and ethical support (4), to provide the formation of physicians and nurses, to establish protocols and the control of the cost-benefit ratio. The unit consists in a 40-bed ward for inpatients, a day hospital service for 10 outpatients, an outpatient clinic, and a laboratory. The staff in the unit consists of two full-time neurologists, two full-time geriatricians, one full-time psychiatrist, one full-time neuro-psychologist, six full-time medical fellows, 12 full-time nurses, one full-time social worker, two full-time physical therapists, 6 full-time occupational therapists, 16 full-time hospital attendants, 4 full-time and 2 part-time biologists. Patients are referred to the outpatient clinic by their family doctors or by others specialist (mainly neurologists, geriatricians or psychiatrists), and undergo a pre-admission visit. Only part (about 20%) of patients observed in the outpatient clinic needing accurate diagnostic evaluation, or hospital care and rehabilitation, are admitted to the inpatient clinic or to the day hospital.

During their stay in the ward, patients undergo a complete clinical evaluation including:

1. Comprehensive personal and family history, collected partially from the patients, and mainly from the patients' relatives by a medical fellow;
2. Somatic and neurological examination performed by a neurologist and a geriatrician, respectively;
3. Routine laboratory tests including blood cells count, erythrocyte sedimentation rate, urinalysis, determination of serum creatinin, urea nitrogen, electrolytes, glucose, bilirubin, vitamin B12 and folic acid levels, thryroid function tests (triiodothyronin, thyroxin, and thyrotropin levels), liver function tests (aspartate

and alanine aminotransferase), serologic test for syphilis (VDRL), hepatitis B antigens and hepatitis C antibody determination;
4. Electrocardiography;
5. Electroencephalography;
6. Chest radiography;
7. Brain CT scan;
8. Clinical neuropsychological testing performed by a neurologist, and formal neuropsychological testing by a psychologist, as previously described (5). In particular, MMSE (6) was administered to all patients, while Logical Memory Test (7), Rey-Osterreith Figure Copy and Recall (8), Digit Span Forward and Backward (9), Clock Drawing Test (10), Raven's Progressive Matrices (11), Letter and Category Word Fluency Test (12), Token Test (7) and Wisconsin Card Sorting Test (13) were administered whenever allowed by dementia severity;
9. Other laboratory tests and instrumental examinations such as lumbar puncture, brain magnetic resonance imaging, single photon emission tomography with 99Tc-HM-PAO or 123I-IBZM performed when the standard clinical evaluation is not enough for the diagnostic definition of neurological disease causing the cognitive impairment;
10. Echography, endoscopy, 24-hour electrocardiography recording, echocardiography, and computed tomography or magnetic resonance imaging of organs other than the brain were performed as needed for a more accurate diagnosis of the somatic diseases associated with cognitive impairment.

Diagnosis of dementia is made according to DSM-IV criteria (14), and of probable Alzheimer's disease (AD), Vascular dementia (VaD), Dementia with Lewy Body (DLB), Frontotemporal dementia (FTD), Slowly progressive aphasia, Creutzfeldt-Jakob's disease, Alcohol induced persisting dementia, according to NINCDS-ADRDA (15), NINDS-AIREN criteria (16), Lund and Manchester criteria (17), report of the consortium on DLB international workshop (18), Mesulam criteria (19,20), Masters et al. criteria (21), and DSM-IV criteria (14), respectively.

Severity of cognitive impairment is assessed with Clinical Dementia Rating scale (22), scoring from 0 (no cognitive impairment) to 5 (greatest severity of cognitive and functional impairment).

Basic activities of daily living are collected with the Barthel index (23), and directly evaluated with the Brief Assessment of Nursing Severity Scale (BANSS) (24,25), having a greater sensitivity in recognition of different level of severity in the latest stages of dementia.

Gait and balance are assessed with the Tinetti Scale (26)

Behavioral disturbances are quantified with UCLA Neuro Psychiatry Inventory (NPI) scale (27), assessing presence, frequency and severity of: delusions, hallucinations, agitation, depression, anxiety, apathy, disinhibition, euphoria, irritability, abnormal motor behavior, sleeping disturbances, and eating disturbances. Frequency of each disturbance is computed with a score ranging from 1 (presence of disturbance less than once a week) to 4 (presence of disturbance at least once a day); severity with a score ranging from 1 (lowest severity) to 3 (highest severity). Total score for each symptom is the product of frequency and severity; total score for the scale is the sum of total scores of all the 12 symptoms.

Subjective physical health is evaluated with a scale assessing 12 somatic domains (28): 1. hands, arms, shoulders; 2. feet, legs, hips; 3. back and neck; 4. head and face; 5. lungs and breath; 6. heart and vessels; 7. mouth and mastication; 8. guts and digestion; 9.

kidneys and urinary function; 10. eyes and sight; 11. ears and hearing; 12. other. Complain of somatic symptoms is recorded, and successively pain and discomfort are assessed for each other domain. For each domain pain and discomfort, functioning, and impact on daily activities (i.e. the degree of impairment in daily activities due to pain and discomfort or to malfunctioning of a given apparatus) are assessed. Two scores (each with a 0–12 range) are then obtained according to: 1) number of domains spontaneously reported as causing pain and discomfort (Symptoms Spontaneously Reported, SSR), and 2) number of domains causing pain and discomfort reported only after explicit inquiry (Symptoms Reported After Inquiry, SRAI).

Non-pharmachologic interventions carried out on patients were thus categorized: cognitive rehabilitation (Global Remotivation Therapy), formal or informal occupational therapy, and physical rehabilitation.

Subjects of the study were 193 consecutive patients with cognitive impairment admitted to the inpatient ward of the Dementia Evaluation and Rehabilitation Unit, Sacro Cuore Fatebenefratelli Hospital, Brescia, Italy, between June 1, and December 31, 1996.

We defined outcomes as changes of clinical status and perception of quality of life during the stay in the ward, evaluated in 4 domains: global cognition, physical function, behavior, and complain of somatic symptoms (markers of well-being and subjective physical health). Therefore:

1. Mini Mental State Examination (6), as measure of global cognitive function, was administered on the day of admission, and on the day before the discharge by the same clinician;
2. Barthel index (23) as marker of physical function was collected by a clinician from a relative (the principal caregiver, when possible) on admission, and from nurses caring the patient on discharge;
3. Brief Assessment of Nursing Severity Scale (24,25), as measure of physical function, was evaluated on admission and on discharge by the same nurses and clinicians staff;
4. Tinetti Scale (26) was performed on admission and 1 or 2 days before the discharge by a rehabilitation therapist;
5. UCLA Neuro Psychiatry Inventory (NPI) scale (27) was administered by the same clinician to a relative on admission, and to the nurses staff on discharge;
6. Complain of somatic symptoms was evaluated on the day of admission, and on the day of the discharge by the same clinician.

Since misdiagnosis of dementia syndrome can cause inappropriate management of patients affected by dementia, diagnostic definition of cognitive disturbance, can be considered both a process and an outcomes of our ward. Cognitive diagnosis on admission and on discharge were, therefore, kept into account.

Other variables were collected to provide better description of the sample:

1. Socio-demographic characteristics: gender, age, education (years of formal schooling), disease duration, computed in months, and defined from the time of onset of memory disturbances that exceeded the episodic forgetfulness that might have been regarded as usual for the patient, or of other disturbances (language, praxis, orientation, visuo-spatial skills) clearly related to the disease;
2. Principal cause of admission in the ward;
3. Length of stay in the ward (in days) computed from the day of the admission, excluding the day of the discharge;

4. Somatic health was operationalized as number of chronic diseases among a list of the 15 most frequent chronic conditions by Greenfield et al. (heart diseases of ischemic or organic pathogenesis, primary arrhytmias, congestive heart failure of pathogenesis other than ischemic or organic, hypertension, stroke, peripheral vascular diseases, diabetes mellitus, anemia, gastroenteric diseases, hepatobiliary diseases, renal diseases, respiratory diseases, parkinsonism and non-vascular neuroorganic diseases, muscoloskeletal disorders, malignancies) (29), and as other chronic conditions not included in the 16 considered by Greenfield (e.g. cognitive and psychiatric diseases, skin diseases, ear and eye diseases, malnutrition). Acute diseases potentially causing pain and discomfort were also detected.
5. Number of drugs on discharge.

Statistical analysis was made using SPSS 6.0.1 package (30). The "Δ" scores of MMSE score, Barthel index, BANSS, Tinetti scale, UCLA-NPI scale are the difference of the score on discharge and the score on admission.

The study was approved by the local ethics committee.

RESULTS

The principal socio-demographic and clinical features of the whole sample of 193 consecutive patients under study are shown in Table 1. The most frequent cause of admission was the first diagnosis of a cognitive disturbance, followed by therapy of behavioral disturbances; a quarter of patients were admitted because of onset of acute somatic diseases or needing physical rehabilitation, whereas only about 6% were admitted in the ward to undergo follow up of clinical picture. About half of patients were diagnosed affected by Alzheimer's Dementia, about another quarter by Vascular Dementia or Vascular cognitive Impairment (12 cases) (31), and about 10% was affected by other forms of dementia. The great majority of subjects came from home, and only 12 patients came to our observation from a nursing home. In contrast, on discharge 25 patients were institutionalized.

On admission only less than one third of the patients had a diagnosis of cognitive disturbance (see Table 2) confirmed after complete assessment. About half of patients were admitted in the ward without a cognitive diagnosis nor diagnostic hypothesis, and about a quarter had an aspecific diagnosis of cognitive disturbance (e.g. "Cognitive impairment", "Senile psycho-organic disturbance", "Aterosclerotic dementia"), or a diagnostic definition that was not confirmed after the assessment. Taking into account that the greatest majority of subjects admitted with a correct diagnosis have been previously admitted in our Dementia Evaluation and Rehabilitation Unit, it can be argued that only 10% of patients received a correct diagnosis of a cognitive disturbance in a traditional hospital or by their family doctors. Therefore, the diagnostic definition of the cognitive disturbances appear to have great importance, and must be considered one of the primary skills of our Dementia Evaluation and Rehabilitation Unit.

Global cognitive status, basic activities of daily living, physical function, behavioral disturbances, and subjective physical health (spontaneously reported and evoked somatic pain and discomfort) improved in the whole sample (see Table 3, part A). Excluding patients without dementia, only the improvement of spontaneously reported somatic pain and discomfort was not confirmed (see Table 3, part B). In particular, demented patients improved 1.5 points on MMSE score; about 5 points on Barthel index; about 2 points on BANS scale; about 2.5 points on Tinetti Scale, highly reducing the risk of fall; 20 points

Table 1. Socio-demographic features of 193 consecutive patients

	Proportion or mean ± SD
Gender (females)	136 (70.5)
Age	77.3 ± 8.1
Education (years)	5.3 ± 2.8
Disease duration (months)	41.0 ± 34.7
Coming from	
Home	89.7%
Nursing home	6.2%
Other ward	4.1%
Principal cause of admission	
Diagnosis of cognitive disturbance	47.3%
Behavioral disturbances	23.7%
Somatic disease	13.1%
Physical rehabilitation	10.0%
Follow-up	5.8%
Mean length of stay	34.9 ± 20.6
Diagnosis	
Probable or possible AD	50.3%
Probable or possible VaD, or VCI	23.8%
FTD or Pick's disease	4.2%
Parkinson dementia	2.1%
Dementia with Lewy body (DLB)	1.1%
Slowly progressive aphasia	1.1%
Alcohol induced persisting dementia	0.5%
Creutzfeldt-Jakob's disease	0.5%
Other dementias*	3.2%
Delirium	3.2%
Depression or other psychiatric disease	3.7%
Other neurological or somatic diseases without dementia**	6.3%
Dementia severity	
CDR 0	7.3%
CDR 0.5	14.0%
CDR 1	13.0%
CDR 2	16.6%
CDR 3	37.8%
CDR 4–5	11.4%
Formal cognitive rehabilitation	2.2%
Formal occupational therapy	34.6%
Formal physical rehabilitation	35.7%
Number of diagnosis on discharge	5.7 ± 3.0
Number of drugs on discharge	3.5 ± 2.0
Placement at discharge	
Home	80.5%
Nursing home	13.1%
Other ward	3.8%
Dead	2.7%

*"Other dementia" include: progressive sopranuclear palsy, cerebral tumor, luetic dementia, paraneoplastic dementia, Huntinghton's disease.

**"Other neurological or somatic diseases without dementia" include: Parkinson's disease, multiple system atrophy, previous neurosurgical intervention for cerebral tumor, subjective memory disturbance, Wernicke encephalitis, subdural hematoma, and ventriculo peritoneal shunt for normal pressure hydrocephalus, post-traumatic extrapyramidal syndrome.

Table 2. Diagnosis on discharge formulated in 193 consecutive patients subdivided in three groups according to the presence and the accuracy of the diagnosis on admission, in comparison with diagnosis formulated on discharge, after the diagnostic assessment

Diagnosis	Proportion
Correct # diagnosis on admission (30.5%)	
Probable or possible AD	56.0%
Probable or possible VaD/VCI	22.1%
FTD/pick	6.8%
DLB	—
Parkinson dementia	—
Creutzfeldt–Jakob's disease	—
Alcohol induced persisting dementia	—
Other dementia*	5.1%
Delirium	1.7%
Cognitive impairment due to depression or psychiatric disease	5.1%
Other neurological or somatic diseases without dementia**	3.4%
Absent diagnosis on admission (41.5%)	
Probable or possible AD	57.1%
Probable or possible VaD/VCI	23.4%
FTD/pick	2.6%
DLB	—
Parkinson dementia	1.3%
Creutzfeldt–Jakob's disease	—
Alcohol induced persisting dementia	1.3%
Other dementias*	2.6%
Delirium	1.4%
Cognitive impairment due to depression or psychiatric disease	5.2%
Other neurological or somatic diseases without dementia**	6.5%
Vague or wrong # diagnosis on admission (28.0%)	
Probable or possible AD	33.9%
Probable or possible VaD/VCI	26.5%
FTD/pick	3.8%
DLB	3.8%
Parkinson dementia	5.7%
Creutzfeldt–Jakob's disease	1.9%
Alcohol induced persisting dementia	—
Other dementias*	5.7%
Delirium	9.4%
Cognitive impairment due to depression or psychiatric disease	—
Other neurological or somatic diseases without dementia**	9.4%

#Diagnosis was defined "correct" when confirmed, and "wrong" when changed after the diagnostic assessment during the stay in the Dementia Evaluation and Rehabilitation Unit.

*"Other dementia" include: slowly progressive aphasia, progressive sopranuclear palsy, cerebral tumor, luetic dementia, paraneoplastic dementia, Huntington's disease.

**"Other neurological or somatic diseases without dementia" include: Parkinson's disease, multiple system atrophy, previous neurosurgical intervention for cerebral tumor, subjective memory disturbance, Wernicke encephalitis, subdural hematoma, and ventriculo peritoneal shunt for normal pressure hydrocephalus, post-traumatic extrapyramidal syndrome.

Table 3. Outcome measures in the whole sample and in 160 demented patients

	Admission mean ± SD	Discharge mean ± SD	p
Part A: Whole sample (n=193)			
Cognition			
MMSE	10.7 ± 8.4	12.6 ± 9.4	.000
Physical function			
Barthel index	59.5 ± 33.3	66.2 ± 31.1	.000
BANS scale	14.1 ± 5.2	12.0 ± 4.6	.000
Tinetti scale	15.8 ± 8.8	18.7 ± 8.2	.000
Behavior			
Behavioral disturbances (NPI scale)	34.1 ± 24.4	9.6 ± 9.5	.000
Complain of somatic symptoms			
Symptoms reported after inquiry	1.7 ± 1.8	1.1 ± 1.6	.000
Symptoms spontaneously reported	0.9 ± 1.1	0.7 ± 1.0	.025
Part B: Demented patients (n=160)			
Cognition			
MMSE	9.5 ± 8.0	11.0 ± 8.8	.000
Physical function			
Barthel index	59.3 ± 33.6	64.4 ± 31.2	.000
BANS scale	14:2 ± 5.3	12.4 ± 4.7	.000
Tinetti scale	15.9 ± 9.1	18.3 ± 8.5	.000
Behavior			
Behavioral disturbances (NPI scale)	33.4 ± 24.8	10.2 ± 9.7	.000
Complain of somatic symptoms			
Symptoms reported after inquiry	1.6 ± 1.8	1.1 ± 1.6	.001
Symptoms spontaneously reported	0.7 ± 0.8	0.6 ± 0.9	ns

on NPI scale, with reduction of behavioral disturbances and reaching of easier management of patients at home or in nursing home; 0.5 somatic symptoms reported after inquiry.

The Table 4 shows changes of Tinetti scale, Barthel index, and BANSS score between admission and discharge within two groups of demented patients: those performing and those not performing physical rehabilitation. Table 5 shows the gain in physical function computed as "Δ" scores (difference of score on admission and score on discharge) between the two groups. Patients of both groups showed significant improvement in basic activities of daily living and physical function. All scores significantly more improved in patients that underwent non-pharmacological intervention. However, it should be noted that patients receiving non-pharmacological interventions were significantly less impaired in physical function and in daily function than those non-receiving treatment.

DISCUSSION

The use of health care outcomes cannot be considered a modern invention: an acta from the code of Hammurabi (20th century before Christ) said that "if a doctor treat a sore in a free man and patient dies, doctor will have amputated hands", underlining the primary importance of the results obtained through procedures and interventions (for both patient and doctor). However, in modern medical science, outcome as measure of the quality of care has made up of interest and importance in the last century in some medical fields (mainly surgery and acute medicine), and only in the last decade in geriatric medicine. For years, geriatricians have lost sight of the relevance of positive outcome measures: the

Table 4. Impact of physical function and basic activities of daily living on admission and discharge of two groups of demented patients (n=160) according to execution of physical rehabilitation

	Admission mean ± SD	Discharge mean ± SD	p**
Tinetti score			
No physical rehabilitation	21.4 ± 5.1	23.1 ± 5.0	.000
Physical rehabilitation (n=52)	8.1 ± 7.6	12.1 ± 7.6	.000
p*	.000	.000	
Barthel score			
No physical rehabilitation	73.2 ± 23.6	77.7 ± 24.7	ns
Physical rehabilitation (n=52)	33.8 ± 30.2	45.5 ± 28.3	.000
p*	.000	.000	
BANSS score			
No physical rehabilitation	11.8 ± 3.8	10.8 ± 3.8	.000
Physical rehabilitation (n=52)	17.8 ± 5.1	14.8 ± 5.0	.000
p*	.000	.000	

*Significance of differences between groups of demented patients according to execution of physical rehabilitation on t-test.

**Significance of differences between admission and discharge within groups on t-test.

main efforts were directed to avoid the worsening of the clinical picture (e.g., prevention of pressure sores, falls, malnutrition). The care of elderly disabled people has been viewed as a social necessity, and nursing homes as custodial institution (32), without rehabilitative aims, or research for reduction of disability, improvement of health status, of global perception of health status, and of quality of life. Recent evidences in literature (32) report a new interest in outcomes in geriatric medicine, supported by the observation that very old disabled subjects can improve when the right treatments are performed.

In the care of irreversible dementia, where the recovery is not a reachable goal, a number of outcomes can be identified: the modification of the natural history of the disease and the delaying of institutionalization, the improvement of social functions, the improvement of symptoms, the satisfaction and the improvement of the quality of life. These latter ambitious outcomes are possible even in subjects affected by non-reversible dementia. However, the slowing of decline of cognition and daily function, and the delaying of institutionalization can be evaluated only in a longitudinal study and need a control group, while the observation of an improvement in social functions require a more echologic setting. On the contrary, the improvement of clinical picture (evaluated as daily function with BANSS and Barthel index, physical function with Tinetti scale, cognition with MMSE, and behavioral disturbances with UCLA-NPI), and of the somatic symptoms and quality

Table 5. Change in physical function, basic activities of daily living, behavioral disturbances, and global cognition, in relation to two non-pharmacological interventions (physical rehabilitation), in the 160 demented patients

	No physical rehabilitation Mean ± SD	Physical rehabilitation Mean ± SD	p*
Δ Tinetti	1.6 ± 2.8	4.0 ± 5.4	.002
Δ Barthel	1.5 ± 7.8	11.7 ± 19.2	.000
Δ BANSS	−1.0 ± 1.5	−3.0 ± 3.2	.000

*Significance of differences of Δ scores between groups of demented patients according to execution of physical rehabilitation on t-test.

of life (evaluated with SSR and SRAI as markers of somatic health and global well-being) can be assessed during a relatively brief stay in a hospital ward.

At least one caveat should be underlined. Notices on behavioral disturbances and on basic activities of daily living were collected by the same physician from a relative (the principal caregiver, when possible) on admission, and from the nursing staff on discharge. Relatives, and overall principal caregivers, might overreport the severity of impairment because of the influence of depression or psychological distress on their judgment, or underreport behavioral disturbances and loss of daily function because of will of minimize the entity of damage. The nursing staff is probably more objective in the observation. Therefore, the two measures might be substantially different.

Our data suggest that even in the care of demented patients (the more disabled among the disabled people) it would be possible to define "positive" outcomes.

After about a 30-day stay, all patients received a diagnostic definition of cognitive impairment. The relevance of diagnosis should be underlined for a number of reasons: first, reversible dementias exist, but patients affected by these forms can recover only if reversibility of disease is recognized; second, misdiagnosis of non-reversible dementia can lead to inappropriate management of demented patients, increasing their mortality and morbidity, and determining worsening of their quality of life; finally, we think that a precise and correct diagnosis is a patients right, even if their disease is a non-reversible form of dementia, and resolutive treatments are lacking. Furthermore, patients showed sensible and clinically evident improvement in all the considered domains: on discharge, they obtained higher MMSE score, had better ability in coping basic activities of daily living, showed improved balance and gait, had less behavioral disturbances, and complained less somatic pain and discomfort after specific inquiry. Non-pharmacological rehabilitative physical interventions were performed on subjects with greater impairment in balance and gait, and at greater risk of fall, keeping into account the Tinetti scale score (about < 18/28). All demented patients had greater scores in scales measuring physical abilities on discharge compared to on admission, but those that underwent physical rehabilitation significantly improved both in balance and gait (Tinetti scale), and in daily function (Barthel and BANSS scores). Since this improvement seems to be spread over all the demented patients (including those with normal physical function, and greater Barthel and BANNS scores), even if more marked in impaired subjects, it could be argued that this effect might be due to the global care, and explainable by a roof effect of the scales. However, physical rehabilitative intervention was carried on with patients at high risk of fall, causing a substantial improvement in gait and balance status. The magnitude of increase in the other patients is significantly lower and with a different meaning, and can be probably associated to a more global and aspecific change. Basic daily function follows the same trend. It should be hypothesize that overall the physical component of the two scales (Barthel and BANSS) was interested in this kind of improvement. Behavioral disturbances also decreased during the stay, and global cognitive performance (MMSE) increased, but these improvements do not seem to be related to any specific intervention, and appear to be consequences of the global evaluation, treatment, and non-formal interventions included in the care plan. The significant reduction of the SRAIs on discharge was also not related to any specific intervention. It is reasonable to hypothesize that the complain of somatic symptoms is a proxy of the domain "quality of life", and is therefore influenced by factors more complex than a single intervention. SSR did not change on discharge. It could suppose that to evoke spontaneously symptoms require a relatively intact memory: therefore, in demented patients this scale is able to assess only the momentary pain and discomfort, and is less reliable as marker of global well-being.

The achievement of these results justify the role of our Dementia Evaluation and Rehabilitation Unit Patients with a correct diagnosis of cognitive impairment can be treated with specific interventions, determining positive outcomes in physical and daily functions.

REFERENCES

1. Evans DA, Funkenstein HH, Albert MS et al. Prevalence of Alzheimer's disease in a community population of older persons. JAMA 262:2551–2556, 1989.
2. Rocca W, Amaducci L, Schoenberg BS: Epidemiology of clinically diagnosed Alzheimer's disease. Ann Neurol. 19:415–424; 1986.
3. Clarfield AM. The reversible dementias: do they reverse? Ann Intern Med 1988;109:476–486.
4. Bianchetti A, Scuratti A,Zanetti O, Binetti G, Frisoni GB, Magni E, Trabucchi M. Predictors of mortality and institutionalization in Alzheimer disease patients 1 year after discharge from an Alzheimer dementia unit. Dementia 1995;6:108–112.
5. Binetti G, Magni E, Padovani A, Bianchetti A, Trabucchi M. Neuropsychological heterogeneity in mild Alzheimer's disease. Dementia 1993;4:321–326
6. O- Folstein MF, Folstein SE, McHugh PR. "Mini Mental State": a pratical method for grading the cognitive state of patients for the clinician. J Psych Res 1975;12:189–198.
7. Spinnler H, Tognoni G. Standardizzazione e taratura italiana di test Neuropsicologici. Ital J Neurol Sci 1987;Supplement 8.
8. Rey A. Reattivo delle figure complesse A e B. 1983;Firenze: Organizzazioni Speciali.
9. Orsini A, Grossi D, Capitani E, Laiacona M, Papagno C, Vallar G. Verbal and spatial immediate memory span: normative data from 1355 adults and 1112 children. 1987; Ital J Neurol Sci 8, 539–548.
10. Wolf-Klein G P, Silverstone F A, Levy A P, Brod M S. Screening for Alzheimer's disease by Clock Drawing. J Am Geriatr Soc 1989;37:730–734.
11. Basso A, Capitani E, Laiacona M. Raven's Coloured Matrices: normative values on 305 adult normal controls. Func Neurol 1987;11:189–194.
12. Novelli G, Papagno C, Capitani E, Laiacona M, Vallar G, Cappa SF. Tre test clinici di ricerca e produzione lessicale: taratura su soggetti normali. Arch Psicol Neurol Psichiatr 1986;47:477–506.
13. Berg EA. A simple objective test for measuring flexibility in thinking. J Gen Psychol 1948;39:15–22.
14. American Psychiatric Association. Diagnostic and statistical manual of mental disorders (III edition revised). Washington (DC): American Psychiatric Association, 1987.
15. McKhann G, Drachman D, Folstein M F, Katzman R, Price D Stadlan E M. Clinical diagnosis of Alzheimer's disease: report of the NINCDS-ADRDA Work Group. Neurology 1984;34:939–944.
16. Roman GC, Tatemichi TK, Erkinjuntti T, Cummings JL, Masdeu JC, Garcia JH, Amaducci L, Orgogozo JM, Brun A, Hofman A, et-al. Vascular dementia: diagnostic criteria for research studies. Report of the NINDS-AIREN International Workshop. Neurology 1993;43:250–260
17. Clinical and neuropathological criteria for frontotemporal dementia. The Lund and Manchester Groups. J Neurol Neurosurg Psychiatry 1994;57:416–418
18. McKeith IG, Galasko D, Kosaka K, et al. Consensus guideline for the clinical and pathologic diagnosis of dementia with Lewy bodies (DLB). Report of the consortium on DLB international workshop. Neurology 1996;47:1113–1124.
19. Mesulam M M. Slowly progressive aphasia without generalized dementia. Ann Neurol 1982;11:592–598.
20. Duffy J R, Petersen R C. Primary progressive aphasia. Aphasiol 1992;6:1–15.
21. Masters CL, Harris JO, Gajdusek DC et al. Creutzfeldt-Jakob disease: patterns of worldwide occurrence and the significance of familial and sporadic clustering. Ann Neurol 1979; 5:177–188.
22. Hughes CP, Berg L, Danziger WL, et al. A new clinical scale for the staging of dementia. Brit J Psychiat 1982;140:566–572.
23. Mahoney FI, Barthel DW. Functional evaluation: the Barthel Index. Maryland State Medical Journal 1965;14:61–65.
24. Volicer L, Hurley A, Lathi DC, Kowall NW. Measurement of severity in advanced Alzheimer's disease. J Gerontol 1994;49:M223–226.
25. Bellelli G, Frisoni GB, Bianchetti A, Trabucchi M. The Bedford Alzheimer Nursing Severity Scale for the Severely Demented: Validitation Study. Alzh Dis Assoc Dis, in press.
26. Tinetti M. Performance-oriented assessment of mobility problems in elderly patient. J Am Geriatr Soc 1986;34:119–126.

27. Cummings JL, Mega M, Gray K, Rosenberg Thompson S, Carusi DA, Gornbein J. The Neuropsychiatric Inventory: comprehensive assessment of psychopathology in dementia. Neurology 1994;44:2308 2314
28. De Leo D, Frisoni GB, Rozzini R, Bernardini M, Dello Buono M, Trabucchi M. The Profile of Elderly Quality of Life (PEQOL): a quick package to assess general health conditions in old age. 5th Congress of the International Psychogeriatric Association, Rome, 1991.
29. Greenfield S, Blanco DM, Elashoff RM, et al. Development and testing of a new index of comorbidity. Clin Res 1987;335–346.
30. Statistical Pakage for the Social Sciences, SPSS Inc., Chicago, Illinois.
31. Hachinski V. Vascular dementia: a radical redefinition. Dementia 1994;5:130–132
32. Kane RL. Improving the quality of long-term care. JAMA 1995;273:1376–1380.

21

THERAPY OF ALZHEIMER'S DEMENTIA

Past, Present, and Future

P. Mecocci, M. C. Polidori, A. Cherubini, and U. Senin

Sezione di Gerontologia e Geriatria
Dipartimento di Medicina Clinica, Patologia e Farmacologia
Università degli Studi di Perugia

1. INTRODUCTION

Alzheimer's dementia, one of the most important causes of severe disability in the elderly, fourth cause of death in adults in Western Countries (Bush et al., 1994), represents a dramatic health problem, especially for social and economic implications, whose risk factors are, at present, only age (Herbert et al., 1995), lower education (Ganguli et al., 1991), ApoE genotype (Feskens et al., 1994; Locke et al., 1995), and, possibly, head trauma (Fratiglioni, 1993). The issue "Alzheimer" has been efficaceously synthetized by Khachaturian and collegues with the formula $\mathbf{P}_{AD} = \mathbf{N} \times \mathbf{D} \times \mathbf{C}$, where **N** represents the total number of affected individuals, **D** the lenght in time of the disease, **C** the costs of diagnosis, treatment and assistance (Khachaturian et al., 1994). The solution of such a problem requests therefore an articulate approach, able to influence each of the above factors.

Due to the intense research activity of the past recent years, that poses various biologic and neurochemical deficits as the basis of cognitive disturbances associated to aging brain and dementia, and Alzheimer's dementia in particular, many molecules have been synthetized capable to interact with the systems responsible of neurodegenerative disorders. Some of these molecules have already been proposed as drugs useful in dementia on the basis of the results of clinical trials, while an important therapeutic potential has been shown for others whose trials are still ongoing. Thus, from a strictly medical point of view, Alzheimer's dementia treatment is based on the use of drugs that ameliorate disturbances which characterize the pathology, or at least slow their progression.

Furthermore, it is important to establish adequate enviromental strategies to reduce the risk of appearance of severe behavioural alterations and to make more tolerable the assistential duties of the caregiver. In fact, it is important to underline that up-to-date drugs are not the cure of Alzheimer's disease. The treatment of such a condition, that involves the whole life of the patient, his family and/or other caregivers, cannot be regardless of appropriate behavioural strategies and of a careful treatment of non-cognitive disturbances (delirium, agitation, aggressiveness, insomnia). With respect to this problem, it is impor-

Recent Advances in Geriatrics, edited by Barbagallo, Licata, and Sowers.
Plenum Press, New York, 1998.

tant to identify at the beginning of the disease the less impaired cognitive functions and those already lost, in order to be able to limit the request on the latters, stimulating and ameliorating the preserved functions. In case the patient is assisted at home, it is key to define a strategy capable of stimulating the residual functions of the patient and of reducing potentially dangerous enviromental factors, even modifying internal and/or external spaces of the house (Hiatt, 1986). The family needs to know that certain ways to act of the patient are consequences of the disease, in order to be able to understand and tolerate them. The risk of potential behavioural disturbances can also arise from noise, crowds, confusion (Knopman and Sawyer-DeMaris, 1990), and this is something the family can certainly avoid. Everything the patient tends to do worse and worse over time, has to be highly simplified, but at the same time the caregiver cannot substitute himself to the patient, situation which most of the times anticipates a state of complete disability. In a similar manner, difficulties in expression and comprehension of the verbal language can be overcome with gestures and other non-verbal forms of communication (Mace and Rabins, 1991). Only after having tried all these solutions, it is appropriate to decide a pharmacological treatment, although not all behavioural disturbances respond to drugs. For example, non-aggressive, repetitive behaviour, continuous walking, confabulations do not seem to respond to drug treatment. Other disturbances, including delirium (which needs treatment with neuroleptic agents with lower incidence of extrapiramidal effects, such as chlorpromazine), agitation, insomnia (which can be treated with benzodiazepines with short half-life, such as temazepam or lorazepam) and depression (which very often accompanies dementia in its early stages and can be treated with second generation antidepressive drugs, such as fluoxetine, paroxetine, trazodone), seem to respond, unfortunately with a big interindividual variability (Cummings and Victoroff, 1990).

The aim of this chapter is to review the most important categories of drugs, classified on the basis of the different etiopathogenetic pathways they affect -including deficits of cholinergic, monoaminergic and/or peptidergic neurotransmission, free radical-induced neuronal damage, neuronal damage caused by disturbances in calcium omeostasis, neurotoxicity caused by excitatory aminoacids and neurotoxicity caused by deposition of amiloid protein.

2. DEFICIT OF NEUROTRANSMISSION

The new era of neurobiochemical research in the field of Alzheimer's disease started with the finding of a *deficit of cholinergic neurotransmission* in the cerebral cortex and hyppocampus (Bowen et al., 1976; Davies and Maloney, 1976; Perry et al., 1977). The initial deficit shown was a selective reduction of choline-acetyltransferase (CAT), enzyme of critical importance for the synthesis of acetylcholine. Correlations between the severity of the disease and the density of senile amyloid plaques and neurofibrillary tangles, together with the depletion of CAT, evidentiated the role of cholinergic neurons in Alzheimer's dementia physiopatology (Perry et al., 1978).

The idea of an important involvement of cholinergic neurons in Alzheimer's disease was then confirmed by the observation that the administration, in young healthy adults, of scopolamine, that interferes with cerebral cholinergic transmission, produced memory impairment similar to that of early Alzheimer's disease (Dunne and Hartley, 1986; Warburton and Rusted, 1993). Furthermore, this disturbances ameliorated with physostigmine, that easily crosses the blood brain barrier, although this drug is not useful in Alzheimer's dementia due to its many side effects (nausea, vomiting, diarrhea, bradycardia). Nevertheless, carefully considering these data, peripherally administered scopolamine has been suggested not to primarily and/or selectively affect learning performance and memory processes, but rather sensory/attentional processes (Hagan and Morris, 1988; Kirk et al., 1988; Schurtleff et al., 1992).

Most importantly, a reduced choline uptake (Sims et al., 1983) and a reduced acetylcholine syntesis (Bowen et al., 1983) were shown in cerebral tissue of Alzheimer patients, and, on the basis of the results showing a role of cholinergic neurons and pathways in Alzheimer's disease, the "cholinergic hypothesis" was made (Bartus et al., 1982; Coyle et al., 1983; Davies, 1981; Drachman and Glosser, 1981), and the first therapeutical trial in agreement with the biochemical results has been sostitutive cholinergic therapy, similarly to what happened in Parkinson's disease with levodopa.

During the past years, numerous interventions with cholinergic drugs that cross the blood brain barrier had the purpose of stimulating the production of acetylcholine and its release at a *presynaptic level*, like *choline*, *lecitine*, or *phosphatidylcholine* (Bartus et al., 1984; De Feudis, 1988; Goodnick and Gershon, 1984; Johns et al., 1985), but the results have been rather disappointing. *Oxiracetam*, a nootropic agent similar to *piracetam* (the first drug syntetized in the family of nootropics), has been shown to be able to ameliorate learning and memory functions in both healthy and brain injured animals (Banfi e Dorigotti, 1984), due to its ability to increase the high-affinity choline uptake also in the hippocampus (Spignoli et al., 1986). Similarly, *aniracetam* has been shown to significantly improve cognitive performance in demented patients over a 6-months study with respect to patients receiving placebo, with a good tolerability consistent with the known pharmacological profile of the pyrrolidinone drugs (Senin et al., 1991).

Another group of drugs that release acetylcholine are *gamma-amino-butyric acid (GABA) antagonists*. Rationale for their use is based on data which showed that acetylcholine release and high-affinity choline uptake depend upon inhibitory control of GABA-benzodiazepine receptors located on cerebral cholinergic neurons (Sarter et al., 1988). The problem with GABA-antagonists is that they can exacerbate insomnia and hyperactivity in patients with Alzheimer's dementia, eliminating the physiological sedative effect of GABAergic system (Jansen, 1988).

Other studies involving drugs favoring the release of choline showed that molecules which stimulate the maintenance of the morphofunctional integrity of the neural cell, like *phosphatidylserine* and *citicholine*, have the effect, among others, of incorporating polyunsaturated free fatty acids in phosphatidylcholine and phosphatidylinositole, with a subsequent protective effect on cell membranes (Milan et al., 1986).

Acetyl-l-carnitine is also involved in free fatty acid metabolism and was shown to increase choline-acetyltransferase activity, acetyl-coenzyme A bioavailability, choline uptake and synthesis and release of acetylcholine (Dolezal and Tucek, 1981; Markowska et al., 1990; Spagnoli et al., 1991; Vecchi et al., 1991). At a neuronal level, acetyl-l-carnitine appears to influence numerous functions including DNA transcription (through the acetylation of H4 histones), maintenance of cytoscheletal stability, improvement of the phosphorilative chain reactions (favoring the turnover of the proteins of the mitochondrial membrane). The efficacy of this drug was shown in several recent trials in which acetyl-l-carnitine was demonstrated to be useful in the initial stages of degenerative dementia, ameliorating selective attention, verbal ability, logic intelligence and Blessed Dementia Scale scores (Spagnoli et al., 1991). Acetyl-l-carnitine plasma concentrations have been shown to be higher in treated patients, indicating an active crossing of the molecule through the blood brain barrier (Parnetti et al., 1992), and other studies confirmed these characteristics of the drug (Cucinotta et al., 1988; Senin et al., 1996). A recent multicentric, double-blind and placebo-controlled study on patients with mild-moderate Alzheimer's dementia treated for one year with acetyl-l-carnitine has shown that the drug has a higher efficacy in subjects younger than 65 with respect to the older ones. In fact, although significant differences were not shown between the two treatment groups, young patients treated with acetyl-l-carnitine have achieved higher scores in cognitive tests than over 65 patients (Thal et al., 1996). Further trials are ongoing to assess the real efficacy of acetyl-l-carnitine.

The best approach for an increase in cholinergic transmission and bioavailability of acetylcholine has been shown to be, so far, the blockade, at a *synaptic level*, of acetylcholine catabolism. This can be done by acetylcholine esterase (which hydrolizes acetylcholine in acetic acid and choline) inhibitors (ChEI), of which the above cyted *physostigmine* (very short-acting, with a half-life of 30 minutes to one and a half hours) is hystorically the first example. The main pharmacological effects of ChEIs that constitute the theoretical basis for therapy in Alzheimer's disease are a) the functional improvement of central cholinergic synapses mediated through muscarinic and nicotinic mechanisms (Summers et al., 1994; Cuadra and Giacobini, 1994); b) protection against neuronal degeneration mediated through nicotine receptor activation (Sjak-shie et al., 1990; Janson and Moller, 1993); c) the modification of APP processing mediated through muscarinic M_1 receptor activation (Buxbaum et al., 1992; Nitsch et al., 1993); and d) the regional enhanced synthesis of neuronotrophic molecules such as nerve growth factor (NGF) and brain-derived nerve factor (BDNF) via muscarinic receptor stimulation (Lindfors et al., 1992; Berzaghi et al., 1993).

The best documented studies of ChEI clinical efficacy in Alzheimer's disease are related to the effect of administration of *tacrine* (1,2,3,4-tetrahydro-aminoacridine) for periods of up to 30 weeks. Tacrine has a longer half-life (about three hours) compared to physostigmine. Six major double-blind, placebo-controlled trials using similar methods of assessment of cognitive function in 1905 patients were carried out during the period 1990–1994 (Summers et al., 1986; Eagger et al., 1991; Davis et al., 1992; Farlow et al., 1992; Wilcock et al., 1993; Knapp et al., 1994). These studies showed that tacrine, if administered at high doses (Knapp et al., 1996) is capable of ameliorating cognitive performances in Alzheimer's patients with a mild-moderate impairment (it is possible to anticipate this improvement in 20–30% of treated patients). Up-to-date, tacrine is approved in 23 Nations including US and 9 european States (Austria, Belgium, Finland, France, Germany, Greece, Luxemburg, Spain an Switzerland), and recently (1996) a consensus on the clinical use of tacrine was formulated, restating that 1) there is a considerable heterogeneity in the response of patients to tacrine in terms of both treatment efficacy and tolerability; 2) since there are no predictive criteria for differentiating patients before treatment, all patients with mild to moderate Alzheimer's disease who have no other contraindications should be considered for tacrine therapy; 3) in order to be maximally effective, tacrine should be taken four times daily between meals; 4) a dose tritration regimen should be followed in order to reduce the incidence of adverse effects (40 mg qd for 6 weeks, followed by 80 mg qd for 6 weeks, then 120 mg qd for 6 weeks, increasing up to 160 mg qd); and finally 5) in the presence of a hepatic ALT increase (hepatic toxicity varies between 20 and 42% of the cases) more than three-fold the upper limit of normal, treatment should be continued according to the dose tritration regimen. If elevation is higher (three- to five-fold), the daily dose should be reduced by 40 mg qd, restarting the dose tritration when ALT levels return to normal, and, if a clinical jaundice appears, the drug should definitively be discontinued.

Negative effects of tacrine on acetylcholine synthesis and release have been shown in vitro in cerebral tissue of rats stimulated for the cellular liberation of neurotransmitters

(Tucek and Dolezal, 1991), and this effect could be due to the fact that tacrine-induced long-term increase of synaptic concentrations of acetylcholine activates autoreceptors M_2, resulting in a feed-back inhibition of presynaptic acetylcholine synthesis (Hallack and Giacobini, 1989). For this reason, the use in association of a selective antagonist of M2 autoreceptors has been suggested, while the combination with choline has not shown a distictly better response than ChEI alone (Schwartz et al., 1991b).

After approval of tacrine by the US Food and Drug Administration (October 1993), many ChEI are currently being tested clinically throughout the world. On the basis of the inhibitory mechanism, these compounds can be divided into 3 classes: I, reversible inhibitors (aminoacridines, like tacrine); II, pseudo-irreversible inhibitors (carbamates); and III, irreversible inhibitors (organophosphorous compounds).

Second generation ChEI are characterized by high penetration through the blood-brain barrier, potent, long-lasting and selective inhibition of acetylcholinesterase and mild peripheral cholinergic adverse effects, although these drugs have been recently shown to have haematological side effects such as neutropenia or agranulocytosis. This finding, together with the possibility of hepatotoxicity, needs to be carefully taken into consideration, and new compounds are currently being designed to produce higher central nervous system acetylcholinesterase inhibition at low levels of adverse effects and toxicity. Using recent clinical data, Becker et al. (1991) proposed a hypothetical therapeutic window for red blood cells, i.e. acetylcholinesterase inhibition in the range of 30 to 60% with an average of 40%, producing at least a 50% clinical improvement in cognitive functions.

One of the most important second-generation ChEIs is *eptastigmine* (heptyl-physostigmine tartrate, MF201), derived from physostigmine. Compared with tacrine, eptastigmine has a longer duration of action both in brain and red blood cells and lower cholinomimetic or hepatic toxicity. Phase I studies have demonstrated that eptastigmine is absorbed in a linear fashion, producing a dose-dependent and long-lasting acetylcholinesterase inhibition with good cholinergic tolerability in healthy volunteers (Imbimbo and Lucchelli, 1994; Canal et al., 1994; Canal and Imbimbo for the Eptastigmine Study Group, 1996). Phase II studies employing high doses of the drug (up to 120 mg qd) have revealed reversible neutropenia in two patients with Alzheimer's disease. Further trials are ongoing to evaluate the long-term clinical efficacy of eptastigmine in Alzheimer's disease patients.

Velnacrine, donepezil and exelon are three other important acetylcholinesterase inhibitors. *Velnacrine* (HP-029) acts biochemically as a potent acetylcholinesterase inhibitor. Pharmacodynamic trials with single doses of this drug in both healthy, young individuals and patients with Alzheimer's disease demonstrated statistically significant effects on attention, short-term memory and recent memory as compared to placebo (Siegfred, 1993). Two phase III trials have been completed, the first in Europe (Eagger et al., 1994), the second in US (Moore and Clipp, 1994). In the "Caregiver Activities Time Survey", the comparison of week 24 of treatment with baseline revealed marked differences between treatment groups; in the velnacrine study, time spent on care was reduced by 45% (3.2 hours per day) as compared to the baseline, whereas in the placebo group a nonsignificant reduction of only 25 minutes was observed.

Donepezil (E-2020) is a piperidine-based ChEI which is structurally different from other agents. It has a very low toxicity and a dose-dependent activity, and it is maybe more selective for acetylcholinesterase than either pseudo-irreversible carbamate ChEI, physostigmine or tacrine (Rogers and Friedhoff, 1996). The results on a total of 750 patients treated with E2020 in different trials have been reported. Although final data are not available yet, it looks like the molecule is very well tolerated and has a good efficacy—even in improving quality of life- in patients with mild-moderate Alzheimer's disease.

Exelon (SDZ-ENA-713) is an acetylcholinesterase inhibitor of the carbamate type which is in phase II/III of development. The initial trials indicated some evidence of efficacy (Enz et al., 1993), while several international multicentric trials are still ongoing. With respect to this, a very important project from Sandoz is currently ongoing, called ADENA (Alzheimer's Disease Treatment with ENA-713). It includes 4 multicentric, double-blind, placebo-controlled studies, that have already randomized 2000 patients. The instruments used to assess the efficacy of the drug are the ADAS-cog (Alzheimer's Disease Assessment Scale for cognitive impairment), the CIBIC-plus (Clinician's Interview Based Impression of Change) and the PDS (Progressive Deterioration Scale), validated by DeJong and collegues (DeJong et al., 1989).

At a *postsynaptic level*, some drugs were developed in consideration of the described integrity of muscarinic receptors M1 in Alzheimer's disease, acting as direct muscarinic agonists. Unfortunately, non-selective muscarinic agonists such as *betanecole* (Schwartz et al., 1991a) are associated with not acceptable central and peripheral cholinomimetic side effects, including syncope, epileptic seizures, broncospasm and GI distress, while selective M_1 agonists, such as FKS 508, are more promising from a clinical outcome point of view (Brandeis et al., 1990; Fisher et al., 1990).

Nicotinic receptors are also important in Alzheimer's disease, because they are decreased in the cerebral cortex of patients deceased with this dementing disorder (Nordberg and Winblad, 1986). A loss of nicotinic receptors of the brain has been shown in vivo with positron-emission tomography (PET) (Nordberg, 1992), studies on tacrine treatment have demonstrated that this drug increases the number of nicotinic receptors in the temporal and frontal cortex, and that this effect correlates with neurophysiological data (Nordberg, 1992). Similar regulatory effects on nicotinic receptors of the brain can be obtained when the nerve growth factor is administered for a 3-month period by intraventricular infusion (Olson et al., 1992).

If, from these data, a deficit of the cholinergic system of the brain can be considered of fundamental importance in the etiopathogenesis of memory impairment in Alzheimer's dementia, it has also to be underlined that Alzheimer's dementia is a multisystemic degenerative process that shows, furthermore, large interindividual variabilities. Both of these factors must be taken into account when deciding therapeutical strategies for this disease.

Reduced levels of noradrenaline, dopamine and serotonine and altered concentrations of their metabolites in the cerebral tissue and cerebrospinal fluid of Alzheimer's patients clearly indicate a *deficit of monoaminergic neurotransmission* (Gottfries, 1990), that could have some links with the increase of MAO-B activity, a key enzyme for the catabolism of serotonine and catecolamines (Oreland and Gottfries, 1986). Monoaminergic neurotransmission, in Alzheimer's disease, is damaged also at a receptorial level. Morgan and Finch recently studied various receptorial sites (acetylcholine, serotonine, noradrenaline, dopamine, GABA, glutamate, aspartate, somatostatine), and found, rather constantly, a reduction of serotoninergic and dopaminergic reduction (Morgan and Finch, 1988).

The importance of serotoninergic neurotransmission gained importance especially with respect to some common symptoms of demented patients, like affective and sleep disorders (Gottfries, 1990). A classical example of a drug with a regulatory action on alterations of monoaminergic transmission is a derivate of the synthesis of ergotamine, *hydergina* (dihydroergotoxine mesilate). It has been largely used in geriatric practice to treat patients with cognitive impairment (Yesavage, 1990), and for this indication hydergine was approved by US FDA already in 1971. The beneficial effect of hydergine is not due to cerebral vasodilation, as originally thought, but to a regulatory action on cerebral monoaminergic transmission. Hydergina interferes with noradrenaline, serotonine and dopamine receptors (Markstein, 1989) and has a positive effect on the energy metabolism of the brain, as indicated by the increase in glucose utilization (Meyer-Ruge, 1986) and by the reduction of lipofuscine deposits in animal models (Amenta et al., 1988). Hydergine has also a very good tolerability, and for this reason has been proposed and used as an "anti-aging" drug (Koberle and Spiegel, 1984). More than hydergine, nicergoline, another ergot alkaloid with metabolic, antithrombotic and vasoactive action has been shown to improve vigilance and information processing at a neurophysiological level, leading to an improvement in behaviour both in degenerative and vascular dementia (Saletu et al., 1995; Saletu et al., 1996; Herrmann et al., 1997).

With the aim of ameliorating serotoninergic neurotransmission in Alzheimer's disease a selective blocker of serotonine reuptake, *citalopram*, has been used in clinical trials which have shown beneficial effects mostly on emotional disturbances, irritability and panic attacks (Gottfries, 1990).

The increase of MAO-B activity is the base for the use, in dementia, of another important compound, *selegiline* (l-deprenyl), an irreversible inhibitor of MAO-B. This drug has been tested in long-term experiments in animal models, and it has been shown to prolong life of treated animals and to slow the age-related impairment of cerebral functions (Knoll, 1988). Double-blind, placebo-controlled clinical trials have demonstrated efficacy in treatment of dementia (Tariot et al., 1987; Piccinin et al., 1990; Agnoli et al., 1992). The improvement in cognitive performance seems to depend upon an increase of attention and consciousness. Interestingly, the main metabolite of selegiline is l-anphetamine (the less active isomer of d-anphetamine, a psychostimulating drug), that exerts a stimulating effect on learning identical to that of selegiline (Gelowitz et al., 1994).

Many studies on Alzheimer's dementia showed neurobiochemical alterations involving cerebral neuropeptides and their functions of neurotransmission and neuromodulation, mainly in the cortex and in the hyppocampus. The importance of *deficits of peptidergic neurotransmission* arises from alterations regarding the corticotropin releasing factor (CRF) (De Souza et al., 1986; Whitehouse et al., 1987) and somatotropin release-inhibiting factor, SRIF) (Bissette and Myers, 1992; Cervera-Pierot et al., 1992).

Altered concentrations of SRIF have been described on post-mortem studies of Alzheimer's disease patients (Davies et al., 1980; Rossor et al., 1980; Beal et al., 1985) and, in vivo, in the cerebrospinal fluid of demented patients (Minthon et al., 1991). A positive correlation was shown between liquoral concentrations of SRIF and cognitive performances of Alzheimer patients and depressed elderly patients (Sunderland et al., 1987), but this finding, like the finding that pituitary peptidal hormones (like vasopressine and ACTH) could act as neurotransmitters, has not been confirmed (De Wied, 1989), although many drugs similar to these hormons but without endocrine effects have been synthetized. Examples of these compounds which did not reach so far positive results as nootropics are *Org 5667* (analogue of vasopressine), *Org 2766* (analogue of corticotropin), *alaptide* (a fragment of oxytocine) (Benesova et al., 1991b), while a TRH-analogue, *posatireline* (l-pyro-2-aminoadipyl-l-leucyl-prolinamide) has been used in late-onset Alzheimer's dementia, and showed a significant improvement of affective and cognitive functions, of orientation and memory, of ability in executing activities of daily living and depressive symptoms (Parnetti et al., 1995).

Since nerve growth factor has been shown to have receptors on cholinergic terminals of cortex and hippocampus (Whittemore and Seiger, 1987; Dreyfus et al., 1989), and it is necessary for the survival, regeneration and maintenance of specific neuronal functions, human recombinant NGF has been administered by intraventricular injection, and it has been shown to prevent atrophy and degeneration of brainstem neurons (Koliatsos et al.,

1991; Tuszynski et al., 1991), and to improve performance in spatial memory tests (Hefti et al., 1989).

3. ROLE OF MITOCHONDRIA AND OXIDATIVE DAMAGE IN ALZHEIMER'S DISEASE: POTENTIAL APPROACHES

Findings of region-specific decreases in glucose utilization in a number of neurodegenerative disorders in humans led to the suggestion that compromised energy metabolism in neurons may contribute to the pathogenesis of degenerative processes (Beal, 1992). The largest body of evidence suggesting an impairment of energy metabolism in AD has come from studies of glucose metabolism using positron emission tomography. The major difficulty with these studies is determining whether alterations play a role in the disease process or are merely secondary to neuronal loss. Studies of cerebral blood flow, oxygen utilization, and glucose metabolism show consistent decreases in AD in a temporo-parietal pattern (Duara et al., 1986; Haxby et al., 1986). Comparing patients with early and more advanced dementia, it was shown that a substantial decrease in cerebral glucose metabolism may precede cognitive impairment.

Neurochemical studies (Sims et al., 1993) and electronmicroscopic studies (Saraiva et al., 1985) on cerebral cortical biopsies have also suggested that energy metabolism may be impaired in AD, showing mitochondrial dysfunctions (Schöffener, 1993; Sorbi et al., 1993; Parker et al., 1994). Consequences of impaired mitochondrial function may be the generation of free radicals and excitotoxic processes mediated by glutamate receptors.

In the past decads, it has been largely recognized that oxygen-based free radicals (reactive oxygen species, ROS) are involved in the aging process (Harman, 1956; Harman, 1993), and in a variety of age-related pathologies, including atherosclerosis, cancer, cataract. The role of free radicals has been claimed also for a variety of neurodegenerative diseases, such as ALS, Huntington's disease, Parkinson's disease (Southorn and Powis, 1988) and Alzheimer's dementia (Volicer and Crino, 1990).

In biological systems, ROS are generated by a variety of normal metabolic processes. In normal conditions, the interaction of these compounds with molecules critical for cellular viability is prevented by endogenous antioxidant defense systems, which include enzymatic (superoxide dismutases, catalases, glutathione peroxidases) and non-enzymatic substances (ascorbic acid, uric acid, tochopherols, thiols, ubiquinol-10). In situations where antioxidant defenses are inadequate, free radicals are able to produce damage to the cell membrane, enzymes, nucleic acids, proteins and lipids. It was recently found a significant 50% increase in oxidative damage to nuclear DNA and a threefold increase in oxidative damage to mitochondrial DNA in AD brain tissue (Mecocci et al., 1994). Increases in protein oxidation products (carbonyl groups) occur in aged controls and AD brain samples as compared with young controls (Smith et al., 1991), and there is also evidence that lipid peroxidation is increased in AD cerebral cortex (Hajimohammadreza and Brammer, 1990; Subbarao et al., 1990). It is important to mention that since free radical-induced damage to lipids leads invariably to membrane alteration and damage, treatment with gangliosides has been tried in Alzheimer's disease (*siagoside*). After treatment, patients showed increased activity and more syntonous mood (Augustinsson et al., in press).

Furthermore, there is increased staining of senile plaques and neurofibrillary tangles with antibodies to SOD and catalase (Pappolla et al., 1992). Neurons containing glycated neurofibrillary tangles show evidence of oxidative stress as shown by colocalization with malondialdehyde and heme oxygenase epitopes (Yan et al., 1994).

Another mechanism which might putatively account for the slow neurodegeneration seen in Alzheimer's disease is the enhancement of excitotoxicity caused by an impairment of mitochondrial function, which in turn leads to disturbances of ionic pumping and partial cell depolarization. The excitotoxicity is mediated by the N-metyl-D-aspartate (NMDA) subtype of glutamate receptors (Novelli et al., 1988; Beal, 1992) that are activated by the alleviation of the voltage-dependent Mg^{++} blockade of NMDA-receptor-associated channels, with subsequent increased Ca^{++} influx into neurons which constitutes itself a trigger to further production of free radicals. In support of this process, a number of studies have shown that ambient, and usually non-toxic levels of excitatory aminoacids become toxic in the presence of inhibitors of oxidative phosphorylation (Novelli et al., 1988; Zeevalk and Niklas, 1991), inhibitors of the Na^+/K^+-pump (Novelli et al., 1988), or partial cell-membrane depolarization by K^+ (Zeevalk and Niklas, 1991). Furthermore, a number of in vivo studies in rats have shown that cerebral lesions induced by mitochondrial toxins such as amino-oxyacetic acid, 1-methyl-4-phenyl-pyridinium (MPP^+) and malonate can be blocked by excitatory aminoacids antagonists (Greene et al., 1993; Schulz et al., 1994). Alzheimer's disease patients have been shown to have increased levels of liquoral glutammate with respects to young adults (Pomara et al., 1992).

In light of the evidence of impaired energy metabolism and oxidative damage in neurodegenerative disorders, it has been attempted to investigate the efficacy of agents which putatively ameliorate these events, as potential therapeutic strategies. One approach is to determine whether agents which enhance activity of the electron-transport-chain enzymes can inhibit lesions produced by mitochondrial toxins. Coenzyme Q10 potentiates the activity of some complexes of the electron-transport-chain, hence increasing ATP production, and has been shown to protect against glutamate-induced neurotoxicity in cerebellar cultures (Favit et al., 1992). Human studies have shown that administration of coenzyme Q10 significantly ameliorates the cerebral lactate levels seen in Huntington's disease (Koroshetz et al., 1993). Other agents used to counteract excitatory aminoacid-mediated neuronal damage in Alzheimer's dementia are *dizocilpine* (MK801) (Collins, 1986; Vasar et al., 1993) and *memantine* (CAS41100–52–1) (Bormann, 1989; Kornhuber et al., 1989), which has been shown to be useful in treatment of dementing syndromes (Gortelmeyer and Erbler, 1992).

An alternative approach to try to prevent oxidative damage is to ameliorate the effects of free radicals. Free radical formation can be reduced by administration of free radical scavengers such as the spin trapping agent N-tert-butyl-alpha-phenyl-nitrone (Carney et al., 1991), and in fact spin-trapping agents have been shown significantly attenuate lesions produced in rats by intrastriatal injection of the excitotoxines NMDA, kainic acid and malonate (Schulz et al., 1994).

Several molecules with antioxidant properties have been proposed as treatment modalities in Alzheimer's dementia. *Idebenone* is a synthetic compound which has been tested in various experimental studies and has been shown to be particularly effective in old-age degenerative (Senin et al., 1992; Nappi et al., 1992) and vascular (Nappi et al., 1992; Marigliano et al., 1992; Bergamasco et al., 1992) dementias. In patients with moderately severe impairment from Alzheimer's disease, treatment with selegiline or α-tocopherol has been shown to slow the progression of the disease (Sano et al., 1997).

An extremely interesting class of potentially useful drugs is represented by 21-aminosteroids, also called *lazaroids*, which are potent inhibitors of lipid peroxidation. One of these compounds, tirilazad mesylate, has shown high efficacy in different models of brain injury (Hall, 1993), while U78517F, has been shown to be able to protect hippocampal neurons from beta-amyloid toxicity, and its l-isomer, U83836E, has been demonstrated to prevent the elevation of intracellular calcium produced by beta amyloid 25–35 in cultured PC 12 cells (Richardson et al., 1994).

Mitochondrial dysfunctions also lead to increased production of potentially amyloidogenic fragments in cultured neurons (Gabuzda et al., 1994), and free radicals and metal-catalyzed oxidation systems may cause aggregation and deposition of beta-amyloid (Dyrks et al., 1993). This effect is inhibited by free radical scavengers (Dyrks et al., 1992; Dyrks et al., 1993). In addition, it has been demonstrated that the toxicity of APP fragments is inhibited by vitamin E and propyl gallate, another antioxidant, and that oxidative stress may lead to increased binding of amyloid to apolipoprotein E, an important risk factor for sporadic AD (Strittmatter et al., 1993), and to tau polymerization, that appears to facilitate dimerization and polymerization into filaments.

Of course, there are other approaches to prevent damage due to amyloid protein, such as the prevention of amyloid formation by stimulating non-amyloidogenic APP processing (with selective muscarinic and serotoninergic agonists), interfering with ApoE production and by blocking the dysregulation of Ca^{++} balance induced by amyloid (Ca^{++} channel blockers).

As mentioned above, the rised intracellular levels of calcium due to increased neuronal depolarization can lead to cell death (Siesjo, 1988), and this constitutes the rationale for the use of drugs able to mantain calcium omeostasis, i.e. calcium channel blockers such as nimodipine. Nimodipine has been shown to protect neurons against excitotoxic processes (Weiss and Choi, 1991), and it has been used mainly in vascular dementia (Schmage and Bergener, 1992; Parnetti et al., 1993).

It is also important to mention the interest that continues in elucidating the precise role played by aluminium in Alzheimer's disease, although it is unlikely that excessive exposure to aluminium is the cause of this disorder. Aluminium ions are known to be neurotoxic, aluminosilicates have been identified at the cores of senile plaques, and aluminium has been found within neuron bearing neurofibrillary tangles, thus it may be hypothesized that Alzheimer's disease leads to an impaired blood-brain barrier, increasing the accumulation of aluminium within the brain. Some or all of this aluminium may enter attached to transferrin, which binds aluminium with high affinity. Gutteridge et al. (1985) showed that aluminium ions alone cannot promove membrane lipid peroxidation, but that they accelerate Fe^{++}-dependent peroxidation under certain circumstances. McLachlan et al. (1993; 1994) reported that intramuscular injections of the powerful ion chelator *deferoxamine* in patients with Alzheimer's disease led to a significant reduction in the rate of decline of "daily living skills", but this compound should be used with caution.

4. ANTI-INFLAMMATORY AND ESTROGEN-REPLACEMENT THERAPY

Results from epidemiologic retrospective studies that, in the late '80s, showed the lower incidence of Alzheimer's disease among people treated with anti-inflammatory drugs for other reasons (McGeer et al., 1990; McGeer et al., 1992), proposed the hypothesis of the inflammatory treatment for Alzheimer's dementia. This proposal was also suggested by the finding, in the cerebral tissue of Alzheimer's patients, of elevated levels of acute phase proteins, complement and various cytokines, all conditions favoring amyloid deposition and aggregation. A clinical trial with indomethacin in Alzheimer's dementia has in fact shown better cognitive performances in treated patients with respect to the placebo group, while other studies on patients on chronic treatment with non-steroidal anti-inflammatory drugs have shown better performances on memory tests (Rich et al., 1995) and a minor risk of developing Alzheimer's dementia (Andersen et al., 1995) with respect to individuals who never took anti-inflammatory drugs.

Another epidemiological observation is the base of the rationale for estrogen-replacement therapy. Alzheimer's disease occurs mainly in post-menopausal women, when estrogens, which have been also shown to have a neurotrophic action, are highly reduced. Thus, it has been hypothesized that estrogen replacement therapy in women may exert a protective effect on their risk of developing Alzheimer's disease. this relationship was investigated in the Baltimore Longitudinal Study of Aging (BLSA), a prospective multidisciplinary study of normal aging conducted by the National Institute on Aging. The sample consisted of 472 post- or perimenopausal women followed for up to 16 years in the BLSA. Approximately 45% of the women in the cohort had used estrogen-replacement therapy, and, in this group, a reduced risk of Alzheimer's disease was shown (relative risk in users vs. non-users=0.46) (Kawas et al., 1997). This finding obviously offers additional support for a protective influence of estrogens in Alzheimer's dementia, although randomized trials will be necessary to confirm this association.

5. CONCLUSIONS

Continuous improvements in Alzheimer's research contribute each year to a better understanding of the etiopathogenesis of this dementing disorder, thus favoring the opening of new horizons in the large field of therapeutical approaches. In particular, in the past recent years highly promising therapies have resulted, such as nonsteroidal (indomethacin and antimalarials) and steroidal (prednisone) anti-inflammatory drugs, and also estrogens (Robinson et al., 1994; Kawas et al., 1997), which have been used in several recent trials (Fillit et al., 1986; Honjo et al., 1989; Ohkura et al., 1994; Ohkura et al., 1995), and have been shown to significantly improve several global measures of cognitive functions in most of the patients studied, although currently available epidemiologic data are still limited.

Despite increasing knowledge of the pathological processes underlying Alzheimer's disease, there are at present no effective treatments to slow down its progression or to substantially ameliorate its clinical symptoms.

An increased understanding of factors that influence beta-amyloid aggregation might provide other strategies for intervention. Another interesting strategy would be to counteract the formation of paired helical filaments (Iqbal et al., 1989; Papasozomenos and Su, 1995), while a deeper knowledge of different phosphatases and kinases involved in this process will be needed.

REFERENCES

Agnoli A, Fabbrini G, Fioravanti M, Martucci N. CBF and cognitive evaluation of Alzheimer type patients before and after IMAO-B treatment: a pilot study. Eur. Neuropsychopharmacol. 2:31–35, 1992.

Amenta D, Ferrante F, Franch F, Amenta F. Effects of long-term Hydergine administration on lipofuscin accumulation in senescent rat brain. Gerontologist 34:250–256, 1988.

Andersen K, Launer LJ, Ott A, et al. Do nonsteroidal antiinflammatory drugs decrease the risk for Alzheimer's disease? The Rotterdam Study. Neurology, 45: 1441, 1995.

Augustinsson LE, Blennow K, Blomstrand C, et al. Intracerebroventricular administration of GM1 ganglioside to presenile Alzheimer patients. Dementia (in press).

Banfi S, Dorigotti L. Experimental behavioural studies with oxiracetam on different types of chronic cerebral impairment. Clin. Neuropharmacol. 7 (Suppl. 1):768–769, 1984.

Bartus RT, Dean RL, Beer B. Cholinergic precursor therapy for geriatric cognition: its past, its present and a question of its future. In: Nutrition in gerontology, Orsy et al. (eds.) Raven Press, New York, pp. 191–225, 1984.

Bartus R.T., Dean R.L., Beer B., Lippa A.S. The cholinergic hypothesis of geriatric memory disfunction. Science 217: 408–417, 1982.

Beal M.F. Does impairment of energy matabolism result in excitotoxic neuronal death in neurodegenerative illnesses? Ann. Neurol. 31: 119–130, 1992.

Beal MF, Mazurek MF, Tran VT, et al. Reduced numbers of somatostatin receptors in the cerebral cortex in Alzheimer's disease. Science 229:289–291, 1985.

Becker R, Moriearty P and Unni L: The second generation of cholinesterase inhibitors: clinical and pharmacological effects. In: Cholinergic Basis for Alzheimer Therapy, Becker RE and Giacobini E, eds. Boston: Birkhauser, pp 263–296, 1991.

Benesova O, Kristofikova Y, Tejkalova H. Experimental study of long-term administration of cholinesterase inhibitors in aging rats. Homeostasis 33:170–172, 1991b.

Bergamasco B, Villardita C, and Coppi R: Idebenone in the treatment of multi-infarct dementia: a randomised, double-blind, placebo controlled multicentre trial. Arch Gerontol Geriatr, 15: 271–2378, 1992.

Berzaghi M, Cooper J, Castren E, Zafra F, Sofroniew M, Thoenen H and Lindholm D: Cholinergic regulation of brain-derived neurotrophic factor and nerve growth factor but not neurotrophin-3 mRNA levels in the developing rat hippocampus. J Neurosci 13: 3818–3826, 1993.

Bissette G, Myers B. Somatostatin in Alzheimer's disease and depression. Life Sci. 51:1389–1410, 1992.

Bormann J: Memantine is a potent bloker of N-methyl-D-aspartate (NMDA) receptor channels. Eur. J. Pharmacol. 166: 591–594, 1989.

Bowen DM, Allen SJ, Benton JS, et al. Biochemical assessment of serotonergic and cholinergic dysfunction and cerebral atrophy in Alzheimer's disease. J. Neurochem. 41:226–272, 1983.

Bowen DM, Smith CB, White P, Davison AN. Neurotransmitter-related enzymes and indices of hypoxia in senile dementia and other abiotrophies. Brain 99:459–496, 1976.

Brandeis R, Dachir S, Sapir M, Levy A, Fisher A. Reversal of age-related cognitive impairment by an M_1 cholinergic agonist, AF102B. Pharmacol. Biochem. Behav. 36:89–95, 1990.

Bush TL, Miller SR, Criqui MN, et al. Risk factors for morbidity and mortality in older population: an epidemiological approach. In: Hazzard WR, Bierman EL, Blass JP, et al., editors: Principles of geriatric medicine and gerontology. New York, McGraw Hill, 153–166, 1994.

Buxbaum JD, Oishi M, Chen HI, Pinkas-Kramarski R, Jaffe EA, Gandy SE and Greengard P: Cholinergic agonists and interleukin 1 regulate processing and secretion of the Alzheimer β/A4 amyloid protein precursor. Proc Natl Acad SCI USA 89: 10075–10078, 1992.

Canal N, Franceschi M and the Italian Eptastigmine Investigators: Eptastigmine (MF-201). A double-blind, placebo-controlled, clinical trial in Alzheimer disease patients. In: Alzheimer Disease: Therapeutic Strategies, eds E. Giacobini and R. Becker, Birkhäusser Boston, pp 108–112, 1994.

Canal N, Imbimbo B, for the Eptastigmine Study Group. Clinical trial and therapeutics: relationship between pharmacodynamic activity and cognitive effects of eptastigmine in patients with Alzheimer's disease. Clin. Pharmacol. Ther. 60: 218–228, 1996.

Carney JM, Starke-Reed PE, Oliver CN, Landum RW, Cheng MS, Wu JF,and Floyd R. Proc. Natl. Acad. Sci. U.S.A. 88, 3633–3636, 1991.

Cervera-Pierot P, Hirsch EC, Javoz-Agid F, et al. Hippocampal and parahippocampal somatostatin 28 and neuropeptide Y containing neurons in Alzheimer's disease. Dementia 3:282–298, 1992.

Collins RC: elective vulnerability of brain: new insights from the excitatory synapse Metab. Brain Dis. 1: 231–240, 1986

Coyle JT, Price DL, De Long MR. Alzheimer's disease: a disorder of cortical cholinergic innervation. Science 219:1184–1190, 1983.

Cuadra G, Summeers K and Giacomini E: Cholinesterase inhibitors effects on neurotransmitters in rat cortex in vivo. J Pharmacol Exptl Therapeutics 270, 1994 (in press).

Cucinotta D, Passeri M, Ventura S, et al. Mulcenter clinical placebo-controlled study with acetyl-l-carnitine (LAC) in the treatment of mildly demented elderly patients. Drug Dev. Res. 14:213–216, 1988.

Cummings J.L., Victoroff J. Noncognitive neuropsychiatric syndromes in Alzheimer's disease. Neuropsychiatry Neuropsychol. Behavioral Neurol. 2: 140, 1990.

Davies P. Theoretical treatment possibilities for dementia of the Alzheimer's type. The cholinergic hypothesis. In: Strategies for the development of an effective treatment for senile dementia, Crook & Gershon (eds.) M. Powley Ass., Madison, pp. 19–34, 1981.

Davies P, Katzman R, Terry RD. Reduced somatostatin-like immunoreactivity in cerebral cortex from cases of Alzheimer's disease and Alzheimer senile dementia. Nature 288:279–280, 1980.

Davies P., Maloney A.J.F. Selective loss of central cholinergic neurons in Alzheimer's disease. Lancet ii: 1403, 1976.

Davis KL, Thal LJ, Gamzu ER et al.: A double-blind, placebo-controlled multicenter study of tacrine for Alzheimer's disease. N Engl J Med 327: 1253–1259, 1992.

De Feudis FV. Central cholinergic system, cholinergic drugs and Alzheimer's disease - an overview. Drugs Today 24:473–490, 1988.

De Jong R, Osterlund OW, Roy GW: Measurement of quality of life change in patients with Alzheimer's disease. Clin. Ther. 11:545, 1989.

De Souza EB, Whitehouse PJ, Kuhar MJ, Price DL, Vale WW. Reciprocal changes in corticotropin-relaising factor (CRF)-like immunoreactivity and CRF receptors in cerebral cortex of Alzheimer's disease. Nature 319:593–595, 1986.

De Wied D. Effects of peptide hormones on behaviour. In: Frontiers in neuroendocrinology, Oxford University Press, London, pp. 97–140, 1989.

Dolezal V, Tucek S. Utilization of citrate, acetylcarnitine, acetate, pyruvate and glucose to the synthesis of acetylcholine in rat brain slices. J. Neurochem. 36:1323–1330, 1981.

Drachman DA, Glosser G. Pharmacologic strategies in aging and dementia: the cholinergic hypothesis. In: Strategies for the development of an effective treatment for senile dementia, Crook & Gershon (eds.) M. Powley Ass., Madison, pp. 35–51, 1981.

Dreyfus CF. Effects of nerve growth factor on cholinergic brain neurons. Trends Pharmacol. Sci. 10:145–149, 1989.

Duara R, Grady C, Haxby J, Sundaram M, Cutler NR, Heston L, Moore A, Schlageter N, Larson S, Rapoport SI. Positron emission tomography in Alzheimer's disease. Neurology 36: 879–887, 1986.

Dunne MP, Hartley LR. Scopolamine and the control of attention in humans. Psychopharmacology 89: 94–97, 1986.

Dyrks T, Dyrks E, Hartmann T, et al. Amyloidogenicity of β-A4 and βA4-bearing amyloid protein precursor fragments by metal-catalyzed oxidation. J Biol Chem, 267: 18210–17, 1992.

Dyrks T, Dyrks E, Masters CL, et al. Amyloidogenicity of rodent and human βA4 sequences. FEBS Lett. 324: 231–236, 1993.

Eagger SA, Levy R, Sahakian BJ: Tacrine in Alzheimer's disease. Lancet 337: 989–992, 1991.

Eagger SA, Richards M, Levy R: Long-term effects of tacrine in Alzheimers disease: an open study. Int. J. Geriatr. Psychiatry. 9: 643–647, 1994.

Enz A, Amstutz R, Boddeke H, et al. Brain selective inhibition of acetylcholinesterase: a novel approach to therapy for Alzheimer's disease. Progr. Brain Res., 98: 431–438, 1993.

Farlow M, Gracon SI, Hershey LA et al.: A controlled trial of tacrine in Alzheimer's disease. JAMA 268: 2523–2529, 1992.

Favit A, Nicoletti F, Scapagnini U, et al. Ubiquinone protects cultured neurons against spontaneous and excitotoxin-induced degeneration. J. Cereb. Blood Flow Metab. 12. 638–645, 1992.

Feskens EJM, Havekes LM, Kalmijn S, et al. Apolipoprotein E4 allele and cognitive decline in elderly men. Br. Med. J. 309: 1202–1206, 1994.

Fillit H, Weinreb H, Cholst I. Observations in a preliminary open trial of estradiol therapy for senile dementia (Alzheimer's type). Psychoneuroendocrinology 2: 337–345, 1986.

Fisher A, Brandeis R, Karton I, et al. AF102B: rational treatment strategy for Alzheimer's disease: recent advances. In: Advances in neurology, Wurtman et al. (eds.) Vol. 51 Alzheimer's Disease, Raven Press, New York, pp. 257–259, 1990.

Fratiglioni L. Epidemiology of Alzheimer's disease: issues of etiology and validity. Acta Neurol. Scand. 87: 1–912, 1993.

Gabuzda DH, Busciglio J, Chen LB, Matsudaira P, Yankner BA. Inhibition of energy metabolism alters the processing of amyloid precursor protein and induces a potentially amyloidogenic derivative. J. Biol. Chem. 6: 13623–13628, 1994.

Ganguli M, Ratcliff G, Huff FJ, et al. Effects of age, gender, andeducation on cognitive tests in a rural elderly commuity sample: norms from the Monongahela Valley Independent Elders Survey (MoVIES). Neuroepidemiology 10: 42–52, 1991.

Gelowitz DL, Richardson JS, Wishart PH, Yu PH, Lai CT. Chronic L-deprenyl or D-amphetamine: equal cognitive enhancement unequal MAO inhibition. Pharmacol. Biochem. Behav. 47:41–45, 1994.

Goodnick P, Gershon S. Chemotherapy of cognitive disorders in geriatric subjects. J. Clin. Psychiatry 45:196–209, 1984.

Görtelmeyer R, Erbler H: Mementine in the treatment of mild to moderate dementia syndrome: a double-blind placebo controlled styudy. Arzneimittel-Forschung. 42: 904–913, 1992.

Gottfries CG. Neurochemical aspects of dementia disorders. Dementia 1:56–64, 1990.

Greene JG, Porter RHP, Eller RV, et al. Inhibition of succinate dehydrogenase by malonic acid produces an "excitotoxic" lesion in rat striatum. J. Neurochem. 61: 1151–1154, 1993.

Gutteridge JMC, Quinlan GJ, Clark I, Halliwel B: Aluminum salts accelerate peroxidation of membrane lipids stimulated by iron salts. Biochimica Biophysica Acta. 835: 441–447, 1985.

Hagan JJ, Morris RGM. The cholinergic hypothesis of memory: a review of animal experiments. In: Iversen LL, Iversen SD, Snyder SH (Eds.), Handbook of Psychopharmacology, Plenum Press, New York, 237–305, 1988.

Hajimohammadreza I, Brammer M. Brain membrane fluidity and lipid peroxidation in Alzheimer's disease. Neurosci Lett, 112: 333–7, 1990.

Hall ED. Cerebral ischemia, free radicals and antioxidant protection. Biochem Soc Trans, 21: 334–9, 1993.

Hallak M, Giacobini E. Physostigmine, tacrine and metrifonate: the effect of multiple doses on acetylcholine metabolism in rat brain. Neuropharmacology 28:199–206, 1989.

Harman D. Aging: a theory based on free radical and radiation chemistry. J. Gerontol. 11:298–300, 1956.

Harman D. Free radical involvement in aging: pathophysiology and therapeutic implications. Drugs & Aging 3:60–80, 1993.

Haxby JV, Grady CL, Duara R, Sclageter NL, Berg G, Rapoport SI. Neocortical metabolic abnormalites precede nonmemory cognitive deficits in early Alzheimer type dementia. Arch. Neurol. 43: 882–885, 1986.

Hefti F, Hartikka J, Knusel B. Function of neurotrophic factors in the adult and aging brain and their possible use in the treatment of neurodegenerative diseases. Neurobiol. Aging 10:515–533, 1989.

Herbert LE, Scherr PA, Beckett LA, et al. Age-specific incidence of Alzheimer's disease in a community population. JAMA 273: 1354–1359, 1995.

Herrmann WM, Stephan K, Gaede K, Apececche M: Multicenter randomized double-blind study on the efficacy and safety of nicergoline in patients with multi-infatct dementia. AADE Ed J. 8:9–17, 1997.

Hiatt L.G. Environmental design and mentally impaired older people. In: Haltman H.J., (Ed.) Alzheimer's disease and dementia, New York, Plenum Press; 214, 1986.

Honjo H, Ogino Y, Naitoh K, et al. In vivo effects by estrone sulfate in the central nervous system-senile dementia (Alzheimer's type). J. Steroid Biochem. 34: 521–525, 1989.

Imbimbo PB, Lucchelli PE. A pharmacodynamic strategy to optimize the clinical response to eptastigmine (MF-201). In: Alzheimer disease: therapeutic strategies, E. Giacobini, R. Becker, Birkhäuser, Boston, pp. 103–107, 1994.

Iqbal K, Grundke-Iqbal I, Smith AJ, et al. Identification and localization of a tau peptide to paired helical filaments of Alzheimer's disease. Proc Natl Acad Sci USA, 86: 5646–50, 1989.

Jansen KLR. Is treating memory impairment in Alzheimer's disease an objective? Trends Neurosci. 11:210, 1988.

Janson AM and Moller A: Chronic nicotine treatment counteracts nigral cell loss induced by a partial mesiodiencephalic hemitransection: an analysis of the total number and mean volume of neurons and glia in substantia nigra of the male rat. Neuroscience 57 (4): 931–941, 1993.

Johns CA, Haroutunian V, Greenwald BS, et al. Development of cholinergic drugs for the treatment of Alzheimer's disease. Drug Dev. Res. 5:77–96, 1985.

Kawas C, Resnick S, Morrison A et al. A prospective study of estrogen replacement therapy and the risk of developing Alzheimer's disease: The Baltimore Longitudinal Study of Aging. Neurology, 48: 1517–1521, 1997.

Khachaturian Z.S., Phelps C.H., Buckholtz N.S.: The prospect of developing treatments for Alzheimer disease. In: Alzheimer Disease, edited by Terry R.D., Katzman R., Bick K.L., Raven Press, New York, 445–457, 1994.

Kirk RC, White KG, McNaughton N. Low dose of scopolamine affects discriminability but not rate of forgetting in delayed conditional discrimination. Psychopharmacology 96: 541–546, 1988.

Knapp M.J., Knopman D.S., Solomon P.R., Pendlebury W.W., Davis C.S., Gracon S.I. for the Tacrine Study Group: A 30-week randomized controlled trial of high-dose tacrine in patients with Alzheimer's disease. JAMA 27, 985, 1996.

Knapp MJ, Knopman DS, Solomon PR et al.: A 30-week randomized controlled trial of high-dose tacrine in patients with Alzheimer's disease. JAMA 271: 985–991, 1994.

Knoll J. The striatal dopamine dependency of life span in male rats. Longevity study with (-)deprenyl. Mech. Ageing Dev. 46:237–262, 1988.

Knopman D.D., Sawyer-DeMaris S. Practical approach to managing behavioural problems in dementia patients. Geriatrics 45: 27, 1990.

Köberle S, Spiegel R. A long-term study with co-dergocrine mesylate (Hydergine) in healthy pensioners. Gerontology 30–237–262, 1984.

Koliatsos VE, Clatterbuck RE, Nauta HJW, et al. Human nerve growth factor prevents degeneration of basal forebrain cholinergic neurons in primates. Ann. Neurol. 30:831–840, 1991.

Kornhuber J, Bormann J, Retz W, Huber M, Riederer P: Mementine displaces [H] MK-801 at therapeutic concentrations in postmortem human frontal cortex. Eur. J. Phatrmacol. 166: 589–590, 1989.

Koroshetz W, Jenkins B, Rosen B, et al. Ubiquinone lowers occipital lactate levels in patients with Huntington's disease. Neurology 43 (suppl. 2): A334, 1993.

Lindfors N, Ernfors P, Falkenberg T and Persson H: Septal cholinergic afferents regulate expression of brain-derived neurotrophic factor and beta-nerve growth factor mRNA in rat hippocampus. Exp Brain Res 88: 78–90, 1992.

Locke PA, Conneally PM, Tanzi RE, et al. Apolipoprotein E4 allele and Alzheimer's disease: Examination of allelic association and effect on age at onset in both early- and and late-onset cases. Genet. Epidemiol. 12: 83–92, 1995.

Mace N., Rabins P. The 36-Hour Day. Revised Edition, The John Hopkins University Press, 1991.

Marigliano V, Abate G, Barbagallo-Sangiorgi G et al.: Randomized, double-blind, placebo-controlled, multicentre study of idebenone in patients suffering from multi-infarct dementia., Arch Gerontol Geriatr 15: 239–248, 1992.

Markowska AL, Ingram DK, Barnes CA, et al. Acetyl-l-carnitine: I. Effects on mortality, pathology and sensory-motor performance in aging rats. Neurobiol. Aging 11:491–498, 1990.

Markstein R. Pharmacological approaches in the treatment of senile dementia. Eur. Neurol. 29 (Suppl.):33–41, 1989.

McGeer PL, Harada N, Kimura H, et al. Prevalence of dementia amongst elderly Japanese with leprosy: apparent effect of chronic drug therapy. Dementia, 3: 146, 1992.

McGeer PL, McGeer EG, Rogers J, et al. Antiinflammatory drugs and Alzheimer's disease (letter). Lancet, 335: 1037, 1990.

McLachlan DR, Kruck TPA, Smith WL. Aluminum chelation therapy of Alwheimer's disease. In: Giacobini E, Beker R, editors. Alzheimer disease: therapeutic strategies. Boston: Birkhauser, 328–33, 1994.

McLachlan DR, Smith WL, Kruck TPA. Desferrioxamine and Alzheimer's disease: video home behavior assessment of clinical course and measures of brain aluminum. Ther Drug Monit. 15:602–607, 1993.

Mecocci P, MacGarvey U., Beal MF. Oxidative damage to mitochondrial DNA is increased in Alzheimer's disease. Ann Neurol, 36: 747–51, 1994.

Meyer-Ruge W. Effects of prolonged co-dergocrine mesylate (Hydergine) treatment on local cerebral glucose uptake in aged Fisher 344 rats. Arch. Gerontol. Geriatr. 5:65–67, 1986.

Milan F, Nunzi MG, Guidolin D. Age related loss of dendritic spines in rat hippocampus: effects of phosphatidylserine administration. In: Senile dementias: early detection, A. Bes, J. Cahn, R. Cahn (eds.) John Libbey Eurotext, p. 408, 1986.

Minthon L, Edvinsson L, Ekman R, Gustafson L. Reduced lumbar cerebrospinal fluid somatostatin levels in Alzheimer's disease and dementia with frontotemporal degeneration. Dementia 2:273–277, 1991.

Moore MJ and Clipp EC: Alzheimer's disease and caregiver time. Lancet 343 (8891): 239–240, 1994.

Morgan DG, Finch CE. Neurotransmitter receptors in Alzheimer's disease and nonpathological aging. In: Molecular neuropathology of aging, Banbury Report 27, Cold Spring Harbor Laboratory, pp. 21–35, 1988.

Nappi G, Bono G, Merlo P et al.: Long-term idebenone treatment of vascular and degenerative brain disorders of the elderly. Arch Gerontol Geriatr 15: 261–269, 1992.

Nitsch RM, Farber SA, Growdon JH and Wurtman RJ: Release of amyloid β-protein precursor derivatives by electrical depolarization of rat hippocampal slices. Proc Natl Acad Sci USA 90: 5191–5193, 1993.

Nordberg A. Neuroreceptor changes in Alzheimer disease. Cerebr. Brain Metab. Rev. 4:303–328, 1992.

Nordberg A, Winblad B. Reduced number of 3h-nicotine and 3H acetylcholine binding sites in the frontal cortex of Alzheimer brains. Neurosci. Lett. 72:115–119, 1986.

Novelli A, Reilly JA, Lysko PG, et al. Glutamate becomes neurotoxic via the N-methyl-D-aspartate receptor when intracellular energy levels are reduced. Brain Res. 451: 205–212, 1988.

Ohkura T., Isse K., Akazawa K., et al. Evaluation of estrogen treatment in female patients with dementia of Alzheimer's type. Endocrine J. 41: 361, 1994.

Ohkura T., Isse K., Akazawa K., et al. Long-term estrogen replacement therapy in female patients with Alzheimer's type dementia: seven case reports. Dementia 6: 99, 1995.

Olson L, Nordberg A, von Holst H., et al. Nerve growth factor affects 11C-nicotine binding, blood flow, EEG and verbal episodic memory in an Alzheimer patient (case report). J. Neural Transm. 4:79–95, 1992.

Oreland L, Gottfries CG. Platelet and brain monoamine oxidase in aging and in dementia od Alzheimer's type. Prog. Neuropsychopharmacol. Biol. Psychiatry 10:533–540, 1986.

Papasozomenos S Ch, and Su Y. Rapid dephosphorylation of τ in heat-shocked fetal rat cerebral explants: prevention and hyperphosphorylation by inhibitors of protein phosphatases PP1 and PP2A. J Neurochem, 65: 396–406, 1995.

Pappolla MA, Omar RA, Kim KS, et al. Immunohistochemical evidence of antioxidant stress in Alzheimer's disease. Am. J. Pathol 140: 621–628, 1992.

Parker WD Jr, Parks J, Filley CM, Kleinschmidt-DeMasters BK. Electron transport chain defects in Alzheimer's disease brain. Neurology 44: 1090–1096, 1994.

Parnetti L, Ambrosoli L, Abate G, et al. Posatirelin for the treatment of late-onset Alzheimer's disease: a double-blind multicentre study vs citicoline and ascorbic acid. Acta Neurol. Scand. (in press).

Parnetti L., Gaiti A., Mecocci P., Cadini D., Senin U. Pharmacokinetics of IV and oral acetyl-L-carnitine in a multiple dose regimen in patients with senile dementia of Alzheimer type. Eur. J. Clin. Pharmacol. 42: 89–93, 1992.

Parnetti L, Senin U, Carosi M, Baasch H, and The Nimodipine Study Group. Mental deterioration in old age: results of two multicenter, clinical trials with nimodipine. Clin. Ther. 15:394–406, 1993.

Perry EK, Gibson PH, Blessed G, Perry RH, Tomlinson BE. Neurotransmitter enzyme abnormities in senile dementia. J. Neurol. Sci. 34:247–265, 1977.

Perry EK, Tomlinson BE, Blessed G, et al. Correlation of cholinergic abnormalities with senile plaques and mental test scores in senile dementia. BMJ 2:1457–1459, 1978.

Piccinin GL, Finali G, Piccirilli M. Neuropsychical effects of l-deprenyl in Alzheimer's type dementia. Clin. Neuropharmacol. 13:147–163, 1990.

Pomara N, Singh R, Deptula D, et al: Glutamate and other CSF amino acids in Alzheimer's disease. Am. J. Psychiatry . 149: 251–254, 1992.

Rich JB, Rasmusson DX, Folstein MF et al. Nonsteroidal antiinflammatory drugs in Alzheimer's disease. Neurology, 45: 51, 1995.

Richardson JS, Kumar U, Kala SV, et al. In vitro evidence for the use of antioxidants in Alzheimer's dissease.In: Giacobini E, Becker R, editors. Alzheimer Disease: Therapeutic Strategies. Birkhäusser Boston, 334–9, 1994.

Robinson D, Friedman L, Marcus R, et al. Estrogen replacement therapy and memory in older women. J. Am. Geriatr. Soc. 42: 919–922, 1994.

Rogers S.L., Friedhoff L.T. and the Donepezil Study Group: The efficacy and safety of Donepezil in patients with Alzheimer's disease: results of a US multicentre randomized, double-blind, placebo-controlled trial. Dementia, 7: 293, 1996.

Rossor MN, Emson PC, Mountjoy CQ, Roth SM, Iversen LL. Reduced amounts of immunoreactive somatostatin in the temporal cortex in senile dementia of Alzheimer type. Neurosci. Lett. 20:373, 1980.

Saletu B, Paulus E, Linzmayer L, Anderer P: Nicergoline in senile dementia of Alzheimer type and multi-infarct dementia: a double-blind, placebo controlled, clinical and EEG/ERP mapping study. Folha Med. 113, 103, 1996.

Saletu B, Paulus E, Linzmayer L, Anderer P, Semlitsch HV: Grunberger J, Wicke L, Neuhold A, Podreka I: Nicergoline in senile dementia of Alzheimer type and multi-infarct dementia: a double-blind, placebo controlled, clinical and EEG/ERP mapping study. Psychopharmacology, 117: 385–395., 1995.

Sano M, Ernesto C, Thomas RG, et al. A controlled trial of selegiline, alpha-tocopherol, or both as treatment for Alzheimer's disease. N Engl J Med, 336: 1216–1222, 1997.

Saraiva AA, Borges MM, Madeira MD, Tavares MA, Paula-Barbosa MM. Mitochondrial abnormalities in cortical dendrites from patients with Alzheimer's disease. J. Submicrosc. Cytol 17: 459–464, 1985.

Sarter M, Schneider HH, Stephens DN. Treatment strategies for senile dementia: antagonist beta carbolines. Trends Neurosci. 11:13–17, 1988.

Schmage N, Bergener M. Global rating, symptoms, behavior and cognitive performance as indicators of efficacy in clinical studies with nimodipine in elderly patients with cognitive impairment syndromes. Int. Psychogeriatr. 4 (suppl. 1):89–99, 1992.

Schulz JB, Henshaw DR, Jenkins BG, et al. 3-acetylpyridine produces age-dependent excitotoxic lesions in rat striatum. J. Cereb. Blood Flow Metab. 14: 1024–1029, 1994.

Schwartz RD, Coughenour LL, Davis RE, et al. Novel muscarinic agonists for the treatment of Alzheimer's disease. In: Cholinergic basis for Alzheimer therapy, Becker & Giacobini (eds.), Birkhäuser, New York, pp. 347–353, 1991a.

Schwartz RD, Davis RE, Gracon S, et al. New generation tacrine. Neurobiol. Aging 12:185–187, 1991b.

Senin U, Abate G, Fieschi C, Gori G, Guala A, Marini G, Villardita C, Parnetti L: Aniracetam (Ro 13–5057) in the treatment of senile dementia of Alzheimer type (SDAT): Results of a placebo controlled multicenter clinical study. Eur Neuropsychopharmacology 1: 511–517, 1991.

Senin U, Cherubini A, Mecocci P. I farmaci per i disturbi cognitivi: fra presente e futuro. Giorn. Geront., 1996 (in press).

Senin U, Parnetti L, Barbagallo-Sangiorgi G et al.: Idebenone in senile dementia of Alzheimer type: A multicentre study. Arch Gerontol Geriatr 15: 249–260, 1992.

Shoffner JM, Brown MD, Torroni A, Lott MT, Cabell P, Mirra SS, Beal MF, Yang C-C, Gearing M, Salvo R, Watts R, Juncos JL, Hanson LA, Crain BJ, Fayad M, Wallace DW. Mitochondrial DNA mutations associated with Alzheimer's and Parkinson's disease. Genomics 17: 171–184, 1993.

Shurtleff D, Raslear TG, Genovese RF, Simmons L. Perceptual bisection in rats: the effects of physostigmine, scopolamine and pirenzipine. Physiol. Behav. 51: 381–390, 1992.

Siegfred K: The pharmacodynamics of velnacrine: results and conclusion from clinical studies in ealthy subjects and patients with Alzheimer's disease. In: The Management of Alzheimer's disease, Wilcock GK, ed. Wrightson Biomedical Publishing Ltd., pp. 189–201, 1993.

Siesjo BK. Historical overview: calcium, ischemia and death of brain cells. Ann. N Y Acad. Sci. 522:638–661, 1988.

Sims NR, Bowen DM, Allen SJ, et al. Presynaptic cholinergic dysfunction in patients with dementia. J. Neurochem. 40:503–509, 1983.

Sims NR, Bowen DM, Neary D, Davison AN. Metabolic processes in Alzheimer's disease: Adenine nucleotide content and production of 14CO2 from [U-14C] glucose in vitro in human neocortex. J. Neurochem. 41: 1329–1334, 1993.

Sjak-shie NN, Burks JN and Meyer EM: Long-term actions on nicotinic receptor stimulation in nucleus basalis lesioned rats: blockade of trans-synaptic cell loss. In: Advances in Behavioral Biology, Vol 2, Nagatsu T, Fisher A and yoshida M, eds. New York: Plenum Press, pp 471–475, 1990.

Smith CD, Carney JM, Starke-Reed PE, et al. Excess brain protein oxidation and enzyme dysfunction in normal aging and Alzheimer disease. Proc Natl Acad Sci USA, 88: 10540–43, 1991.

Sorbi S, Bird ED, Blass JP. Decreased pyruvate dehydrogenase complex activity in Hungtington and Alzheimer brain. Ann. Neurol. 13: 72–78, 1993.

Southorn P, Powis G. Free radicals in medicine: I. Chemical nature and biologic reactions. Mayo Clin. Proc. 63:381–389, 1988a.

Spagnoli A., Lucca U., Menasce G., Bandera L., Cizza G., Forloni G., Tettamanti M., Frattura L., Tiraboschi P., Comelli M., Senin U., Longo A., Petrini A., Brambilla G., Belloni A., Negri C., Cavazzuti F., Salsi A., Calogero P., parma E., Stramba-Badiale M., Vitali S., Andreoni G., Inzoli M.R., Santus G., Caregnato R., Peruzza M., Favareytto M., Bozeglav C., Alberoni M., De Leo D., Serraiotto L., Baiocchi A., Scoccia S., Culotta P., Ieracitano D.: Long-term acetyl-L-carnitine treatment in Alzheimer's disease. Neurology 41, 1726, 1991.

Spignoli G, Pedata F, Giovannelli L, Banfi S, Moroni F, Pepeu G. Effects of oxiracetam and piracetam on central cholinergic mechanisms and active-avoidance acquisition. Clin. Neuropharmacol. 9 (suppl. 3):39–47, 1986.

Strittmatter WJ, Saunders AM, Schmechel D, Pericak-Vance M, Enghild J, Salvesen GS and Roses AD: Apolipoprotein E: High avidity binding to β-amyloid and increased frequency of type 4 allele in late-onset familial Alzheimer disease. Proc Natl Acad Sci 90: 1977–1981, 1993.

Subbarao KV, Richardson JS, Ang LC. Autopsy samples of Alzheimer's cortex show increased peroxidation in vitro. J Neurochem, 55: 342–5, 1990.

Summers KL, Cuadra G, Naritoku D and Giacobini E: Effects of nicotine levels on acetylcholine and biogenic amines in rat cortex. Drug Dev Res 31: 108–119, 1994.

Summers WK, Majovski LV, Marsh GM et al.: Orla tetrahydroaminoacridine in long-term treatment of senile dementia, Alzheimer type. N Engl J Med 315: 1241–1245, 1986.

Sunderland T, Rubinow DR, Tariot PN, et al. CSF somatostatin in patients with Alzheimer's disease, older depressed patients and age-matched controls. Am. J. Psychiatry 144:1313–1316, 1987.

Tariot PN, Cohen RM, Sunderland T., et al. L-deprenyl in Alzheimer's disease: preliminary evidence for behavioral changes with monoamine oxidase B inhibitor. Arch. Gen. Psychiatry 44:427–433, 1987.

Thal L.J, Carta A, Clarke WR, Ferris SH, Friedland RP, Petersen RC, Pettegrew JW, Pfeiffer E, Raskind MA, Sano M, Tuszynski MH, Woolson RF:A one year multicneter placebo controlled study of acetyl-L-carnitine in patients with Alzheimer's disease. Neurology ,1996 (in press).

Tucek S, Dolezal V. Negative effects of tacrine (tetrahydroaminoacridine) and methoxytacrine on the metabolism of acetylcholine in brain slices incubated under conditions stimulating neurotransmitter release. J. Neurochem. 56:1216–1221, 1991.

Tuszynski MH, Sang H, Yoshida K, Gage FH. Recombination human nerve growth factor infusions prevent cholinergic neuronal degeneration in the adult primate brain. Ann. Neurol. 30:625–363, 1991.

Vasar R, Harro J, Lang A et al: Anti-exploratory effects of N-methyl-D-aspartate in elevated pls-maze. Involvement of NMDA and CCK receptors. Eur. Neuropsychopharmacol. 3: 63–73, 1993.

Vecchi GP, Chiari G, Cipolli C, Cortelloni C. Acetyl-l-carnitine treatment of mental impairment in the elderly: evidence from a multicentre study. Arch. Gerontol. Geriatr. 10 (suppl. 2):159–168, 1991.

Volicer L, Crino PB. Involvement of free radicals in dementia of the ALzheimer's type hypothesis. Neurobiol. Aging 11:567–571, 1990.

Warburton DM, Rusted JM. Cholinergic control of cognitive resources. Neuropsychobiology 28: 43–46, 1993.

Weiss JH, Choi DW. Dihydropyridines attenuate slow excitatory amino acid neurotoxicity. In: Nimodipine, pharmacological and clinical studies in cerebral ischemia, Scriabine et al. (eds.) Springer Verlag, Berlin, pp. 57–63, 1991.

Whitehouse PJ, Vale WW, Zweig RM, et al. Reduction in corticotropin releasing factor-like immunoreativity in cerebral cortex in Alzheimer's disease, Parkinson's disease and progressive sopranuclear palsy. Neurology 37:905–909, 1987.

Whittemore SR, Seiger A. The expression, localization and functional significance of beta-nerve growth factor in the central nervous system. Brain Res. Rev. 12:439–464, 1987.

Wilcock GK, Surmon DJ, Scott M et al.: An evaluation of the efficacy and safety of tetrahydroaminoacridine (THA) without lecithin in the treatment of Alzheimer's disease. Age and Aging 22: 316–324, 1993.

Yan S-D, Chen X, Schmidt A-M, et al. Glycated tau protein in Alzheimer disease: a mechanism for induction of oxidant stress. Proc. Natl. Acad. Sci. USA 91: 7787–7791, 1994.

Yesavage J. Ergoloid mesylates (Hydergine). In: Alzheimer's disease: treatment and long-term management. Cummings & Miller (eds.) M. Dekker, New York, pp. 45–52, 1990.

Zeevalk GD, Nicklas WJ. Chemically induced hypoglycemia and anoxia: relationship to glutamate receptor-mediated toxicity in retina. J. Pharmacol. Exp. Ther. 253: 1285–1292, 1991.

22

GENETIC POLYMORPHISMS AND ARTERIAL THROMBOSIS

Maurizio Margaglione, Elvira Grandone, Francesco P. Mancini, and Giovanni Di Minno

Unità di Trombosi e Aterosclerosi
IRCCS "Casa Sollievo della Sofferenza" S. Giovanni Rotondo
Istituto di Biochimica e Biotecnologie
Università degli Studi di Napoli, "Federico II"
Cattedra di Gerontologia e Geriatria
Università degli Studi di Palermo, Italy

1. INTRODUCTION

In Western countries, acute myocardial infarction and stroke, are major causes of morbidity and mortality (1). An occlusive coronary thrombus on an ulcerated atherosclerotic plaque in the coronary arteries is the central event in more than 90% of patients with Q-wave myocardial infarction (2). The underlying abnormality in non-Q-wave infarctions is a ruptured atherosclerotic plaque, which acts as a nidus for the deposition and activation of platelets. Atherosclerotic changes in the carotid and vertebrobasilar arteries resemble those of coronary arteries (3). These lesions may progress to local occlusions, but most often do not become symptomatic until embolization to more distal arteries takes place (ischemic stroke). In the cerebral arteries, vessel wall and lumen may be normal until the artery is occluded by an embolus from a more proximal arterial lesion or from the heart (4). Rather than to emboli, occlusion of the small penetrating arteries is often due to degenerative changes of the vessels or to extracranial large-artery disease (5).

2. PREDICTORS OF ISCHEMIC EVENTS

The risk of vascular ischemic disease presents a different distribution pattern throughout the world, mortality for myocardial infarction being lower in Southern than in Northern European Countries, in Japan than in North America (6,7). Excess weight, diabetes mellitus, arterial hypertension, and differences in dietary and smoking habits only account for a limited portion of the future ischemic event (8,9). In the different populations of the WHO/MONICA Core Study, differences in mortality for coronary artery disease among populations presented a correlation with coexistence of hypertension, dyslipidemia

Recent Advances in Geriatrics, edited by Barbagallo, Licata, and Sowers.
Plenum Press, New York, 1998.

and smoking that was around 20% (10). More recently, an increased risk of arterial thrombosis has been associated with high plasma levels of coagulation factors (fibrinogen, factor VII) (9,11), of fibrinolytic variables {tissue plasminogen activator, plasminogen activator inhibitor-1, (PAI-l)} (12,13), and of lipoproteins and apo 1 apoliproteins (LDL-cholesterol, Lp(a), apo B) (14–16). Some of them (e.g. fibrinogen, PAI-1) are acute-phase proteins (17,18). Cigarette smoking, excess weight and diabetes mellitus are known to increase the plasma levels of some acute-phase proteins, including fibrinogen and PAI-1. Moreover. regardless of the risk factor(s) involved, a prolonged treatment with antithrombotic drugs significantly reduces the recurrence of ischemic events (19).

3. GENETIC DETERMINANTS AND ISCHEMIC EVENTS

Observations that young individuals and families lacking major risk factors for thrombosis experience thrombotic episodes, has fostered the search for additional conditions predisposing to ischemic diseases (20–22). On the other hand, the aggregation of ischemic disease in families, ethnic groups and specific subsets of population (23–25), and the observation that the levels of some risk factors are genetically determined, supported the search for genetic factors in the susceptibility to ischemic complications of atherosclerosis. Further support to the role of genetics with respect to the risk of ischemia derived from the following: a) parental history of coronary heart disease is associated with increased risk of myocardial ischemia (26); b) the onset of coronary artery disease in a first degree relative before the age of 55 yrs increases by ten-fold the risk in other family members (27); c) in several twin studies, a strong genetic component in the occurrence of cardiovascular events is documented; (28) d) four studies (29–32) have been devoted to identifying risk factors for stroke events. In three of them (29,30,32), a significant contribution of genetic factors to the development of the cerebral event has been documented; e) a nearly five-fold increase in the prevalence of stroke is present among monozygotic twin pairs as compared to dizygotic ones (33); f) in a large prospective study in Great Britain, an association between history of parental death from stroke and risk of stroke has been documented (34). This association is independent of the presence of risk factors for cerebrovascular events.

4. SUSCEPTIBILITY GENES

In polygenic disorders, a genetic determinant may increase the risk of a disease (susceptibility locus) without being necessary or sufficient for the disease expression. Thus, an allelic form at some locus increases the chances that a person will become ill with a disease, but the presence of that allele is not the determining factor in the disease expression. It merely lowers the threshold for the disease.

Large populations carry an array of alternative forms of genes (polymorphisms) that would never result in or contribute to a disease if not present in the appropriate milieu (35). In most cases, the interaction with environmental factors is needed for common molecular variations (polymorphisms) to regulate protein levels and/or function. This is true for most hemostatic factors whose raised plasma levels are associated with the risk of arterial thrombosis (36–38), for apolipoproteins (39,40), and for the angiotensin converting enzyme (ACE) (41). Moreover, genetic variations within the gene loci of apolipoprotein E (Apo E) (42), of endothelial constitutive nitric oxide synthase (43), and of methylenetetrahydrofolate reductase enzyme (44) affect protein function, thus mediating the risk of ischemic disease. Many pathways are involved in the development of arterial thrombosis. Thus, there may be different mutations and gene combinations contributing to ischemic vascular disease. A strategy for identifying these genes, is to search for intermediate phenotypes (e.g. subjects with dyslipidemia, obesity, diabetes mellitus, and hypertension) at high risk for developing ischemic complications of atherosclerosis. An alternative approach is to investigate phenotypes at high risk for developing thrombosis.

4.1. Fibrinogen

The data so far available support the relevance of genetic determinants in the regulation of plasma fibrinogen concentrations, especially in the youth (45). Recurrent mutations within the gene loci of the fibrinogen chains have been identified, that contribute to genetic differences in fibrinogen gene expression (46). A G-to-A transition at position -455 within the 51 untraslated region of the BB-chain gene locus of the fibrinogen shows a significant correlation with plasma fibrinogen levels especially in smokers (47). Risk factors such as cigarette smoking and a positive family history for ischemic episodes, are strong determinants of plasma fibrinogen levels (48). Similarly to sex, the effect of cigarette smoking on plasma fibrinogen is mediated by polymorphisms that modulate fibrinogen gene expression (49). On the other hand, some gene variations of the BB-chain gene have been related to coronary or peripheral artery thrombosis irrespective of their effect on plasma fibrinogen levels (50,51). This suggests that, in addition to plasma levels, polymorphisms may affect some functional properties of fibrinogen. Because of the weak linkage between the genes coding for the three fibrinogen chains, studies in which their polymorphisms are evaluated in combination, and in conjunction with plasma fibrinogen levels are likely to be more informative than single determinations with respect to the prevention of ischemia.

4.2. Factor VII

Differences in FVII levels have been reported in different ethnic groups (52). However, there is no perspective study aimed at evaluating genotype frequencies in large groups of individuals either at risk for or with a history of ischemic episodes. Among the variations located within the FVII gene locus, a G-to-A substitution that causes the change of a arginine for a glutamine, and a decanucleotide insertion in the promoter have been reported to significantly affect FVII plasma levels (37,53). Due to the strong linkage between these molecular markers, they show similar frequencies and informativeness (54). A case-control study has failed to document raised plasma concentrations of FVII or raised frequency of the Arg/Arg genotype in men with a history of myocardial infarction (55).

4.3. PAI-1

Common genetic variations have been described within the PAI-1 gene, and some of them have been related to different plasma levels of PAI-1 (38,56). In a group of individuals with non insulin dependent diabetes mellitus, insulin sensitivity, the G-675 insertion/deletion (4G/5G) of PAI-1 gene and plasma triglycerides, were the strongest determinants of PAI-1 activity (57). Moreover, the genotype was found to modulate the effects of triglycerides on PAI-1 activity. The frequency of the deletion allele (4G) has been reported to be significantly higher than normal in patients with a previous myocardial infarction (58), and in those with non-insulin dependent diabetes mellitus with coronary artery disease (59). We have found similar data in a population of subjects with previous ischemic stroke, being the genotype a strong determinant of plasma PAI-1 levels (60). In addition, healthy subjects whose first-degree relatives suffered from myocardial ischemia carry a significant higher frequency of the 4G allele than controls (Margaglione et al., unpublished). A large case-control study (61), has confirmed the association between plasma PAI-1 and the 4G/5G genotype, while it did not find allele or genotype differences between patients with or without a history of myocardial infarction.

4.4. ACE

Plasma ACE levels are stable in a given subject, and show an intrafamilial correlation largely related to a major gene effect (62). A common gene variation has been found to account for up to 50% of the variance of plasma and tissue ACE concentrations, higher levels being related to the homozygosity for the deletion genotype (DD) (41). Several case-control reports have shown a raised frequency of the DD genotype in groups of individuals with myocardial infarction (63,64), with idiopathic and ischemic-dilated cardiomyopathy (65), with sudden death in hypertrophic cardiomyopathy (66), and with restenosis after percutaneous transluminal coronary angioplasty (67). We found a raised frequency of the DD genotype in a subset of individuals with previous ischemic stroke (68). In addition, an association between the D allele and the occurrence (69), as well as a parental history (70), of ischemic stroke has been found in Japanese hypertensive subjects. Recent case-control (71,72) and perspective (73,74) studies have challenged the conclusions of these reports. Differences in the genetic background (75); in criteria used to select the groups examined; the low informativeness of the marker used, and the low statistical power of some studies may account for these discrepancies.

4.5. Apo E

Population studies show that the highest plasma LDL-cholesterol are found in carrers of a molecular variation of the apoprotein E, E4, the lowest being found in carriers of another variation, Apo E2 (42,76). This difference is more pronounced in women after menopause, implying that estrogen status and Apo E alleles may concurrently affect lipid levels. on the other hand, both Apo E2 and E4 are associated with hypertriglyceridemia (77). A series of reports have pointed to the relationships between Apo E alleles and early development of atherosclerosis and its ischemic complications (78,79). Cross-sectional studies report a lower than normal frequency of the apo E2 allele in a group of subjects with coronary heart disease, and an excess of this allele among octogenarians and centenarians (80). However, lower ischemic cardiovascular event rates have not been reported in individuals carrying this allele. Apo E4 allele, on the other hand, is strongly and consistently correlated with the risk of cardiovascular ischemic events (42,81–83). A metanalysis recently published (84), further strengthens this correlation both in men and in women. The relationship between apo E 4 allele with ischemic cerebrovascular disease is still matter of investigation (85,86).

4.6. Other Genes

In addition to the variations reported above, variations in other gene loci (43,50,87,88) have been shown to correlate with the risk of ischemic events. Their clinical relevance requires further observations.

5. THE BEGINNING OF A JOURNEY

An in-depth analysis of the contribution of a gene variation or a mutation in the propensity to develop common multifactorial disorders (e.g. vascular ischemic events), should take into account several issues. a) If a molecular variation plays only a role in determining arterial thrombosis, why is it so frequent? Most arterial ischemic events develop after or during the reproductive years. A number of strategies are currently available that allow individuals who otherwise would die from arterial thrombosis to live and transmit these genes to offspring. b) The effect of some gene variations requires an interaction with environmental factors. The "westernized" lifestyle (diet, inactivity, pollution, stress) that was uncommon in the past, is now represented in different degrees throughout the world. c) The rate of thrombotic disease increases progressively with age, its risk being highest in the elderly (89,90). Several coagulation and fibrinolytic variables rise with age, suggesting that a hypercoagulable and/or a hypofibrinolytic state contributes to the increased thrombotic tendency in the elderly (91–93). However, an enhanced activity of the coagulation enzymes is present in healthy men up to 80 years of age (94,95); a high coagulation enzyme activity leading to discrete fibrin formation and to secondary hyperfibrinolysis occurs in healthy centenarians in the absence of a history of current thrombotic episodes (96). Are such biochemical findings a marker of physiological aging rather than of an age-dependent molecular derangement predisposing to thrombosis? d) Unlike single-gene disorders, where the relationship is essentially qualitative, multifactorial disorders involve additive effects. A candidate gene or combinations of gene markers may be present in individuals, single families or populations without necessarily implying that the target disease will occur. e) To evaluate the contribution of any individual gene to the incidence of a disorder, potential biases in patient selection, that would obscure positive data and make reproducibility difficult, should be avoided. Only rigorously designed, large, perspective studies meet these requirements, and allow for reliable extrapolations of clinical implications from observational/interventional reports. Most results summarized in the previous paragraphs derive from inadequate (i.e. cross-sectional or case-control) studies.

6. PERSPECTIVES

In some subsets, genotyping has helped clarify the mechanisms leading to fluctuations of some variables, thus leading to the identification of subjects whose plasma levels show large variations over time, approaching the highest values. For example, FVII and PAI-1 plasma levels are related, to some extent, to the interaction of certain gene variations with triglycerides. Presently, genotyping is the method of choice for variables (ACE, Apo E) whose detection by alternative means is complex and not readily available. The latter genotypes help clarify different responses to dietary and pharmacological strategies. ACE-inhibitors slow down renal failure mainly in non-DD individuals (97,98); the lipid-lowering effect of diets, HMG-COA reductase inhibitors, and probucol is more pronounced in carriers of the Apo E4 genotype (99,100). However, whether genetic tests might provide additional information over the measurement of the variables (14); whether to identify high-risk individuals, it would be cheaper and easier to look for these "variable genotypes" than take repeated measures of the protein over a period of time; whether they will replace currently employed measurements of the risk of ischemia associated with high levels of some variables; whether, in the youth, they will identify subjects at risk for future events regardless of the effect of environmental factors (e.g. age, diet, hormonal status etc); whether such information will help interpret the results of future observational and/or interventional studies, and whether this will allow for a more accurate identification of groups of individuals who need appropriate advice on environmental conditions predisposing to thrombotic events, is presently unclear and cannot be inferred from the data available. The long journey of genetics in cardiovascular disease is just beginning (101).

REFERENCES

1. Fuster V, Badimon L, Badimon JJ, Chesebro JH. The pathogenesis of coronary artery disease and acute coronary syndromes. New Engl. J. Med. 1992;326,242~ 250.
2. Mizuno K, Miyamoto A, Satomura K et al. Angioscopic coronary macromorphology in patients with acute coronary disorders. Lancet 1991;337, 809–12.
3. Jorgensen L, Torvik A. Ischemic cerebrovascular diseases in an autopsy series. Part 2: Prevalence, location, pathogenesis, and clinical course of cerebral infarct. J. Neurol. Science 1969; 9:285–320.
4. Olsen TS, Skriver EB, Heming M. Cause of cerebral infarction in the carotid territori. Its relation to the size and the location of the infarct and to the underlying vascular lesion. Stroke 1985; 16:459–466.
5. Millikan C, Futrell N. The fallacy of the lacune hypothesis. Stroke 1990;21:1251–1257.
6. Parra HJ, Arveiler D, Evans AE, Cambou JP, Amouyel P, Bingham A, McMaster D, Schaffer P, Douste-Blazy P, Luc G, Richard JL, Ducimetière P, Fruchart JC, Cambien F. A case-control study of lipoprotein particles in two populations at contrastino risk for coronary heart disease. Arterioscler Thromb 1992;12:701707.
7. Sing CF, Moll PP. Genetics of variabilità of CHD risk. Int. J. Epidemiol. 1989;18 (suppl 1): S183-S195.
8. Kannell WB. Bishop lecture: Contribution of the Framingham study to preventive cardiology. J. Am. Coll. Cardiol. 1990;15, 206–211.
9. Ernst E., Resch KL. Fibrinogen as a cardiovascular risk factor: a meta-analysis and review of the literature. Ann Int Med 1993;118:956–963.
10. The WHO MONICA project. A worldwide monitoring system for cardiovascular disease. World Health Stat Annu. 1989;27.
11. Meade TW, Mellows S, Brozovic M, Miller GJ, Chakrabarti RR, North WRS, Haines AP, Stirling Y, Imeson JD, Thompson SG. Hemostatic function and ischemic heart disease: Principal results of the Northwick Park Study. Lancet 1986;2:533–7.
12. Ridker PM, Vaughan, DE, Stampfer MJ, Manson JE, Hennekens CH. Endogenous tissue-type plasminogen activator and risk of myocardial infarction. Lancet 1993; 341: 1165–1168.
13. Hamsten A, De Faire U, Walldius G, Dahlen G, Szamosi A, Landou C, Blomback M, Wiman B: Plasminogen activator inhibitor in plasma: risk factor for recurrent myocardial infarction. Lancet 1987;2:3–9.
14. Kannel WB. Range of serum cholesterol values in the population developing coronary artery disease. Am. i. Cardiol. 1995;76:69C-77C.
15. Schaefer EJ, Lamon-Fava S, Jenner JL, McNamara JL, Ordovas JM, Davis CE, Abolafia JM, Lippel K, Levy RI. Lipoprotein(a) levels and risk of coronary heart disease in men. The Lipid Research Clinics Coronary Primary Prevention Trial. JAMA 1994, 271: 999–1003
16. Tornvall P, Bavenholrn P, Landou C, de Faire U, Hamsten A. Relation of plasma levels and compogition of apolipoprotein B-containing lipoproteins to angiographically defined coronary artery disease in young patients with myocardial infarction. Circulation 1993;88(part 1):2180–2189.
17. Heinrich PC, Castell JV, Andus T. Interleukin 6 and the acute phase response. Biochem. J. 1990; 265:621–636.
18. Schneiderman J, Loskutoff DJ. Plasminogen Activator inhibitors. Trends Cardiovasc. Med. 1991;1:99–102.
19. Antiplatelet Trialists, Collaboration. Secondary prevention of vascular events by prolonged antiplatelet therapy. BMJ 1988;296:320–331
20. Goldbourt U, Neufeld HN. Genetic aspect of arteriosclerosis. Arteriosclerosis 1986; 6:357–377.
21. Miletich JP, Prescott SM, White R, Majerus PW, Bovill EG. Inherited predisposition to thrombosis. Cell 1993; 72:477–480.
22. Hamsten A, Iselius L, Dahlen G, defaire U. Genetic and cultural inheritance of serum lipids, low and high density lipoprotein cholesterol and serum apoprotein A~I, A-II, and B. Atherosclerosis 1986;60:199–208.
23. Humphries SE. The genetic contribution to the risk of thrombosis and cardiovascular disease. Trends Cardiovasc. Med. 1994;4:8–17.

24. Haverkate F, Samama M. Familial dysfibrinogenemia and thrombophilia. Report on a study of the SSC Subcommitte on fibrinogen. Thromb. Haernost. 1995; le 73:151–161.
25. Deutscher S, Epstein F, Kjelsberg M. Familial aggregation of coronary heart disease. Circulation 1966;33:911–924.
26. Nora J, Lortscher R, Spangler R, Nora A, Kimberling W. Genetic-epidemiological study of early onset ischemic heart disease. Circulation 1980;61:503508.
27. de Faire U. Ischemic heart disease in death discordant twins. A study in 205 male and female pairs. Acta Med. Scand. Suppl. 1974;568:1–109.
28. Berg K. Twin research in coronary heart disease. In Parisi GL, Nance WL. Twin research 3: Epidemiological and Clinical Studies. New York, Alan R Liss, 1981; pp. 117–130.
29. Khaw KT, Barrett CE. Family history of stroke as an independent predictor of ischemic heart disease in men and stroke in women. Am. J. Epidemiol. 1986;123:59–66.
30. Welin L, Svardsudd K, Wilhelmsen L, Larsson B, Tibblin G. Analysis of risk factors for a stroke cohort of men born in 1913. N. Engl i. Med 1987;317:321326.
31. Boysen G, Nyboe J, Appleyard M, Sorensen PS, Boas J, Somnier F, Jensen J, schnohr P. stroke incidence and risk factors for stroke in Copenhagen, Denmark. Stroke 1988;19:1345–1353.
32. Kiely DK, Wolf PA, Cupples A, Beiser AS, Myers RH. Familial aggregation of stroke. The Framingham study. 1993;24:1366–1371.
33. Brass LM, isaacsohn i, Merikangas KR, Robinette CD. A study of twins and stroke. Stroke 1992;23:221–223.
34. Wannamethee SG, Shaper GA, Ebrahim S. History of parental death from stroke or heart trouble and the risk of stroke in middle-aged men. Stroke 1996;27:1492–1498.
35. Wright S. The shifting balance of evolution theory and macroevolution. Ann. Rev. Genet. 1982;16:1–19.
36. Humphries SE, Cook M, Dubovitz M, Stirling Y, Meade TW. Role of genetic variation at the fibrinogen locus in the determination of plasma fibrinogen concentrations. Lancet 1987;1:1452–5.
37. Green F, Kelleher C, Wilkes H, Temple A, Meade T, Humphries S. A common genetic polymorphism associate with lower coagulation factor VII levels in healthy individuale. Arterioscler. Thromb. 1991;11:540–546.
38. Dawson SJ, Wiman B, Hamsten A, Green F, Humphries S, Henney AM: The two allele sequences of a common polymorphism in the promoter of the plasminogen activator inhibitor-1 (PAI-l) gene respond differently to interleukin-1 in HepG2 cells. J. Biol Chem 1993;268:10739–10745.
39. Wade DP, Klarke JC, Lindahl GE, Liu AC Zysow BR, Meer K, Schwartz K, Lawn RM. 51 control regions of the apoprotein(a) gene and members of the related plasminogen gene family. Proc. Natl. Acad. Sci. USA 1993; 90:1369–1373.
40. Hansen PS, Gerdes LU, Klausen IC, Gregersen N, Faergeman 0. Polymorphisms in the apoliprotein B-100 gene contributes to normal variation in plasma lipids in 464 Danish men born in 1948. Hum. Genet. 1993;91:45–50.
41. Cambien F, Poirier O, Lecerf L, Evans A, Cambou JP, Arveiler D, Luc G, Bara L, Ricard S, Tiret L, Amouyel P, Alhenc-Gelas F, Soubrier F. Deletion polymorphism in the gene for angiotensin-converting enzyme is a potent risk factor for myocardial infarction. Nature 1992; 359: 641–344.
42. Cumming AM, Robertson F. Polymorphism at the apo E locus in relation to risk of coronary disease. Clin. Genet. 1984;25:301–313.
43. Wahg XL, Sim AS, Badhenop RF, McCradie RM, Wilcken DEL. A smoking-dependent risk of coronary artery disease associated with a polymorphism of the endothelial nitric oxide synthase gene. Nat. Med. 1996;2:41–45.
44. de Franchis R, Mancini FP, D'Angelo A, Sebastio G, Fermo I, De Stefano V, Margaglione M, Mazzola G, Di Minno G, Andria G. Elevated total plasma homocysteine and 677C->T mutation of the 5,10 Methylenetetrahydrofolate reductase gene in thrombotic vascular disease. Am. J. Hum. Genet. 1996;59:262–264.
45. Livshits G, Schettler G, Graf f E, Bletter M, Wahrendorf J, Brunner D. Tel Aviv-Heidelberg three-generation offspring study: genetic determinants of plasma fibrinogen level. Am. J. Med. Genet. 1996;63:509–517.
46. Margaglione M, Grandone E, Mancini FP, Di Minno G. Genetic modulation of plasma fibrinogen concentrations: possible importance of interleukin-6. i. Thromb. Thrombolysis 1996;3:51–56.
47. Thomas AE, Green FR, Kelleher CH, et al. Variation in the promoter region of the b fibrinogen gene is associated with plasma fibrinogen levels in smokers and non-smokers. Thromb. Haemost. 1991;65: 487–490.
48. Margaglione M, Di Minno G, Grandone E, Vecchione G, Celentano E, Cappucci G, Giordano M, Grilli M, Simone P, Fusilli S, Panico S, Mancini M. Raised plasma fibrinogen concentrations in subjects attendine a metabolic ward. Relation to family history and vascular risk factors. Thromb Haemost 1995;73:579–83.

49. Humphries SE, Ye S, Talmud P, Bara L, Wilhelmsen L, Tiret L, on behalf of the European Atherosclerosis Research Study (EARS) group. European atherosclerosis research study: genotype at the fibrinogen locus (G-455-A b-gene) is associated with differences in plasma fibrinogen levels in young men and women from different regions in Europe. Evidence for gender-genotype-environment interaction. Arterioscler Thromb Vasc Biol 1995;15:96–104.
50. Fowkes FGR, Connor JM, Smith FB, Wood J, Donnan PT, Lowe GDO. Fibrinogen genotype and risk of peripheral atherosclerosis. Lancet 1992;339:693–696.
51. Behague I, Poirier 0, Nicaud V, Evans A, Arveiler D, Luc G, Cambou JP, Scarabin PJ, Bara L, Green F, Cambien F. b-fibrinogen gene polymorphisms are associated with plasma fibrinogen and coronary artery disease in patients with myocardial infarction. The ECTIM study. Circulation 1996; 93:440–9.
52. Lane A, Cruickshank JK, Mitchell J, Henderson A Humphries S, Green F. Genetic and environmental determinants of factor VII coagulant activity in ethnic groups at different risk of coronary heart disease. Atherosclerosis 1992;94:43–50.
53. Marchetti G, Petracchini P, Papacchini M, Ferrati M, Bernardi F. A polymorphism in the 51 region of coagulation factor VII gene (F7) due to an inserted decanucleotide. Hum Genet 1993;90:575–6.
54. Bernardi F, Marchetti G, Pinotti M, Arcieri P, Baroncini C, Papacchini M, Zepponi E, Ursicino N, Chiarotti F, Mariani G. Factor VII gene polymorphisms contributo about one third of the factor VII level variation in plasma. Arterioscler Thromb Vasc Biol 1996;16:72–6.
55. Moor E, Silvera A, vanlt Hooft F, Suontaka AM, Eriksson P, Blomback M, Hamsten A. Coagulation factor VII mass and activity in young men with myocardial infarction at a young age. Role of plasma lipoproteins and factor VII genotype. Arterioscler Thromb Vasc Biol 1995;15:655–64.
56. Dawson **S**, Hamsten A, Wiman B, Hehney A, Humphries S. Genetic variation at the plasminogen activator inhibitor-1 locus is associate with altered levels of plasma plasminogen activator inhibitor-1 activity. Arterioscler. Thromb. 1991;11:183–190.
57. Panahloo A, Mohamed-Ali V, Lane A, Green F, Humphries SE, Yudkin JS. Determinants of plasminogen activator inhibitor 1 activity in treated NIDDM and its relation to a polymorphism in the plasminogen activator inhibitor 1 gene. Diabetes 1995;44: 37–42.
58. Eriksson P, Kallin B, van t'Hooft FM, Bavhenolm P, Hamsten A. Allelic-specific increase in basal transcription of the plasminogen-activator inhibitor 1 gene is associate with myocardial infarction. Proc. Natl. Acad. Sci. USA 1995;92:1851–1855.
59. Mansfield MW, Stickland MH, Grant PJ. Plasminogen activator inhibitor-1 (PAI-l) promoter polymorphism and coronary artery disease in non-insulin-dependent diabetes. Thromb. Haemost. 1995; 74:1032–1034.
60. Margaglione M, Grandone E, Vecchione G, Cappucci G, Giuliani N, Colaizzo N, Celentano E, Panico S, Di Minno G.Plasminogen activator inhibitor-1 (PAI-1) antigen plasma levels in subjects attending a metabolíc ward..Relation to polymorphisms of the PAI-1 and of the angiontensin converting enzyme (ACE) genes. Atrioscler. Thromb. Vasc. Biol. 1997 17: (in press).
61. Ye S, Greeh FR, Scarabin PY, Nicaud V, Bara L, Dawson Si, Humphries SE, Evans A, Luc **G**, Cambou JP Arveiler D, Henney AM, Cambien F. The 4G/5G genetic polymorphism in the promoter of the plasminogen activator inhibitor-1 (PAI-l) gene is associate with differences in plasma PAI-1 activity but not with risk of myocardial infarction in the ECTIM study. Thromb. Haemost. 1995;74:837–841.
62. Cambien F, Soubrier F. The angiotensin-converting enzyme: molecular biology and implication of the gene polymorphism in cardiovascular diseases. In Hypertension, pathophysiology and management. Second Edition. Raven Press LTD, New York, Larg JH, Brenner BM Eds, 1995; pp 1667–1682.
63. Cambien F, Poirier 0, Lecerf L, Evans A, Cambou JP, Arveiler D, Luc G, Bara L, Ricard S, Tiret L, Amouyel P, Alhenc-Gelas F, Soubrier F. Deletion polymorphism in the gene for angiotensin-converting enzyme is a potent risk factor for myocardial infarction. Nature 1992; 359: 641–344.
64. Samani N, Thompson JR, O'Toole L, Channer K, Woods KL. A meta-analysis of the association of the deletion allele of the angiotensin-converting enzyme gene with myocardial infarction. Circulation 1996;94:708–712.
65. Reynolds MV, Bristow MR, Bush EW, Abraham WT, Lowes BD, Zisrnan LS, Taft CS, Perryman MB. Angiotensin-converting enzyme DD genotype in patients with ischaemic or dilated cardiomyopathy. Lancet 1993;342:1073–1075.
66. Marian AJ, Yu QT, Workman R, Greve G, Roberts R. Angiotensin-converting enzyme polymorphism in hypertrophic cardiomyopathy and sudden cardiac death. Lancet 1993;342:1085–1086.
67. Samani NJ, Martin DS, Brack M, Cullen J, Chauhan A, Lodwick D, Harley A, Swales JD, de Bono DP, Gershlick AH. Insertion/deletion polymorphism in the angiotensin-converting enzyme gene and risk of restenosis after coronary angioplasty. Lancet 1995;345:1013–1016.

68. Margaglione M, Celentano E, Grandone E, Vecchionè G, Cappucci G, Giuliani N, Colaizzo D, Panico S, Mancini FP, Di Minno G. Deletion Polymorphism of the angiotensin convertine enzyme gene in patients with a history of ischemic stroke. Arteriosc1. Thrombos Vasc. Biol. 1996; 16: 304–309.
69. Kario K, Kanai N, Saito K, Nago N, Matsuo T, Shimada K. Ischemic stroke and the gene for angiotensin-converting enzyme in Japanese hypertensives. Circulation 1996;93:1630–1633.
70. Maeda Y, Ikeda U, Ebata H, Hojo Y, Seino Y, Hayashi Y, Kuroki S, Shimada. Angiotensin-converting enzyme gene in hypertensive individuale with parental history of stroke. Stroke 1996;27:1521–1523.
71. Bonh, Berge KE, Bakkan A, Erikssen J, Berg K. Insertion/deletion (I/D) polymorphism at the locus for angiotensin I-converting enzyme and myocardial infarction. Clin. Genetics, 1993; 44:298–301.
72. Catto A, Carter AM, Barrett JH, Stickland M, Bamford J, Davis JA, Grant PJ. Angiotensin-converting enzyme insertion/deletion polymorphism and cerebrovascular disease. Stroke 1996;27:435–440.
73. Lindpaintner K, Pfeffer MA, Kreutz R, Stampfer MJ, Grodstein F, LaMotte F, Burig J, Hennekens CH. A prospective evaluation of angiotensin-converting enzyme gene polymorphism and the risk of ischemic heart disease. N. Engl. J Med 1995, 332, 706–711.
74. Lindpainter K, Lee M, larson M, Rao VR, Pfeffer MA, Ordovas JM, Schaefer EJ, Wilson AF, Wilson PWF, Vasan RS, Myers RH, Levy D. Absence of association or genetic linkage between the angiotensin-converting enzyme gene and left ventricular mass. N. Engl. J. Med 1996;334:1023–1028.
75. Bloem LJ, Manatunga AK, Pratt JH. Racial differente in the relationship of an angiotensin-converting enzyme gene polymorphism to serum angiotensin Iconverting enzyme activity. Hypertension 1996;27:62–66.
76. Davignon J. Apolipoprotein E polymorphism and atherosclerosis. In: Born GVR, Schwartz CJ, eds. New horizons in coronary heart disease. London UK: Science Press Ltd. 1993:5.1–5.21.
77. Dallongeville J, Lussier-Cacan S, Davignon J. Modulation of plasma triglyceride levels by apo E phenotype: a meta-analysis. J. Lipid Res. 1992;33:447454.
78. Hixson JE, Pathobiological Determinants of Atherosclerosis in Youth (PDAY) research group. Apolipoprotein E polymorphisms affect atherosclerosis in young males. Arterioscler. Thromb. 1991;11:1237–1244.
79. Pedro-Botet J, Senti M, Nogues X, Rubiès-Prat J, Roquer J, D'Olhaberriague L, Olivé J. Lipoprotein and apolipoprotein profile in men with ischemic stroke. Role of lipoprotein(a), triglyceride-rich lipoproteins, and apolipoprotein E polymorphism. Stroke 1992;23:1556–1562.
80. Schachter F, Faure-Delanef L, Guenot F, Rouger H, Froguel R, Lesueur-Ginot L and Cohen D. Genetic associations with human longevità at the Apo E and ACE loci. Nat Genet 1994; 6: 29–32
81. Utermann G, Hardewig A, Zimmer F. Apo E phenotypes in patients with myocardial infarction. Hum. Genet. 1984;65:237–241.
82. Wilson PWF, myers RH, larson MG, Ordovas JM, Wolf PA, Schaefer EJ. Apolipoprotein E alleles, dyslipidemia, and coronary heart disease. The Framingham Offspring Study. JAMA 1994;272:1666~1671.
83. Stengard JH, Zerba KE, Pekkanen J, Ehnholm C, Nissinen A, Sing CF. Apolipoprotein E polymorphism predicts death from coronary heart disease in a longitudinal study of elderly Finnish men. Circulation 1995;91:265–269.
84. Wilson PWF, Schaefer EJ, Larson MG, Ordovas JM. Apolipoprotein E alleles and risk of coronary disease. A meta-analysis. Arterioscler. Thromb. Vasc. Biol. 1996; 16:1250–1255.
85. Couderc R, Mahieux F, Bailleul S, Fenelon G, Mary R, Fermianan J. Prevalence of apolipoprotein E phenotypes in ischemic cerebrovascular disease. A case-control study. Stroke 1993;24:661–664.
86. Basun H, Corder EH, Guo Z, Lannfelt L, Corder LS, Manton KG, Winblad B, Viitanen N. Apolipoprotein E polymorphism and stroke in a population aged 75 years or more. Stroke 1996;27:1310–1315.
87. Weiss EJ, Bray PF, Tayback M, Schulman SP, Kickler TS, Becker LC, Weiss JL, Gerstenblith G, Goldschmidt~Clermont PJ. A polymorphism of a platelet glycoprotein receptor as an inserite risk factor for coronary thrombosis. N. Engl. J. Med. 1996;334:1090–1094.
88. Ye S, Eriksson P, Hamsten A, Kurkinen M, Humphries SE, Henney AM. Progression of coronary atherosclerosis is associate with a common genetic variant of the human stromelysin-1 promoter which results in reduced gene expression. Biol. Chem. 1996;271:13055–13060.
89. Castelli WP, Garrison RJ, Wilson PWF, Abbott RD, Kalousdian F, Kannell WB. Incidence of coronary heart disease and lipoprotein cholesterol levels in the Framingham Study. JAMA 1986;256:2835–2838.
90. Alberts MJ. Genetic aspects of cerebrovascular disease. Stroke 1991;22:277–280.
91. Hamilton PJ, Allardyce PJM, ogston D, Dawson AA, Douglas AS. The effect of age upon the coagulation system. J. Clin. Pathol. 1974;27:980–989.
92. Meade TW, North WRS, Chakrabarti R, Haines AP, Stirling Y. Population-based distribution of hemostatic variables. Br. Med. Bull. 1977;33:283–288.
93. Meade TW, Chakrabarti R, Haines AP, North WRS, Stirling Y. Characteristics affecting fibrinolytic activity and plasma fibrinogen concentrations. Br. Med. 1979;1:153–156.

94. Bauer KA, Wiess LM, Sparrow D, Vokonas PS, Rosenberg RD. Aging-associated changes in indices of thrombin generation and protein C activation in humans. Normative aging study. J. Clin. Invest. 1987;80:1527–1533.
95. Bauer KA, Kass BL, ten Cate H, Bednareck MA Hawiger JJ, Rosenberg RD. Detection of Factor X in humans. Blood 1989;74:2007–2012.
96. Mari D, Mannucci PM, Coppola R, Bottasso B, Bauer KA, Rosenberg RD. Hypercoagulability in centenarians: the paradox of successful aging. Blood 1995;85:3144–3149.
97. Yoshida H, Mitarai T, Kawamura T, Kitajima T, Miyazaki Y, Nagasawa R, Kawaguchi Y, Kubo H, Ichikawa I, Sakai 0. Role of the deletion polymorphism of the angiotensin convertine enzyme gene in the progression and therapeutic responsiveness of IgA nephropathy. J. Clin. Invest. 1995;96:2162–2169.
98. van Essen GG, Rensma P, de Zeeuw D, Sliter WJ, Apperloo AJ, de Jong PE. Association between angiotensin-converting-enzyme gene polymorphism and failure of renoprotective therapy. Lancet 1996;347:94–95.
99. Cobb MM, Teitlebaum H, Risch N, iekel J, Ostfeld A. Influence of dietary fat, apolipoprotein E phenotype, and sex on plasma lipoprotein levels. Circulation 1992;86:849–857.
100. Carmena R, Roederer G, Mailloux H, Lussier-Cacan S, Davignon J. The response to lovastatin treatment in patients with heterozygous familial hypercholesterolemia is modulate by apolipoprotein E polymorphism. Metabolism 1993;42:895–901.
101. Harrap SB. Genetics and coronary disease: beginning the long journey. Lancet 1994; 344: 901–902

23

FROM THROMBOSIS TO ACUTE INFLAMMATORY REACTION

New Aspects of Unstable Angina

Gian Gastone Neri Serneri,* Pietro Amedeo Modesti, and Ilaria Cecioni

Clinica Medica Generale e Cardiologia
Center for Heart and Thrombosis Research
University of Florence
Viale Morgagni, 85
50134 Florence, Italy

INTRODUCTION

Autoptic studies performed on large number of patients (1,2) have demonstrated that the frequency of raised coronary atherosclerotic lesions in patients died from ischemic heart disease was not significantly different from that of patients who never had suffered from ischemic artery disease. Thus, the severity of coronary artery lesions is not sufficient to cause the occurence of clinical symptoms. Recent angiographic studies have confirmed that the coronary lesions of the patients with unstable angina are not more severe than those of patients with effort stable angina (3) and that the great majority of myocardial infarction occurs in coronary stenosis between 50 and 70% of luminal area reduction (4,5). Thus, one of the most important problems is to investigate the mechanism(s) responsible for the occurrence of the clinical manifestation of coronary artery disease.

In the last years we deal with the pathophysiology of unstable angina and particularly with the mechanisms responsible for the clinical manifestation of this disease. Unstable angina is a syndrome which includes an heterogeneous population of patients (6) among whom patients with angina at rest (or spontaneous angina), that is patients with sudden and unpredictable occurrence of angina at rest or at minimal workloads, who have previously been completely free of symptoms. It is large consensus that the decrease in coronary blood flow plays a major role in the pathogenesis of myocardial ischemia in the patients with spontaneous angina. However, despite many clinical and experimental studies, the true nature of unstable angina and the factors or mechanisms responsible for its

* Corresponding author: Prof. Gian Gastone Neri Serneri, Clinica Medica Generale e Cardiologia, University of Florence, Viale Morgagni 85, 50134 Florence, Italy. Phone: +39 55 411145; fax: +39 55 4378638.

Recent Advances in Geriatrics, edited by Barbagallo, Licata, and Sowers.
Plenum Press, New York, 1998.

occurrence are not yet clarified. For about a decade unstable angina has been considered as a thrombus-related syndrome and many cardiologists still retain that the development of a coronary non-occlusive thrombus is responsible for the disease. However, the recent demonstration that unstable angina is associated with an acute lymphocyte activation (7) indicates that an acute immuno-mediated reaction may be the primary cause of the angina, and that the development of mural thrombosis may be one of the consequences of the inflammatory reaction.

In the present report we will discuss the current opinion about the mechanisms responsible for unstable angina, i.e. the theory of the non-occlusive thrombus, and the findings supporting the hypothesis that unstable angina is associated and probably due to an acute immuno-mediated reaction.

THE THEORY OF NON-OCCLUSIVE THROMBOSIS

Initially unstable angina was regarded as a more severe form of coronary artery disease than effort stable angina. However, angiographic studies clearly demonstrated that unstable and stable angina did not differ in the number of diseased vessels or in the percentage of stenosis in the affected vessels (3). From these observations the theory of non-occlusive thrombosis arose. This theory is founded on several post-mortem, angiographic and angioscopic studies.

Several post-mortem studies (8–10) performed in patients who had suffered from unstable angina, but had died from complicating myocardial infarction, demonstrated non-occlusive thrombus in these patients. However, this high prevalence of coronary thrombosis (90 to 95%) appeared due to the complicating myocardial infarction and not to unstable angina per se. Indeed, when only those patients who died from "pure", i.e. isolated unstable angina, were studied the frequency of coronary thrombosis was less than 40% (11–14). These findings have been confirmed by recent studies on specimens of atherosclerotic plaques obtained from monodirectional atherectomy. Analysis of the atherectomy specimens has revealed the presence of red or mural thrombus in about 40% of patients with unstable angina (15–19).

In angiographic studies clear evidence of thrombosis is infrequent in patients with unstable angina, whereas so-called "complex" lesions have been found in 34 to 68% of patients (3,20,21). These kinds of angiographic images have been postulated as representing a fissured plaque with superimposed thrombus (22). However, post-mortem examinations suggest that these complex lesions do not necessarily indicate coronary thrombosis, but might be due to plaque containing multiluminal channels (23) and recent studies failed to find any relation between culprit lesion morphology and the clinical outcome in unstable angina patients (24).

At angioscopic observation the presence of a nonocclusive thrombus, often very little thrombi, mainly formed by platelets (18,25), frequently associated with plaque fissuring, was detectable in 80 to 90% of patients with unstable angina (26–29). Thus, angioscopic observations provide the major support for the opinion that unstable angina is due to nonocclusive thrombus. However, coronary thrombus so frequency detectable in patients with unstable angina, seems to play a minor pathogenetic role since, differently from myocardial infarction, thrombolysis is substantially ineffective. Interestingly, thrombolytic therapy was ineffective even in the presence of angiographic improvement, thus indicating that the prevailing platelet composition of the thrombi (28) is not enough to explain the ineffectiveness of thrombolytic therapy in unstable angina.

In conclusion, the theory of the nonocclusive thrombus is simple and easily understood; it corresponds to a hemodynamic conception and assimilates the unstable angina to myocardial infarction. However, it is very difficult to sustain it because: 1) angina is present even in the absence of thrombus; 2) thrombolysis is ineffective even in the presence of angiographic improvement; 3) the presence of coronary thrombus is unable to explain several other findings occurring in unstable angina patients (see below). Therefore, mural thrombosis may be of importance in some particular subgroups of patients, but in the majority of patients it does not seem to play a major role in the pathogenesis of unstable angina.

UNSTABLE ANGINA AS A CONSEQUENCE OF AN ACUTE INFLAMMATORY REACTION

The hypothesis that unstable angina was correlated with and probably due to an acute inflammatory reaction superimposed on the chronic inflammatory atherosclerotic process arose both from the observation of the clinical pattern of spontaneous angina and from several studies on thromboxane A2 (TxA2) formation in patients with unstable angina.

TxA2 Formation by Coronary Vascular Wall in Anginal Patients

A sharp increase in plasma TxB2 during both painful and asymptomatic ischemic attacks was found in continuously monitored patients with unstable angina pretreated with aspirin (10 mg/Kg i.v.) (30). This finding suggested that TxB2 was not of platelet origin. However, at that time the opinion that platelets alone were the source of TxA2 was largely predominant and since aspirin administration was unable to cause a 100% platelet inhibition, the increase in plasma TxB2 was considered to be due to insufficient platelet inhibition. However, one year later evidence was given that the endothelium and smooth muscle cells of human arteries and veins of different vascular beds (coronary arteries were not assayed) were able to synthesize TxA2 (31). The results of this study led to investigate the formation of TxA2 and other prostaglandins by human coronary vascular bed in vivo both in control subjects and in anginal patients (32,33). In these studies patients with unstable angina, but not controls or patients with effort stable angina, were found to have a significant TxB2 positive aorta coronary-sinus gradient after cold pressor test (32). All patients were pretreated with aspirin (10 mg/Kg i.v.) (32). The results of this study were particularly important for three reasons: 1) they overcame the objection that the increase in plasma TxB2 was due to the insufficient platelet inhibition, because TxB2 did not increase in controls and patients with effort stable angina; 2) they showed that normal coronary arteries did not form substantial amounts of TxA2 and 3) they indicated that TxA2 formation by the coronary vascular bed was not due to the coronary atherosclerotic lesions themselves, because the angiographic score was not significantly different in the two groups of anginal patients. Thus, TxA2 formation in unstable angina patients appeared to be due to something peculiar which caused the plaques of anginal patients to be qualitatively different from those of patients with effort stable angina or patients with inactive unstable angina.

The Acute Immuno-Mediated Reaction

Beside the studies on abnormal coronary TxA2 formation in patients with active unstable angina, other investigations demonstrated that patients with active unstable angina had increased levels of fibrinopeptide A (FpA) in the plasma (34), i.e. an increased thrombin generation (35). Patients with effort stable angina and patients with inactive unstable angina had plasma FpA levels not significantly different from controls (34). The increased thrombin formation in patients with unstable angina could have two meanings: 1) reflecting the blood clotting activation, or 2) being the expression of an acute immuno-mediated inflammatory reaction, since activated monocytes and macrophages as well as endothelial cells produce tissue factor (36,37), express factor X and are able to activate it (38,39) and to assemble the functional prothrombinase complex (40). The hypothesis that the enhanced levels of FpA in plasma were expression of an acute inflammatory reaction agreed with the abnormal cardio-coronary TxA2 formation found in these patients (32).

The occurrence of an acute immuno-mediated reaction in patients with unstable angina was soon after demonstrated by the observation that circulating mononuclear cells (monocytes and lymphocytes) from patients with active unstable angina produce significant amounts of procoagulant activity, subsequently identified as tissue factor (7,41,42). Mononuclear cells from controls or from patients with effort stable angina were unable to produce procoagulant activity (7,41). The same patients with unstable angina restudied 8–12 weeks later, when they were in the inactive phase of disease (inactive unstable angina), expressed very low amounts of tissue factor, like the controls or patients with effort stable angina (7).

Monocytes from patients with unstable angina incubated with lymphocytes from the same patients also produced significantly higher amounts both of TxA2 (43) and alpha-TNF (44) than mononuclear cells from controls or stable angina.

The in vitro expression of tissue factor or TxA2 formation by monocytes requires a close contact between monocytes and lymphocytes (7,43) and the presence of gamma interferon. In in vivo studies Neri Serneri et al.gave indirect evidence that tissue factor (7) and TxA2 formation (43) occurred inside the atherosclerotic plaque, where monocytes and activated lymphocytes are closely associated with one another (45–49). Recently, Annex et al.(50), using in situ hybridization and immuno-histochemical methods, demonstrated the formation of tissue factor by monocyte-macrophages present in human atherosclerotic plaques.

The activation of monocytes, leading to the formation of tissue factor and TxA2, is a lymphocyte-mediated response. In reconstitution and cross-mixing experiments (7) the addition of pure (98%) lymphocyte preparations from patients with unstable angina induced a significant expression of tissue factor after 4 hours of incubation. Only lymphocytes obtained from patients with active unstable angina were able to induce monocytes to express tissue factor. Lymphocytes from controls, from patients with inactive unstable angina or from patients with effort stable angina were unable to express tissue factor or TxA2. It is worthwhile stressing that lymphocytes from patients with active unstable angina were able to induce tissue factor expression both from control monocytes and monocytes from patients with effort stable angina.

A direct proof that circulating lymphocytes from patients with active unstable angina are activated is given by the observation that patients with active unstable angina have a significantly higher number of circulating lymphocytes which express HLA-DR antigen, a protein of the HLA class II of the histocompatibility system, that is expressed by activated lymphocytes (51). Moreover, in these patients the plasma concentration of the soluble IL-2 receptor is significantly increased (51). Follow-up of these patients showed that the number of DR-positive lymphocytes progressively decreased, and after 8–12 weeks there were no significant differences in comparison to controls or patients with effort angina. A further proof that the outbursts of unstable angina are associated with an acute inflammatory reaction was recently provided by Liuzzo et al.(52), who showed a frequent increase of C reactive protein in plasma, by Ikeda et al. (53), who reported augmented plasma P-selectin concentrations, and by Biasucci et al., who found elevated plasma levels of Interleukin-6 (54).

The Histopathologic Features

The demonstration that outbursts of unstable angina were associated with an acute transient immuno-mediated reaction (7,41) prompted the investigators to look for histopathological findings supporting an inflammatory reaction. Some not very recent autopsy studies (11,12) demonstrated that when a strict definition of unstable angina was applied, the incidence of coronary thrombosis was noticeably lower than that reported in previous autopsy series of unstable angina progressing to myocardial infarction (8–10). More recent autopsy studies (12,13) confirming the previous results (11,12) have further shown that unstable angina-related thrombi are essentially mural and mostly composed of platelets which are firmly attached to plaque tissue, but are rarely layered on plaque ulceration of fissuring (13–15).

The recently-introduced directional coronary atherectomy (DCA) tecnique radically modified in vivo investigation approaches to human coronary artery plaques. In atherectomy samples obtained from patients with unstable angina during coronary by-pass graft surgery, the prevalence of coronary thrombosis was by 32% as compared to 52% in acute myocardial infarction (autopsy) and 12% in effort stable angina (DCA) (15). The same incidence of thrombosis was reported in a recent series of pathologic studies on DCA samples from unstable angina patients (22, 34, and 35%) (16–18). Therefore, the frequency of coronary thrombosis in unstable angina patients is about 35%, a long way from the frequency found in the first autopsy studies (8–10), which had been performed in patients with fatal unstable angina that evolved to myocardial infarction and sudden death (8–10).

In addition to thrombosis, two other histopathologic features characterize the unstable plaques: inflammation and neointimal hyperplasia, initially called accelerated fibrogenesis (13–18,23,51).

It has to be remembered that a chronic quiet inflammatory process is characteristic of atherosclerotic lesions and that rare inflammatory cells are commonly present in the plaques (40,42,55,56). However, plaques of patients with unstable angina are different from those of patients with effort stable angina because they have a much more abundant population of inflammatory cells (lymphocytes and monocyte-macrophages), whereas stable plaques are generally richer in fibrous tissue (15,57). In unstable plaques more than 50% of cells are inflammatory cells, more precisely T-lymphocytes (about 25%) and macrophages (about 30%) whereas in the plaque of patients with stable angina only about 10% of the total plaque cells are T-lymphocytes (about 3%) and macrophages (about 7%) (15).

In unstable plaques, sparse non-clustered inflammatory cells are a common finding in most of the lesions but in these plaques inflammatory cells are specially grouped in clusters forming inflammatory infiltrates which can be isolated or grouped together, usually beside groups of foam cells (14–16). On the other hand, clusters of inflammatory cells are rare in DCA specimens of stable plaques (15). Inflammatory infiltrates in unstable plaques are particularly frequent in lipid-rich plaques, whereas they are rare in fibrous plaques (14,15,17,52,53). Within the unstable plaques, unlike in normal coronary arteries of control subjects, tissue factor (49) alpha-TNF (14,58,59) and IL-2 (15) have been documented, as well as a number of growth factors including acid and basic FGF and PDGF (15). These factors may be present in minimal concentrations in the fibrous plaque

(14,15). Tissue factor and inflammatory cytokines are not related to the presence of thrombus (14,15). The presence of IL-2 within the unstable plaques is indicative of the occurrence of a cell-mediated immunological reaction. This is further supported by the documentation that T-lymphocytes and macrophages express HLA-DR antigens in about 5 times higher percentage than macrophages and T-lymphocytes of the stable angina plaques (11.3±8.7 vs 2.7±9) (18). Likewise, the percentage of cells which are positive for different growth factors (smooth muscle cells and to a lesser extent macrophages) is much higher in unstable than in stable plaques (18). Thus, the marked abundance of inflammatory cells sparse or grouped in clusters, which express HLA-DR antigens, and the presence in the plaque of tissue factor and cytokines represent a distinct inflammatory feature that differentiates the plaques of unstable angina from those of patients with stable angina and very well it agrees both with the presence of activated circulating T-lymphocytes and the augmented plasma levels of soluble IL-2 receptors (7,42,51).

The third relevant histopathologic finding of the unstable plaque is neointimal hyperplasia (17) which is characterized by the occurrence of very loose fibrosis, tissue with abundant matrix, and several plump smooth muscle cells (15,17,18,60,61). Its frequency in plaques of unstable angina patients is about 40% in comparison to about 20% in plaques of stable angina patients (15,17). Neointimal hyperplasia is a type of rapid and highly cellular fibrogenesis which probably results from a particular inflammatory reaction characterized by a high growth potential, as is suggested both by the widespread expression of basic and acid FGF (14) and by the presence of numerous smooth muscle cells which express PDGF AA, PDGF AB, PDGF alpha beta r (15). Since smooth muscle cells and inflammatory cells in unstable plaque are usually adjacent, growth factors produced by inflammatory cells and/or cytokines, such as IL-1, which are able to induce growth factor formation from smooth muscle cells, can play a key role in triggering neointimal hyperplasia.

The three main histopathologic features which characterize unstable plaques, i.e. mural thrombosis, inflammatory reaction and neointimal hyperplasia, do not necessarily occur together, and only 52% of plaques show combined features of thrombosis and/or neointimal hyperplasia and/or clustered inflammatory infiltrates (18).

PECULIARITY AND SIGNIFICANCE OF THE ACUTE INFLAMMATORY REACTION OF THE UNSTABLE ANGINA

The acute inflammatory lymphocyte-dependent reaction characteristic of unstable angina should be separated from the post-perfusional inflammation. This is an acute inflammatory reaction probably due to leukocytes (mainly granulocytes and monocytes) which undergo activation during the passage through previously ischemic cardiac regions. The oxygen-derived free radicals formed by ischemic tissues may contribute to ischemic damage or postischemic damage caused by reperfusion (62). In this condition a cascade of events, which has not so far been well clarified, is activated. The activation is substantially due to the activation of complement and to the release of vasoactive and chemotactic factors (63,64) which cause an endothelial inflammatory reaction. Endothelial cells express adhesion molecules and activated leucocytes may adhere to endothelial cells and cause a decrease in the blood flow of the coronary microcirculation. If endothelial damage is severe, edema and necrosis of myocytes can occur (65–67). The activated leukocytes (leukocytes and/or monocytes) which have not adhered to the endothelium may be found in coronary sinus blood from patients with myocardial infarction or unstable angina

(68–70). The presence of activated leukocytes in coronary sinus blood in comparison to aortic blood reflects a ischemia-reperfusion damage, and is not related to the acute immuno-mediated inflammatory reaction of unstable angina.

The acute reaction of unstable angina is triggered by as yet unknown factor(s) and is sustained by the same cell types (T-lymphocytes and monocyte-macrophages) which represent the customary cell population of the atherosclerotic plaques. The relevant neointimal proliferation which in unstable plaques is as frequent as thrombosis (15,17) indicates that plaque smooth muscle cells participate in the acute inflammatory reaction. The involvement of smooth muscle cells is further indicated by the abundant formation of growth factors and the expression of HLA-DR antigens on smooth muscle cells specially when these are adjacent to activated lymphocytes (71). Thus, all the cell population which characterizes atherosclerotic lesions is involved in the acute reaction. This fact indicates that unstable angina is not due to a different form of atherosclerosis, but is the expression of an acute sudden reaction to some trigger factors. The presence of a large number of cells (T-lymphocytes, macrophages and smooth muscle cells) which express activation antigens and the documented presence of IL-2 in the unstable plaques strongly indicate the immunological nature of the reaction. Although rarely, some aspects of immunological activation may be observed in stable plaques, but this again confirms the common atherosclerotic nature of the unstable and stable lesion.

A fundamental point to be discussed is whether the acute inflammatory reaction, which differentiates unstable angina from effort stable angina, is only a marker of instability and represents the vascular response to endothelial disruption and thrombus formation, or whether it represents a primary peculiar coronary pathologic process in which lymphocyte and monocyte-macrophage activation leads to the formation of different inflammatory mediators and causes myocardial ischemia and the occurrence of unstable angina. The presence of a thrombus in less than 40% of patients makes very unlikely the hypothesis that the local and systemic inflammatory reaction, which characterizes the episodes of unstable angina, is secondary to the vascular disruption and thrombus development. Thus it seems to be a primary pathologic coronary process.

The acute inflammatory reaction of unstable angina, besides representing the common ground of different pathomorphologic aspects including thrombosis, may also explain several peculiar clinical characteristics of unstable angina, such as the recurrent nature of the disease (72,73), the relative unimportance of the extent of stenoses in the outcome of clinical events (74), the increased sensitivity to vasoconstrictor stimuli (75) and the high incidence of complications after angioplasty or directional atherectomy when these revascularization procedures are performed in the first two weeks than later (76–79).

CONCLUSIONS

In the majority of patients, the outbursts of unstable angina are associated and probably due to an acute immunological inflammatory reaction. The first documentations of immunological activation in unstable angina patients have been confirmed by many histopathological studies which have demonstrated that the frequency of non-occlusive thrombus in patients with unstable angina is less than 40%, whereas in the majority of these patients an acute inflammatory reaction is present in unstable plaques. Therefore, the theory of unstable angina as due to non-occlusive thrombus is no longer tenable. Apart from the low frequency of thrombosis, this theory does not explain either the clinical findings of lymphocyte activation documented in almost all the patients, or the other histopathologic findings demonstrated in the unstable plaques, such as inflammation and neointimal hyperplasia. A large number of the T-lymphocytes and macrophages which represent the inflammatory cells of the unstable plaques are activated and express HLA-DR antigens. This finding provides a morphologic basis to the previous observation that the circulating lymphocytes of patients with active unstable angina are activated. Thus, the acute immuno-mediated inflammatory reaction which characterizes unstable angina may represent the common ground of the different histopathologic features of the unstable plaque, including thrombosis, and explain several clinical and biological characteristics of unstable angina which are very difficult to explain with the theory of non-occlusive thrombus. But, overall, the knowledge that unstable angina is due to an acute inflammatory reaction represent a first step on the way of the understanding of the mechanisms responsible for the different clinical manifestations of coronary artery disease.

REFERENCES

1. McGill HC Jr (Ed.). The geographic pathology of atherosclerosis. Baltimore, Md, Waverly Press 1968.
2. Solberg LA, Strong JP. Risk factors and atherosclerotic lesions. A review of autopsy studies. Arteriosclerosis 1983; 3: 187–198.
3. Ambrose JA, Hjemdahl-Monsen CE. Angiographic morphology of unstable plaque. In: JD Rutherford (Ed., New York, M. Dekker): Unstable Angina 1992: 49–68.
4. Little WC, Constantinescu M, Applegate RJ, Kutcher MA, Burrows MT, Kahl FR, Santamore WP. Can coronary angiography predict the site of a subsequent myocardial infarction in patients with mild-to-moderate coronary artery disease? Circulation 1988; 78 (5Pt1): 1157–1166.
5. Hackett D, Verwilghen J, Davies G, Maseri A. Coronary stenoses before and after acute myocardial infarction. Am J Cardiol 1989; 63: 1517–1518.
6. Braunwald E. Unstable angina. A classification. Circulation 1989; 80: 410–414.
7. Neri Serneri GG, Abbate R, Gori AM et al. A transient intermittent lymphocyte activation is responsible for the instability of angina. Circulation 1992; 85: 1200–1220.
8. Davies MJ, Thomas AC. Thrombosis and acute coronary artery lesions in sudden cardiac ischemic death. N Engl J Med 1984; 310: 1137–1140.
9. Davies MJ, Thomas AC. Plaque fissuring: the cause of acute myocardial infarction, sudden death and crescendo angina. Br Heart J 1985; 53: 363–373.
10. Falk E. Morphologic features of unstable atherothrombotic plaques underlying acute coronary syndromes. Am J Cardiol 1989; 63: E114-E120.
11. Guthrie RB, Vlodaver Z, Nicoloff DM et al. Pathology of stable and unstable angina pectoris. Circulation 1975; 51: 1059–1063.
12. Roberts WC, Virmani R. Quantification of coronary arterial narrowing in clinically isolated unstable angina pectoris: an analysis of 22 necroscopy patients. Am J Med 1979; 67: 792–799.
13. Kragel AH, Gertz SD, Roberts WC. Morphologic comparison of frequency and types of acute lesions in the major epicardial coronary arteries in unstable angina pectoris, sudden coronary death and acute myocardial infarction. J Am Coll Cardiol 1991; 18: 810–818.
14. Arbustini E, Grasso M, Diegoli M et al. Coronary atherosclerotic plaques with and without thrombus in ischemic heart syndromes: a morphologic immunohistochemical and biochemical study. Am J Cardiol 1991; 68: B36-B51.
15. Arbustini E, De Servi S, Bramucci E et al. Comparison of coronary lesions obtained by directional coronary atherectomy in unstable angina, stable angina, and restenosis afer either atherectomy or angioplasty. Am J Cardiol 1995; 75: 675–682.
16. Escaned J, van Suylen RJ, McLeod DC et al. Histologic characteristics of tissue excessed during directional atherectomy in stable and unstable angina. Am J Cardiol 1993; 71: 1442–1447.
17. Flugelman MY, Virmani R, Correa R et al. Smooth muscle cell abundance and fibroblast growth factors in coronary lesions of patients with nonfatal unstable angina. A clue to the mechanism of trasformation from the stable to the unstable clinical state. Circulation 1993; 88: 2493–2500.
18. Rosenschein U, Ellis SG, Haudenshild CC, et al. Comparison of histopathologic coronary lesions obtained from directional atherectomy in unstable angina, stable angina, and restenosis after either atherectomy or angioplasty. Am J Cardiol 1995; 75: 675–682.

19. De Servi S, Arbustini E, Marsico F et al. Correlation between clinical and morphologic findings in unstable angina. Am J Cardiol 1996; 77: 128–132.
20. Ambrose JA, Winters SL, Stern A, et al. Angiographic morphology and the pathogenesis of unstable angina pectoris. J Am Coll Cardiol 1985; 5: 609–616.
21. Wilenski RL, Bourdillon PDV, Vix VA, Zeller JA. Intracoronary artery thrombus formation in unstable angina: a clinical, biochemical and angioscopic correlation. J Am Coll Cardiol 1993; 21: 692–699.
22. Ambrose JA, Israel DH. Angiography in unstable angina. Am J Cardiol 1991; 68: B78-B84.
23. Kragel AH, Reddy SG, Wittes FT, Roberts WC. Morphometric analysis of the composition of coronary arterial plaques in isolated unstable angina pectoris with pain at rest. Am J Cardiol 1990; 66: 562–567.
24. Bar FW, Raynaud P, Renkin JP, Vermeer F, de Zwaan C, Wellens HJJ. Coronary angiographic findings do not predict clinical outcome in patients with unstable angina. J Am Coll Cardiol 1994; 24: 1453–1459.
25. Mizuno K, Sotomura K, Miyamoto A et al. Angioscopic evaluation of coronary-artery thrombi in acute coronary syndrome. N Engl J Med 1992; 326: 287–291.
26. Sherman CT, Litvack F, Grundfest W, et al. Coronary angioscopy in patients with unstable angina pectoris. N Engl J Med 1986; 315: 913–919.
27. Hombach V, Hoher M, Kochs M, et al. Pathophysiology of unstable angina pectoris. Correlations with coronary angioscopic imagine. Eur Heart J 1988; 9 (suppl.4): 40–5.
28. Mizuno K, Miyamoto A, Satomura K et al. Angioscopic coronary macromorphology in patients with acute coronary disorders. Lancet 1991; 337: 809–812.
29. De Feyter PJ, Ozaki Y, Baptista J, et al. Ischemia-related lesion characteristics in patients with stable or unstable angina. Circulation 1995; 92: 1408–1413.
30. Neri Serneri GG. Prostaglandins in patients with ischemic heart disease. In: AG Herman, PM Vanhoutte, H Demolin, A Goossen (Eds., Raven Press, New York): Cardiovascular pharmacology of Prostaglandins, 1982: 361–374.
31. Neri Serneri GG, Abbate R, Gensini GF, Panetta A, Casolo GC, Carini M. TxA2 production by human arteries and veins. Prostaglandins 1983; 25: 753–765.
32. Neri Serneri GG, Gensini GF, Abbate R, et al. Abnormal cardiocoronary thromboxane A2 production in patients with unstable angina. Am Heart J 1985; 109: 732–738.
33. Neri Serneri GG, Gensini GF, Abbate R. et al. Impaired cardiac PGI2 and PGE2 biosynthesis in patients with angina pectoris. Am Heart J 1986; 112: 472–478.
34. Neri Serneri GG, Gensini GF, Abbate R et al. Is raised plasma fibrinopeptide A a marker of acute coronary insufficiency? Lancet 1980; 2: 982–983.
35. Nossel HL, Yudelman I, Canfield E, et al. Measurement of fibrinopeptide A in human blood. J Clin Invest 1974; 54: 43–54.
36. Bevilacqua MP, Prober JS, Majean GR et al. Interleukin-1 (IL-1) induces biosynthesis and cell surface expression of procoagulant activity in human vascular endothelial cells. J Exp Med 1984; 160: 618–628.
37. Edwards RL, Rickels FR. Macrophage procoagulants. In: TH Spaet (Ed., Grune & Stratton Inc., New York): Progress in Haemostasis and Thrombosis 1984; 7: 183–209.
38. Altieri DC, Morissey JH, Edgington TS. Adhesive receptor Mac-1 coordinates the activation of factor X on stimulated cells of monocytes and mieloid differentiation: an alternative initiation of the coagulation protease cascade. Proc Natl Acad Sci USA 1988; 85: 7462–7468.
39. McGee PC, Li LC. Functional differences between intrinsic and extrinsic coagulation pathways. Kinetics of factor X on human monocytes and alveolar macrophages. J Biol Chem 1991; 266: 8079–8087.
40. Tracy PB, Rohzbach MS, Mann KG. Functional prothrombinase complex assembly on isolated monocytes and lymphocytes. J Biol Chem 1983; 258: 7264–7269.
41. Neri Seneri GG, Abbate R, Gensini GF, Gori AM, Attanasio M, Martini F. Monocyte activation and increased procoagulant activity in unstable angina. Lancet 1990; 336: 1444–1445.
42. Jude B, Agraou B, McFadden EP et al. Evidence for time-dependent activation of monocytes in the systemic circulation in unstable angina but not in acute myocardial infarction or in stable angina. Circulation 1994; 90: 1662–1668.
43. Neri Serneri GG, Gensini GF, Poggesi L et al. The role of extraplatelet thromboxane A2 in unstable angina investigated through a dual antithromboxane inhibitor. Importance of activated monocytes. Coronary Artery Disease 1994; 5: 137–145.
44. Neri Serneri GG. Fattori immunologici nell'aterogenesi e nella comparsa delle manifestazioni cliniche dell'aterosclerosi coronarica. Relazione al 95°Congresso della Societa' Italiana di Medicina Interna. (L Pozzi Ed., Roma) 1995: 453–597.
45. Libby P, Hansson GK. Involvement of the immune system in human atherogenesis: current knowledge and unanswered questions. Lab Invest 1991; 64: 5–15.

46. Jonasson L, Holm J, Skally O et al. Regional accumulation of T cells, macrophage and smooth muscle cells in the human atherosclerotic plaque. Atherosclerosis 1986; 6: 131–138.
47. Munro JM, Cotran RS. The pathogenesis of atherosclerosis. atherogenesis and inflammation. Lab Invest 1988; 58: 249–261.
48. Ross R. The pathogenesis of atherosclerosis: a perspective for the 1990s. Nature 1993; 362: 801–809.
49. Hansson GK, Geng YJ, Holm J, Stemme S. Immune mechanisms in the pathogenesis of atherosclerosis. In: GG Neri Sermeri, GF Gensini, R Abbate, D Prisco (Eds., Scientific Press, Firenze): Atherosclerosis inflammation and thrombosis 1993: 163–168.
50. Annex BH, Denning S, Channon KM et al. Differential expression of tissue factor protein in directional atherectomy specimens from patients with stable and unstable coronary syndromes. Circulation 1995; 91: 619–622.
51. Neri Serneri GG, Prisco D, Martini F et al. Acute T-cell activation is detectable in unstable angina. Circulation 1997; 95: 1806–1812.
52. Liuzzo G, Biasucci LM, Gallimore JR et al. The prognostic value of C-reactive protein and serum amyloid a protein in severe unstable angina. N Eng J Med 1994; 331: 417–424.
53. Ikeda H, Takajo Y, Ichiki K et al. Increased soluble form of P-selectin in patients with unstable angina. Circulation 1995; 92: 1693–1696.
54. Biasucci LM, Vitelli A, Liuzzo G, et al. Elevated levels of interleukin-6 in unstable angina. Circulation 1996; 94: 874–877.
55. Gown AM, Tsukada T, Ross R. Human atherosclerosis II. Immunocytochemical analysis of the cellular composition of human atherosclerotic lesion. Am J Pathol 1986; 125: 191–207.
56. Lablanche JM, Hamon M, Mc Tadden E, Bauters C, Bertrand ME. Coronary angioscopy. An inner view. 8th Annual International Workshop on Future directions in Interventional Cardiology. Santa Barbara, California 1994.
57. Moreno PR, Falk E, Palacios IS et al. Macrophage infiltration in acute coronary sindromes: implications for plaque rupture. Circulation 1994; 90: 775–778.
58. Barath P, Fishbein MC, Cao J, et al. Detection and localization of tumor necrosis factor in human atheroma. Am J Cardiol 1990; 65: 297–302.
59. Barath P, Fishbein MC, Cao J, et al. Tumor necrosis factor gene expression in human vascular intimal smooth muscle cells detected by in situ hybridisation. Am J Pathol 1990; 137: 503–509.
60. Safian RD, Gelbfish JS, Emy RE, Shnitt SJ, Schmidt DA, Baim DS. Coronary atherectomy. Clinical, angiographic and histological findings and observations regarding potential mechanisms. Circulation 1990; 82: 69–79.
61. Miller MJ, Kuntz RE, Friedrich SP, et al. Frequency and consequences of intimal hyperplasia in specimens retrieved by directional atherectomy of native primary coronary artery stenoses and subsequent restenoses. Am J Cardiol 1993; 71: 652–658.
62. Rossen RD, Swain JL, Michael LH et al. Selective accumulation of the first component of complement and leukocytes in ischemic canine heart muscle. Circ Res 1985; 57: 119–130.
63. Entman ML, Smith CW. Post-perfusion infiammation: a model for reaction to injury in cardiovascular disease. Circ Res 1994; 28: 1301–1311.
64. Kloner RA, Giacomelli F, Alker JK et al. Influx of neutrophils into the walls of large epicardial coronary arteries in response to ischemia/reperfusion. Circulation 1991; 84: 1758–1772.
65. Ma XL, Tsao PS, Lefer AM. Antibody to CD-18 exerts endothelial and cardiac protective effects in myocardial ischemia and reperfusion. J Clin Invest 1991; 88: 1237–1243.
66. Silver MJ, Sutton JH, Hook S et al. Adjunctive selectin blockade successfully reduces infarct size beyond thrombolysis in the electrolytic canine coronary model. Circulation 1995; 92: 492–499.
67. Grangey DN, Benoit JN, Suzuki M, Grisham HB. Leukocyte adherence to venular endothelium during ischemia-riperfusion. Am J Physiol 1989; 257: G683-G688.
68. Dinerman JL, Metha JL, Saldeen TG et al. Increased neutrophil elastase release in unstable angina pectoris and acute myocardial infarction. J Am Coll Cardiol 1990; 15: 1559–1563.
69. Mazzone A, De Servi S, Ricevuti G et al. Increased expression of neutrophil and monocyte adhesion molecules in unstable coronary artery disease. Circulation 1993; 88: 358–363.
70. Biasucci LM, D'Onofrio G, Liuzzo G et al. Intracellular neutrophil myeloperoxidase is reduced in unstable angina and acute myocardial infarction, but its reduction is not related to ischemia. J Am Coll Cardiol 1996; 27: 611–616.
71. Hansson GK, Jonasson L, Holm J, Claesson-Welsh L. Class II MCH antigen expression in the atherosclerotic plaque: smooth muscle cells express HLA-DR, HLA-DQ and the invariant gamma chain. Clin Exp Immunol 1986; 64: 261–268.

72. Maseri A, Chierchia S, L'Abbate A. Pathogenetic mechanisms underlying the clinical events associated with atherosclerotic heart disease. Circulation 1980; 62 (suppl.V): V3-V13.
73. Neri Serneri GG, Gensini GF, Carnovali M, et al. Association between time of increased fibrinopeptide A levels in plasma and episodes of spontaneous angina: A controlled prospective study. Am Heart J 1989; 113: 672–678.
74. Alexander RW. The coronary ischemic syndromes: relationship to the biology of atherosclerosis. In: RC Schalnt, RW Alexander (Eds., McGraw Hill, New York): Hurst's The Heart 1994: 1021–1031.
75. Willerson JT, Yao SK, McNatt J et al. Frequency and severity of cyclic flow alterations and platelet aggregation predict the severity of neointimal proliferation following experimental cronary stenosis and endothelial injury. Proc Natl Acad Sci USA 1991; 88: 10624–10628.
76. De Feyter PJ, Suryapranata H, Serruyus PW et al. Coronary angioplasty for unstable angina: immediate and late results in 200 consecutive patients with identification of risk factors for unfavorable early and late outcome. J Am Coll Cardiol 1988; 12: 324–333.
77. Bauters C, Lablanche JM, Mc Fadden EP, Leroy F, Bertrand ME. Repeat percutaneous coronary angioplasty; clinical and angiographic follow-up in patients with stable and unstable angina pectoris. Eur Heart J 1993; 14: 235–239.
78. Abdelmeguid AE, Ellis S, Sapp SK, Simpfendorfer C, Franco I, Witlow PL. Directional coronary atherectomy in unstable angina. J Am Coll Cardiol 1994; 24: 46–54.
79. de Groote P, Bauters C, McFadden EP, Lablanche JM, Leroy F, Bertrand ME. Local lesion-related factors and restenosis after coronary angioplasty. Evidence from a quantitative angiographic study in patients with unstable angina undergoing double vessel angioplasty. Circulation 1995; 91: 968–972.

24

WHEN AND HOW TO TREAT HYPERCHOLESTEROLEMIA IN THE ELDERLY?

Antonio Capurso and Sabrina A. Capurso

Department of Gerontology
University of Bari
Faculty of Medicine, Policlinico
70124 Bari, Italy

INTRODUCTION

The utility of lowering serum cholesterol in elderly patients has been questioned for a long time and is still a matter of debate (1). The main question concerns the role of hypercholesterolemia in elderly people, whether it represents at this age a risk factor for coronary heart disease (CHD) and myocardial infarction (MI) as in young people. A quite common opinion holds that the risk associated with total cholesterol "*shows a definite waning effect with little impact after age 65*" (2) and that "*total cholesterol levels...are not considered important risk factors* (in elderly patients) (3).

Epidemiological studies in middle-aged men have demonstrated that elevated serum cholesterol is a major risk factor for CHD (4,5). There appears to be no threshold level below which serum cholesterol ceases to predict coronary heart disease and the risk increases markedly when cholesterol values exceed 200 mg/dl (5.17 mmol/L). If the coronary heart disease risk is set at 1 for a cholesterol level of 200 mg/dl, the risk is doubled at 250 mg/dl and increased by four times at 300 mg/dl (5). For every 1% reduction in a serum cholesterol level of over 200 mg/dl the coronary heart disease risk is reduced by 2% (5).

The question of whether hypercholesterolemia is still a CHD risk factor in people aged over 65 years and pharmacological treatment of high serum cholesterol levels is profitable in elderly as it is in middle aged men has had conflicting answers from epidemiological studies and clinical trials.

DATA FROM OBSERVATIONAL STUDIES AND INTERVENTION TRIALS

Several longitudinal studies have evaluated the impact of serum cholesterol levels on CHD morbidity and mortality in middle aged persons and in elderly. The *Los Angeles Veterans Administration Study* (6) was a randomly allocated double-blind intervention

Recent Advances in Geriatrics, edited by Barbagallo, Licata, and Sowers.
Plenum Press, New York, 1998.

study that commenced in 1959 and lasted for 8.5 years. The study cohort consisted of 846 male residents of a domiciliary facility, whose median age was 65.5 years at entry to the study. With the aim of reducing serum cholesterol levels and, thus, CHD events, a fat-modified diet, low in saturated fat and cholesterol and high in polyunsaturated fat, was administered to 424 men of the active treatment group. This diet reduced the mean serum cholesterol by 12.7%, the incidence of CHD by 31.3% and the mortality from atherosclerotic disease by 31.4%. These results clearly demonstrated that the reduction in serum cholesterol levels with a diet can significantly decrease the incidence of coronary events even in an elderly population.

The *Framingham Heart Study* (2,4,7) is an ongoing longitudinal study started in 1948. In this study, 5209 residents of Framingham were enrolled and controlled with biannual surveys. In subjects over 65 years, elevated serum cholesterol levels were significantly associated with CHD only in women, while in men there appeared to be no effect (4). High-density lipoprotein cholesterol levels did maintain a predictive power in men aged over 65 years (7).

In contrast with the *Framingham* data, the *Honolulu* study (8) showed that elevated serum cholesterol levels independently predict CHD in men aged over 65 years. The *Honolulu Heart Program on risk factors for coronary heart disease and stroke (9)* is an ongoing prospective study on the Japanese residents of Oahu (Hawaii) born between 1900 and 1919. The study was started in 1971 and recruited 6860 men, of whom 1480 were aged 65–74 years. In a 12-year follow-up, 136 new cases of CHD developed among the 1480 subjects over 65 who had no demonstrable coronary heart disease at entry to the study. The incidence of new CHD cases showed a significant increase from the lowest (4.92 mmol/L) to the highest (6.20 mmol/L) cholesterol quartile. With a multivariate regression analysis including several variables normally present in an older population (elevated systolic blood pressure, smoking and diabetes), elevated serum cholesterol levels were confirmed to be an independent risk factor for CHD. No significant differences between older and younger age groups were found in the incidence of CHD, according to the serum cholesterol levels.

The discrepancy between these two studies could be in part explained with the different methodologies followed. The *Framingham* study examined subjects biannually and referred the CHD risk to the latest cholesterol value while the *Honolulu* study re-examined the subjects after 12 years and referred the risk to the cholesterol values recorded at the first examination. It must be considered that results obtained at 2-year intervals may not be comparable with those found after a 12-year interval, because changes in medical intervention or in behavior may have occurred over the longer interval. Moreover, the latest measure of a biological parameter in older subjects does not necessarily correspond to life-long exposure values, since the latest values may have been modified by other factors such as the presence of co-morbidity or multiple prescriptions, which are quite common events in elderly people.

Several other studies have evaluated the impact of hypercholesterolemia in elderly. In a study (9) on 65-year-old subjects who were re-examined after 10 years, the serum cholesterol levels predicted significantly the development of CHD. In another cohort study (10), 2746 white men aged 60–79 years had a follow-up of 10.1 years, to determine whether high blood cholesterol was still a risk factor for CHD mortality in aged people. The relative risk for mortality from CHD in the highest serum cholesterol quartile (above 279 mg/dl - 7.21 mmol/L) was 1.5 (95% CI, 1.2 to 2) compared to that of the three lower quartiles combined. The relative risk did not change with age, but the excess risk for such mortality attributable to elevated serum cholesterol levels increased five fold, from 2.2 death per 1000 persons/year to 11.3 death per 1000 persons/year.

A recent observational study on the relationship of total cholesterol and HDL-cholesterol with CHD mortality in people over 71 years has been conducted in East Boston and other US countries (11). The study was a prospective cohort study with a median of 4.4 years of follow-up. A total of 2527 women and 1377 men with no history of CHD was enrolled. The data showed that only HDL-cholesterol predicts CHD mortality and occurrence of new CHD events in persons older than 70 years, while elevated serum cholesterol was not found to be associated with CHD mortality. The data of this study were substantially in agreement with those of the *Framingham* study.

These pooled data suggest that in elderly people high serum cholesterol levels are associated with an increased risk for CHD in women, while in men the data are conflicting. The HDL cholesterol levels appear to be a better predictor of CHD than total cholesterol in elderly population. This uncertain impact of hypercholesterolemia in old people could depend on several factors. One factor could be that hypercholesterolemia in elderly patients is frequently a non-genetic form, but secondary to several metabolic disorders which have been acquired late in the life. The prevalence of genetic hypercholesterolemia in the older population should have been reduced, either by the death of affected subjects or by a decline in serum and low-density lipoprotein cholesterol level which normally tends to occur after the age of 65 years (8). In contrast, the frequency of secondary hyperlipidaemia induced by pathological conditions increases in the old age. Clinical conditions such as hypothyroidism, renal insufficiency and diabetes mellitus, as well as drugs like diuretics and steroids, are frequently responsible for serum lipid elevations in the elderly. These secondary forms of hyperlipidaemia in the elderly probably have only a minor impact on the coronary heart disease risk, since they are late in onset and consequently the patient is exposed to the risk for only a short period of time. Poor survival rates among elderly people contribute to reduce the exposure to this risk and, consequently, to reduce the impact of high cholesterol levels on coronary arteries.

On the other hand, a low serum cholesterol level has been demonstrated to predict a higher mortality rate in old people. In a study on 92 women over 60 years of age living in a Parisian home for elderly people a poor survival was observed in individuals with serum cholesterol levels above 320 mg or below 150 mg/dl. In this study the lowest mortality was found in women with cholesterol levels around 270 mg/dl at entry (12). A similar relationship between total cholesterol and overall mortality was found in a 10-year follow-up study on septuagenarians (13). In another study conducted in nursing home patients, cholesterols level below 160 mg/dl were highly predictive of short term mortality (14). The higher mortality rate can probably be explained by the fact that low serum cholesterol levels in institutionalised people are often related to both, a protein-energy malnutrition (15) or a non-diagnosed cancer (16). On the basis of these data, a moderately elevated serum cholesterol level (200 to 300 mg/dl) in older subjects has been suggested to be most compatible with longevity, especially in elderly with coexisting disease processes (1).

DATA FROM STUDIES WITH HMGCoA REDUCTASE INHIBITORS

More recently, the data from primary and secondary prevention studies with HMGCoA reductase inhibitor, although not specifically aimed to evaluate the benefits in elderly people, have clearly demonstrated that the reduction of high levels of serum and LDL-cholesterol is highly effective in reducing CHD mortality and morbidity and the overall mortality also in the elderly, although the cost-effectiveness data of secondary prevention were somewhat better than those of primary prevention.

Data from Secondary Prevention

A pivotal study on secondary prevention of CHD was the *4S Study* (17). 4444 patients aged 35–70 years affected by angina pectoris or myocardial infarction and with serum cholesterol levels above 240 mg per deciliter were treated with simvastatin or placebo for a median follow-up of 5.4 years. In the group of patients treated with simvastatin a 42% reduction in the relative risk of coronary death and other major coronary events, including the coronary bypass surgery, was found. The risk of major coronary events was reduced significantly by a same amount in all quartiles of total cholesterol, LDL-cholesterol and HDL-cholesterol, as evaluated at entry (18). The NNT, i.e. the number of patients needed to treat to prevent one major coronary event (corresponding to the reciprocal of the absolute risk reduction ARR), was 16 patients. The benefits obtained with pharmacological treatment were the same in middle age and elderly patients: "*Although the observed relative risk reductions produced by simvastatin were somewhat less in the patients aged > 60, they were statistically significant...and the absolute differences between treatment groups were similar in the two age groups*" (17). The cost/effectiveness analysis of this trial (19) showed that the cost of each year of life gained ranged from $3,800 for 70-year-old men with 309 mg per deciliter of cholesterol to $27,400 for 35-year-old women with a serum cholesterol level of 213 mg per deciliter. If the indirect costs were included, the data ranged from a saving in the youngest patients to a cost of $13,300 per year of life gained in 70-year-old women with 213 mg of cholesterol per deciliter.

The *CARE* study was a trial of CHD secondary prevention (20) aimed to evaluate the benefit of serum cholesterol reduction in coronary patients with serum cholesterol levels below 240 mg per deciliter. 4159 patients aged 21–75 years were treated with pravastatin or placebo for a mean duration of 5 years. The patients with base-line LDL-cholesterol levels above 150 mg per deciliter had a 35 percent reduction in major coronary events, compared with a 26 percent reduction in patients with base-line cholesterol 125 to 150 mg per deciliter and a 3 percent increase in patients with base-line levels below 125 mg per deciliter. Unexpectedly, the women treated with pravastatin showed a significantly lower rate of major coronary events (46 percent) compared with men (20 percent). Moreover, men and women treated with pravastatin showed also a significant reduction (31 percent) of stroke and transient ischemic attacks. In agreement with these data, a meta-analysis of pravastatin trials in patients with atherosclerosis has demonstrated a 62 percent reduction in stroke events (21).

The treatment with HMGCoA reductase inhibitor has been shown also to promote a significant regression and a reduced progression of coronary lesions in elderly as well as in middle age patients with CHD. The *LCAS* (22,23) was a randomized double-blind, placebo controlled study on the regression/progression of coronary atherosclerotic lesions, as assessed by coronary angiography. The 429 patients participating in the study were men and women 35 to 75 years of age with LDL-cholesterol > 160 mg per deciliter, treated with fluvastatin 40 mg/die or placebo for 2.5 years. The regression of atherosclerosis occurred in nearly twice as many fluvastatin patients (14.6 versus 8.3 percent) and progression occurred less frequently (28.7 versus 39.1 percent of patients). The results observed in older patients were comparable with those of younger patients.

Data from Primary Prevention

In the primary prevention study "*WOSCOPS*" (24), 6595 subjects aged 45 to 64 years with LDL-cholesterol above 155 mg per deciliter and no history of myocardial infarction or other serious coronary illness were treated with pravastatin 40 mg or placebo for a mean follow-up period of 4.9 years. The reduction of relative risk for nonfatal MI was 31% and for coronary angiography and PTCA or CABG was of 31 and 37%, respectively, but the NNT was of 45 patients to treat for saving one combined end point and 143 patients to treat for saving 1 death from cardiac cause.

In terms of cost/effectiveness, these data show that the primary prevention could be somewhat less convenient than secondary prevention (Table 1). Actually, primary prevention has a wide range of cost-effectiveness depending on the individual baseline CHD risk, as discussed in the following paragraph.

The Overall Risk Global Assessment

Although the findings of *4S* (17,18,19) and *CARE* (20) studies substantially have shifted the balance of benefits in favor of the secondary prevention, the management of hypercholesterolemia in primary prevention, i.e. in patients with no overt CHD, should be better targeted at overall risk and not simply at cholesterol or other single risk factors. It has been published a table (27) based on the overall risk evaluation that demonstrates the predominant effect of advancing age on coronary risk. According to this global assessment of the risk factors, a 28-year-old woman with systolic blood pressure of 160 mm Hg, no diabetes, no left ventricular hypertrophy and non-smoker but with serum cholesterol 8.6 mmol/L (320 mg per deciliter), has an estimated risk of a coronary event of only 0.3% in 10 years. By contrast, a 69-year-old man with systolic blood pressure 160 mm Hg, presence of left ventricular hypertrophy, diabetes and smoking but serum cholesterol level of only 5.5 mmol/L (210 mg per deciliter), has an estimated risk of a coronary event of 58.1% in 10 years. The old patients would not be a candidate for lipid lowering drug therapy according to the current guidelines, while his estimated risk clearly indicates the necessity of an aggressive lipid-lowering therapy.

DATA FROM STUDIES ON ENDOTHELIAL FUNCTION

The treatment of hypercholesterolemia with drugs in elderly patients affected by CHD is recommended also for other aspects of coronary atherosclerosis. Elevated serum cholesterol levels have been demonstrated to inhibit several endothelial functions, particularly the production of the nitric oxide (NO), a potent vasodilator secreted by endothelium that induces a relaxation of arterial smooth muscle cells. The infusion of acetylcholine in normal coronaries dilates these vessels while in atherosclerotic coronaries it induces a potent vasoconstriction, due to the presence of a severe endothelial cell dysfunction in atherosclerotic

Table 1. Comparison of benefits obtained by primary and secondary prevention of CHD

	Primary prevention (WOSCOPS)	Secondary prevention (4S study)
Subjects	6595	4444
Relative reduction of CHD death	33%	42%
Absolute reduction of CHD death	7%	33%
Non-fatal myocardial infarction	20%	58%
PTCA	8%	50%

coronaries which impairs the NO production (25). The same vasoconstrictor effect has been observed in patients with hypercholesterolemia or hypertension. The treatment of hypercholesterolemia with HMGCoA reductase inhibitor improves significantly the endothelium mediated response of coronary arteries to acetylcholine in patients with CHD (26). Such improvement in the local regulation of coronary arterial tone potentially relieves ischemic symptoms. These data suggest that patients with angina pectoris can greatly relieve their coronary symptoms and improve significantly the quality of life by pharmacological treatment of hypercholesterolemia. For these reasons, the pharmacological treatment of hypercholesterolemia should be considered as mandatory in elderly patients affected by CHD, in order to reduce CHD mortality and improve coronary symptoms.

CONCLUSIONS

Hypercholesterolemia is still an uncertain risk factor for CHD in elderly men, while in women it appears to be more predictive of CHD. HDL cholesterol level is probably the most predictive index of CHD.

Formal analysis of the most recent clinical trials with the HMGCoA reductase inhinbitor (statins) show that secondary prevention of CHD is very cost-effective while primary prevention has a wide range of cost-effectiveness depending on the individual baseline CHD risk.

In elderly patients with previous CHD (i.e. secondary prevention), the pharmacological treatment of hypercholesterolemia must be considered mandatory for at least two reasons: first, because it reduces mortality and morbidity also in people over 70 years; second, because it can restore a normal coronary response to vasodilator stimuli reducing the symptoms of angina pectoris.

In absence of an overt CHD (i.e. primary prevention), the decision of treating hypercholesterolemia with drugs in elderly people must be made on the basis of the overall risk evaluation, which must take into account also hypertension, diabetes mellitus, smoking and left ventricular hypertrophy.

ACKNOWLEDGMENTS

Supported by Italian MURST, 40% and 60%, 1996 and 1997, and by Consiglio Nazionale delle Ricerche, Roma, Italian Longitudinal Study on Aging, Grant 9400419 PF40.

REFERENCES

1. Kaiser FE, Morley JE. Cholesterol can be lowered in older persons. Should we care? J Am Geriatric Soc 1990; 38:84–85.
2. Kannel WB, Gordon T. Cardiovascular risk factors in the aged: The Framingham Study. In: Haynes SG, Feinleib M. eds. Proceedings of the Second Conference on the Epidemiology of Aging. Bethesda, Maryland: National Institute of Health; 1977:65–89.
3. Moser M. The management of cardiovascular disease in the elderly. J Am Geriat Soc 1982; 30(suppl):SS20-S29.
4. Kannel WB, Castelli WP, Gordon T, McNamara PM. Serum cholesterol, lipoproteins, and the risk of coronary heart disease: the Framingham Study. Ann Intern Med 1971, 74:1–12.
5. Multiple Risk-Factor Intervention Trial: risk factor changes and mortality results. JAMA 1982, 248:1465–1477.

6. Dayton S, Pearce ML, Hasimoto S, Dixon WJ, Tomiyasu U. A controlled clinical trial of a diet high in unsaturated fat in preventing complications of atherosclerosis. Circulation 1969; 39 and 40(suppl II):1–63.
7. Castelli WP, Garrison RI, Wilson PWF, et al. Incidence of coronary heart disease and lipoprotein cholesterol levels: the Framingham Study. JAMA 1986, 256:2835–2838.
8. Benfante R, Deed D: Is elevated serum cholesterol level a risk factor for coronary heart disease in the elderly? JAMA 1990, 263: 393–396.
9. Harris T, Cook EF, Kannel WB, Goldman L. Proportional hazard analysis of risk factors for coronary heart disease in individuals aged 65 or older. J Am Geriatr Soc 1988, 36: 1025–1028.
10. Rubin SM, Sidney S, Black DM, Browner WS, Hulley SB, Cummings SR. High blood cholesterol in elderly men and the excess risk for coronary heart disease. Ann Intern Med 1990; 113, 916–920.
11. Corti MC, Guralnik JM, Salive ME, Harris T, Field TS, Wallace RB, Berkman LF, Seeman TE, Glyn RJ, Hennekens CH, Havlik RJ. HDL Cholesterol Predicts Coronary Heart Disease in Older People. JAMA 1995; 274:539–544.
12. Forette B, Tortrat D, Wolmark Y. Cholesterol as risk factor for mortality in elderly women. Lancet 1989; 1:868–870.
13. Agner E, Hansen PF. Fasting serum cholesterol and triglycerides in a ten- year prospective study in old age. Acta Med Scand 1983; 214:33–61.
14. Rudman JD, Mattson DE, Nagraj HS, Caindec N, Rudman IW, Jackson DL. Antecedents of death in the men of a Veteran Administration nursing home. J Am Geriatr Soc 1987; 35:496–502.
15. Morley JE. Nutritional status of the elderly. Am J Med 1986; 81:679–695.
16. Isles CA, Hole DJ, Gillis CR, et al. Plasma cholesterol, coronary heart disease and cancer in the Renfrew and Paisley survey. Br Med J 1989; 298:920–924.
17. The Scandinavian Simvastatin Survival Study Group. Randomized trial of cholesterol lowering in 4444 patients with coronary heart disease: the Scandinavian Simvastatin Survival Study (4S). Lancet 1994; 344:1383–1389.
18. Scandinavian Simvastatin Survival Study Group. Baseline serum cholesterol and treatment effect in the Scandinavian Simvastatin Survival Study (4S). Lancet 1995; 345:1274–1275.
19. Johannesson M, Jonsson B, Kjekshus J, Olsson AG, Pedersen TR, Wedel H, for the Scandinavian Simvastatin Survival Study Group. Cost effectiveness of simvastatin treatment to lower cholesterol levels in patients with coronary heart disease. N Engl J Med 1997; 336:332–336.
20. Sacks FM, Pfeffer MA, Moye LA, Rouleau JL, Rutheford JD, Cole TG, Brown L, Warnica W, Arnold MO, Wun CC, Davis BR, Braunwald E, for the Cholesterol and Recurrent Events Trial Investigators. The effect of pravastatin on coronary events after myocardial infarction in patients with average cholesterol levels. N Engl J Med 1996; 335:1001–1009.
21. Byington RP, Jukema JW, Salonen JT, et al. Reduction in cardiovascular events during pravastatin therapy: pooled analysis of clinical events of the Pravastatin Atherosclerosis Intervention Program. Circulation 1995; 92:2419- 2425.
22. Herd JA, Ballantyne CM, Farmer JA, Ferguson JJ, Gould KL, Jones PH, West MS, Gotto AM Jr. The effect of fluvastatin on coronary atherosclerosis: the lipoprotein and coronary atherosclerosis study (LCAS). 69th Scientific Session of the Americam Heart Association, New Orleans, November 11–13, 1996. Abstract book p. I-597, n.3496.
23. Herd JA, West MS, Ballantyne CM, Farmer JA, Ferlic LL, Jonas PH, Gotto AM. Clinical cardiac and all fatal events in the lipoprotein and coronary atherosclerosis study (LCAS). 4th International Symposium on Multiple Risk Factors in Cardiovascular Disease, Washington, April 23–25, 1997. Abstract book, p.76.
24. Shepherd J, Cobbe SM, Ford I, Isles CG, Lorimer AR, Macfarlane PW, Mckillop JH, Packard CJ, for the West of Scotland Coronary Prevention Study Group. Prevention of coronary heart disease with pravastatin in men with hypercholesterolemia. N Engl J Med 1995; 333:1301–1307.
25. Vita JA, Treasure CB, Nabel EG, McLenachan JM, Fish RD, Yeung A, Vekshten VI, Selwyn AP, Ganz P. Coronary vasomotor response to acetylcholine relates to risks factors for coronary artery disease. Circulation 1990; 81:491–498.
26. Treasure CB, Klein JL, Weintraub WS, Talley JD, Stillabower ME, Kosinski AS, Zhang J, Boccuzzi SJ, Cedarholm JC, Alexander RW. Beneficial effects of cholesterol-lowering therapy on the coronary endothelium in patients with coronary artery disease. N Engl J Med 1995; 332:481–487.
27. Haq IU, Jackson PR, Yeo WW, Ramsay LE. Sheffield risk and treatment table for cholesterol lowering for primary prevention of coronary heart disease. Lancet, 1995; 346:1467–1471.

ANGIOGENESIS IN MULTIPLE MYELOMA

Angelo Vacca, Monica Minischetti, Antonio Pellegrino, and
Franco Dammacco

Department of Biomedical Sciences and Human Oncology
Section of Internal Medicine and Clinical Oncology
University of Bari Medical School
Piazza Giulio Cesare, 11, I-70124 Bari, Italy

1. GENERAL

Angiogenesis, the new vessel formation, occurs during embryo development and in postnatal life, in wound repair and cyclically in the female genital system (1). In these situations, it is limited in time and characterized by very low proliferation of the endothelial cells. It develops through five steps (2): a) basement membrane degradation by proteolytic enzymes secreted by the endothelial cells, resulting in the facilitation of tiny sprouts; b) migration toward the stimulus of endothelial cells at the sprout tip; c) proliferation of the endothelial cells below the sprout; d) canalization, branching and formation of vascular loops, resulting in a functioning circulatory network; e) perivascular apposition of pericytes, and neosynthesis of basement membrane constituents by both the endothelial cells and the pericytes.

In tumors, it goes through the same steps, but is uncontrolled and unlimited in time, and characterized by a 30- to 40-fold proliferative activity of endothelial cells (3). It is essential for tumor progression in terms of growth, invasion and metastasis because these develop through the transition from the avascular to the vascular phase.

2. THE AVASCULAR AND VASCULAR PHASES OF TUMORS

The avascular phase has been studied by using tumor spheroids in agar (4) and tumor implants into the anterior chamber of rabbit eye (5); the human counterpart is *in situ* carcinoma and melanoma (6). In the spheroid, the volume increases with the cube of the radius, whereas the surface area in proportion to its square. Its growth reaches a steady state when the area becomes too small to allow nutritional material to be supplied to its deep regions and the removal of metabolites. The spheroid is nourished solely by diffusible substances in the culture medium and thus reaches a steady state when its mass is very small (volume: ~1 mm^3; cells: $2\times10^5 - 1\times10^6$, as many cells enter the system at the surface as are lost in depth by apoptosis and necrosis). Proliferative activity is slow and

Recent Advances in Geriatrics, edited by Barbagallo, Licata, and Sowers.
Plenum Press, New York, 1998.

balanced by the apoptosis ("dormant" phase). The tumor has no metastatic potential and may remain in this phase indefinitely.

The vascular phase has been studied by using tumor implants onto the rabbit iris (5), which is a site with high angiogenic potential. The tumor is soon permeated by new vessels, its proliferative activity becomes exponential, while the apoptosis rate declines, its mass grows rapidly, and reaches the steady state at 4,000 to 16,000 times the original volume. The vascular phase corresponds to locally invasive and metastatic tumors (6): indeed, the ingrowth of new capillaries provides the conditions for tumor growth, invasion, intravasation and metastasis. To proceed, the metastasis must be capable of inducing a further angiogenic response (7). If not, it will behave like "dormant" micrometastasis (8). The vascular phase also parallels tumor progression in terms of neoplastic transformation (9). In all these systems, the neoplastic or preneoplastic cell capable of inducing angiogenesis is responsible for the transition from the avascular to the vascular phase.

3. TUMOR PROGRESSION IN MULTIPLE MYELOMA SUGGESTS THE EXISTENCE OF THE VASCULAR PHASE

3.1. Cell Kinetics in Multiple Myeloma: The Gompertzian Growth

In multiple myeloma (MM), the neoplastic population consists of 3 clonally related compartments (10): a) a small stem cell compartment, containing totipotent cells that are self-maintaining and supply cells to the downstream compartments; b) an expansion compartment or "growth fraction" (GF), whose proliferative activity expands the small population entering from the above compartment; c) a differentiation compartment (the largest) where proliferation stops and differentiation into mature plasma cells takes place, and where cell loss by apoptosis and necrosis also occurs.

The kinetics of the stem-cell compartment is unknown, but should be quite negligible, given its very small size. The GF, the basic proliferative nucleus, contains cells in the G1, S, G2 and M phases, as well as resting G0 cells, i.e., cells outside the proliferative cycle, but capable of joining it again following different stimuli. The balance between GF cell production and cell loss from the differentiation compartment determines growth, steady state or reduction of the MM cell mass.

GF proliferative activity is measured by the labeling index (LI)%, which identifies the S-phase cell fraction (11). At diagnosis, the LI%, calculated on the basis of the overall neoplastic population, is usually low (median = 1%; range 0–5). However, if it is solely related to the GF, which is generally small (mean <1%, range <1–3.7), it is much higher (median = 30%, range 15–100), indicating a very lively proliferation. This is confirmed by the fact that the MM cell mass doubling time is relatively short (5–15 months), though a huge cell loss (>90%, given the large size of the differentiation compartment) occurs, indicating that cell production by the GF is quite high.

MM is clinically diagnosed when the cellular mass is $>10^{12}$ cells—a stage reached following Gompertzian growth (12). The initial growth is exponential, and then progressively reduced (LI% and GF decrease) according to a lag factor, just as cell density continues to increase, until the steady state is reached (about 5–25 months after neoplastic transformation). The length of this factor differs from one patient to another and determines the cell mass level of the steady state.

At diagnosis, the MM plasma cell proliferative activity is extremely varied, depending on the steady state level (11): a) if the steady state has been reached, further growth is moderate (low LI% and GF, balanced by the apoptosis), and the disease is poorly aggressive (non-active); b) if the steady state is still a long way ahead, even though the cell mass is large enough (>10^{12} cells) to elicit clinical symptoms, growth is exponential (high LI% and GF, low apoptosis rate and cell loss), the tumor mass expands rapidly, and the disease is aggressive (active). In relapse (11), which is usually diagnosed when the cell mass is <10^{12} cells, growth is exponential because the steady state is distant, and the disease is active. In the post-treatment stable remission ("plateau phase": >50% reduction of the M component for at least 6 months), the cell mass and the steady state have been reduced to a level allowing no further reduction, most cells are in G0 and growth is therefore limited (LI <1%, GF ≤0.5%), resulting in quiescent (non-active) disease (11). While on treatment, responsive patients display growth conditions close to the plateau phase and the disease is non-active (11). In agreement with the Gompertzian growth, the neoplastic population in monoclonal gammopathies of undetermined significance (MGUS) reaches the steady state at very low cell mass levels (10^{10}–10^{11} cells) and LI is very low (LI <1%) (11).

The Gompertzian model relates active MM (exponential growth phase) to experimental solid tumors in the vascular phase, and non-active MM and MGUS (slow growth phase) to their avascular ("dormant") phase.

4. BONE MARROW ANGIOGENESIS IN ACTIVE MULTIPLE MYELOMA

4.1. *In Situ* Findings

We selected (13): a) 28 patients with active MM, of whom 11 were in the active state when diagnosed (symptomatic disease with a progressive increment of the M-component in the three months preceding the study), 9 in relapse, and 8 in progression during chemotherapy; b) 18 patients with non-active MM, of whom 6 were in the plateau phase and 12 in post-treatment complete/objective response; c) 21 patients with MGUS.

Microvessels were quantitated planimetrically on frozen bone marrow biopsies as microvessel area % inside a cellular area, by their highlighting through immunoperoxidase and factor VIII (14). The LI% of plasma cells aspirated from the biopsy site was assessed by immunofluorescence and autoradiography (15).

The microvessel area in active MM patients was significantly higher than in non-active MM and MGUS patients. The increment was both real and related to the larger cellular area (Figure 1).

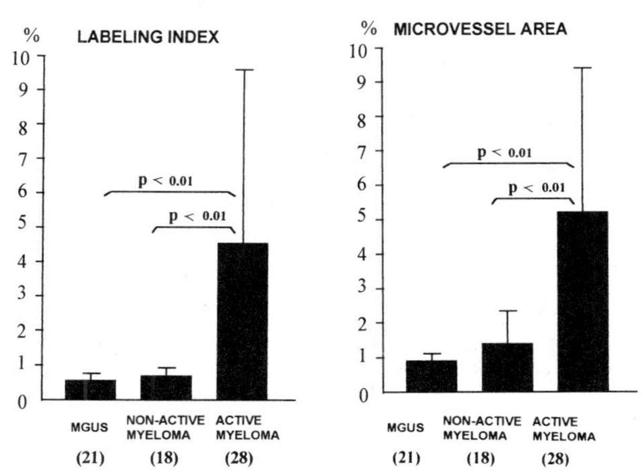

Figure 1. Symmetric variations of microvessel area and plasma cell labeling index in the bone marrow of patients. The cellular area was 0.042±0.007 mm^2 (x400 fields of 0.062 mm^2) for MGUS; 0.044±0.01 for non-active myeloma and 0.054±0.006 for active myeloma. Number of patients between brackets.

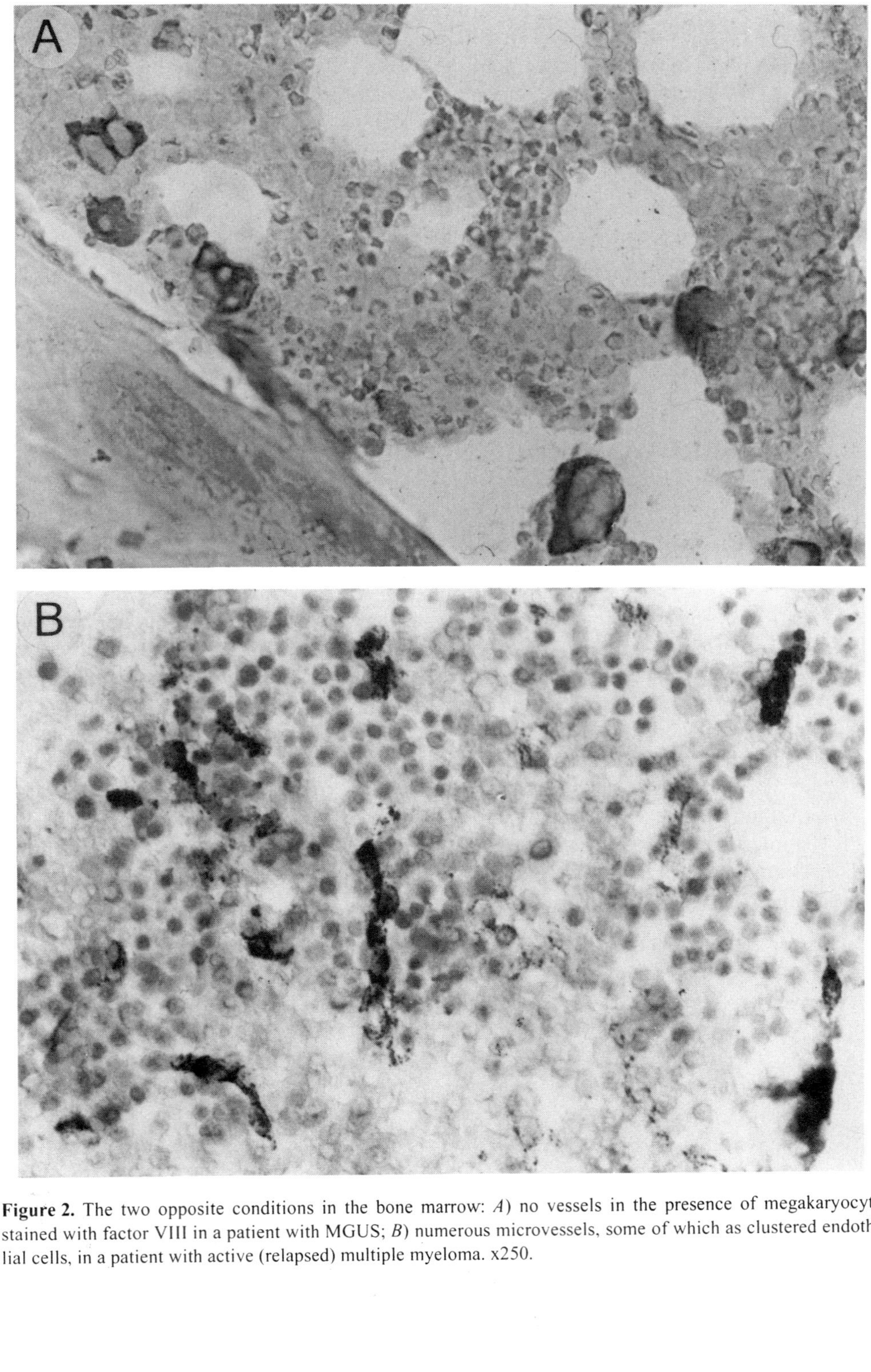

Figure 2. The two opposite conditions in the bone marrow: *A*) no vessels in the presence of megakaryocytes stained with factor VIII in a patient with MGUS; *B*) numerous microvessels, some of which as clustered endothelial cells, in a patient with active (relapsed) multiple myeloma. x250.

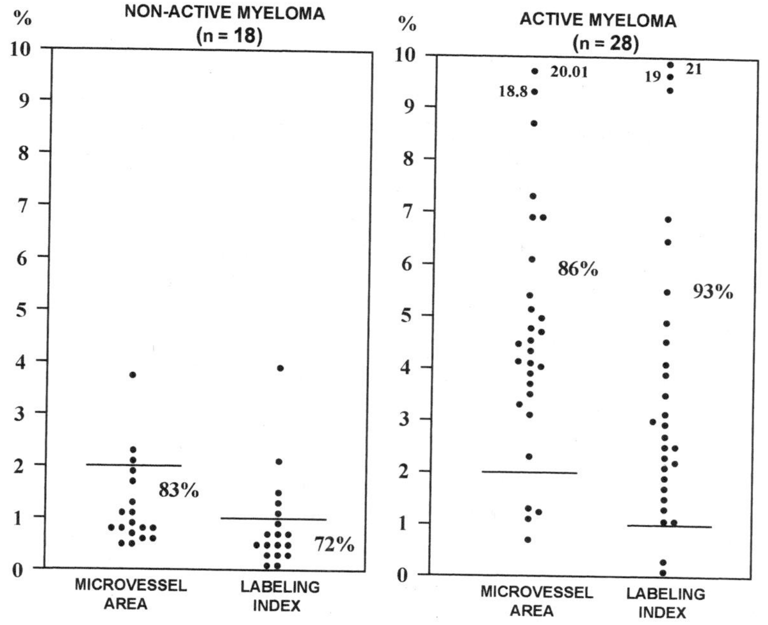

Figure 3. The 2% microvessel area and 1% labeling index cutoffs discriminate 83% and 72% non-active from 86% and 93% active myeloma patients respectively. When combined, they discriminate 83% non-active from 93% active myeloma patients.

A great many small clusters of endothelial cells, or individual endothelial cells, were scattered in the bone marrow tissue of these patients, though not in that of the others (Figure 2).

The microvessel area varied in agreement with the LI% (Figure 1) and both parameters were correlated (active MM, $R^2=0.94$; non-active MM, $R^2=0.78$; MGUS, $R^2=0.73$, $p<0.01$). Conversely, the microvessel area was not correlated with plasmacytosis. The microvessel area 2% cutoff discriminated patients with active and non-active MM with a degree of precision similar to that of the LI 1% cutoff already applied (11). Discrimination was more precise when both cutoffs were combined (Figure 3).

4.2. Functional Studies

The *in situ* findings prompted us to investigate the mechanisms underlying the induction of angiogenesis in the bone marrow of MM patients (Vacca A., Dammacco F., submitted for publication). Enriched bone marrow plasma cells were subjected to *in situ* hybridization for the matrix metalloproteinase-2 (MMP-2) and MMP-9. These proteinases are primarily involved in tumor invasion because they degrade type IV, V, VII and X collagens and fibronectin (16), major components of the interstitial stroma and subendothelial basement membrane, that are hindrance to be traversed by tumor cells during invasion and metastasis (16). Plasma cells expressed the MMP-2, whereas the expression of MMP-9 was less intense and inconstant (Figure 4).

Expression was associated to the secretion of the enzyme into the serum-free culture medium (conditioned medium, CM): when this was run in SDS-PAGE gelatin zymography, it produced gelatinolytic bands with an apparent Mr of 62 kDa and 88 kDa (Figure 5), corresponding to the activated form of MMP-2 and MMP-9, respectively (17). According

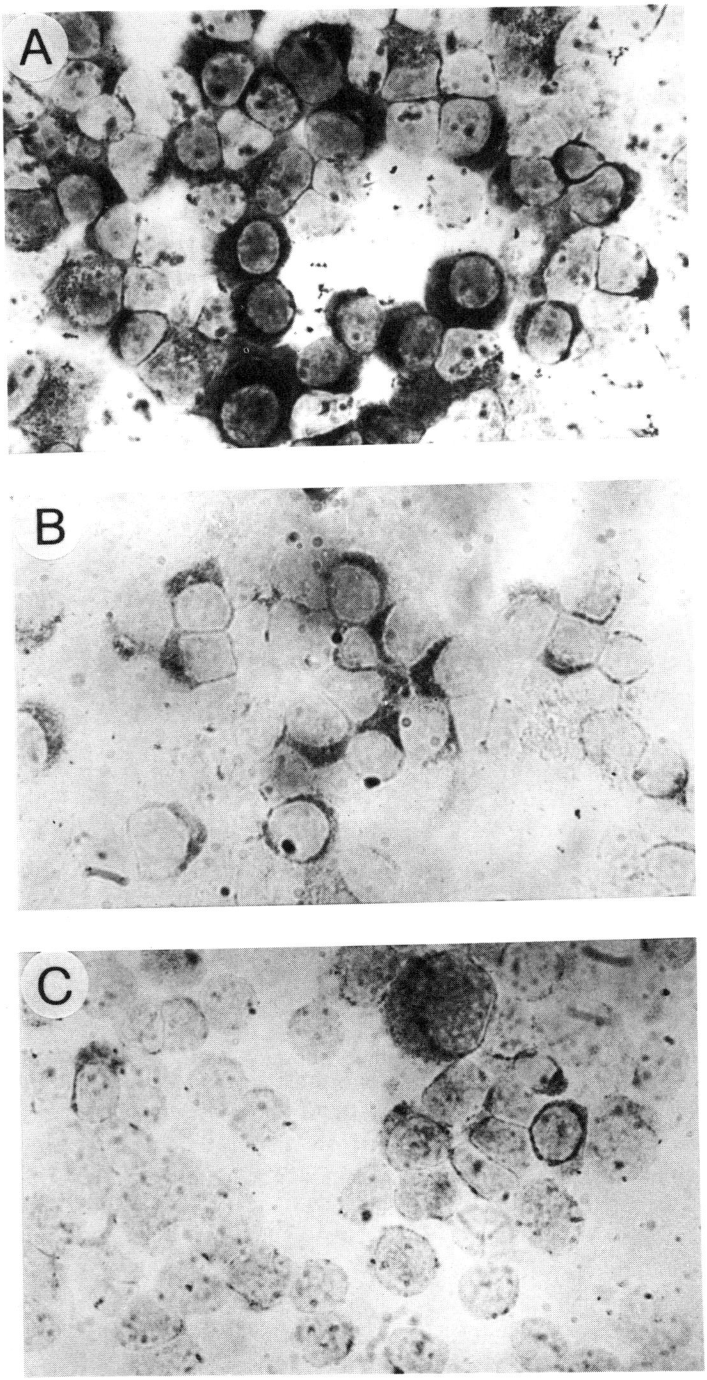

Figure 4. *In situ* hybridization for A) matrix metalloproteinase-2 (MMP-2) and B) MMP-9 mRNA in bone marrow plasma cells of a patient with active multiple myeloma. C) The mRNAse-treated negative control for MMP-2.

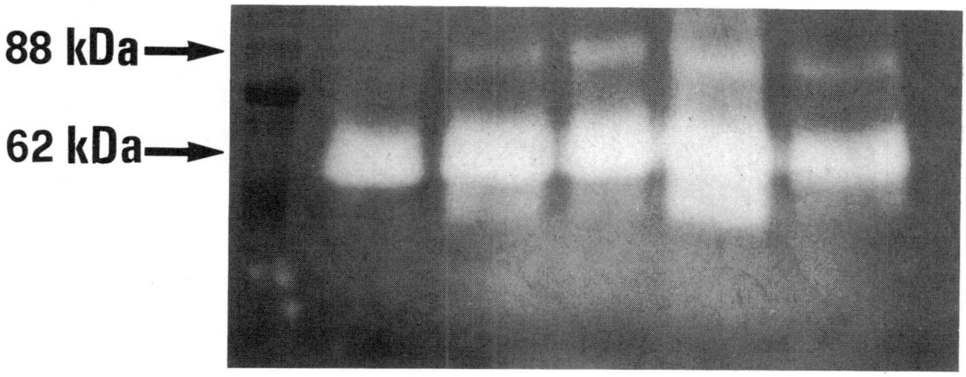

Figure 5. SDS-PAGE gelatin zymography of the conditioned medium of bone marrow plasma cells from patients with multiple myeloma. Note the white bands against a dark background with an apparent Mr of 62 kDa and 88 kDa, corresponding to the gelatinolytic regions of the matrix metalloproteinase-2 (MMP-2) and MMP-9 activity.

to the *in situ* hybridization, the levels of the MMP-9 enzyme activity were always lower, if not absent, than those of MMP-2 (Figure 5).

The CM of plasma cells was also assessed for its angiogenic potential *in vitro* and *in vivo*. *In vitro*, it was evaluated for the capacity to induce morphogenesis in EA.hy926 endothelial cells seeded on Matrigel, a reconstituted basement membrane. As shown in Figure 6, endothelial cells incubated with negative control medium remained spherical and isolated, or clustered in few clumps. By contrast, endothelial cells seeded in the presence of the plasma cell CM spread throughout the Matrigel surface, enlongated and aligned reciprocally to form branching, anastomosing capillary-like structures. The CM also induced proliferation and chemotaxis of EA-hy926 cells. Overall, results indicate that CM of MM plasma cells induces several aspects of the angiogenic phenotype in cultured endothelial cells.

In a second series of *in vivo* experiments, the Matrigel was loaded with the plasma cell CM, injected subcutaneously into mice, and evaluated after 9 days for the angiogenic response. The CM induced angiogenesis into the Matrigel: this was pierced by numerous branching capillary-like structures connecting with one another and originating a thin vascular plexus (Figure 6).

5. TUMOR ANGIOGENESIS IS REGULATED BY THE TUMOR ITSELF AND ITS INFLAMMATORY CELLS

Regulatory elements (Figure 7) are:

1. Secretion by tumor cells of angiogenic factors (18) that: a) stimulate proliferation, chemotaxis and chemoinvasion of endothelial cells, namely the basic fibroblast growth factor (bFGF), the vascular endothelial growth factor (VEGF), the placental growth factor (PlGF) and the hepatocyte growth factor (HGF); or that: b) induce vessel differentiation, namely the transforming growth factor-α (TGF-α) and TGF-β. Human tumors may synthesize more than one factor.
2. Inflammatory cell recruitment on the part of chemotactic factors (chemokines) (19) released by the tumor cells and their activation for the release of angiogenic factors (20). Specifically, activated macrophages release TNF-α and IL-8, and inflammatory cells also release the IL-6, G-CSF and GM-CSF.

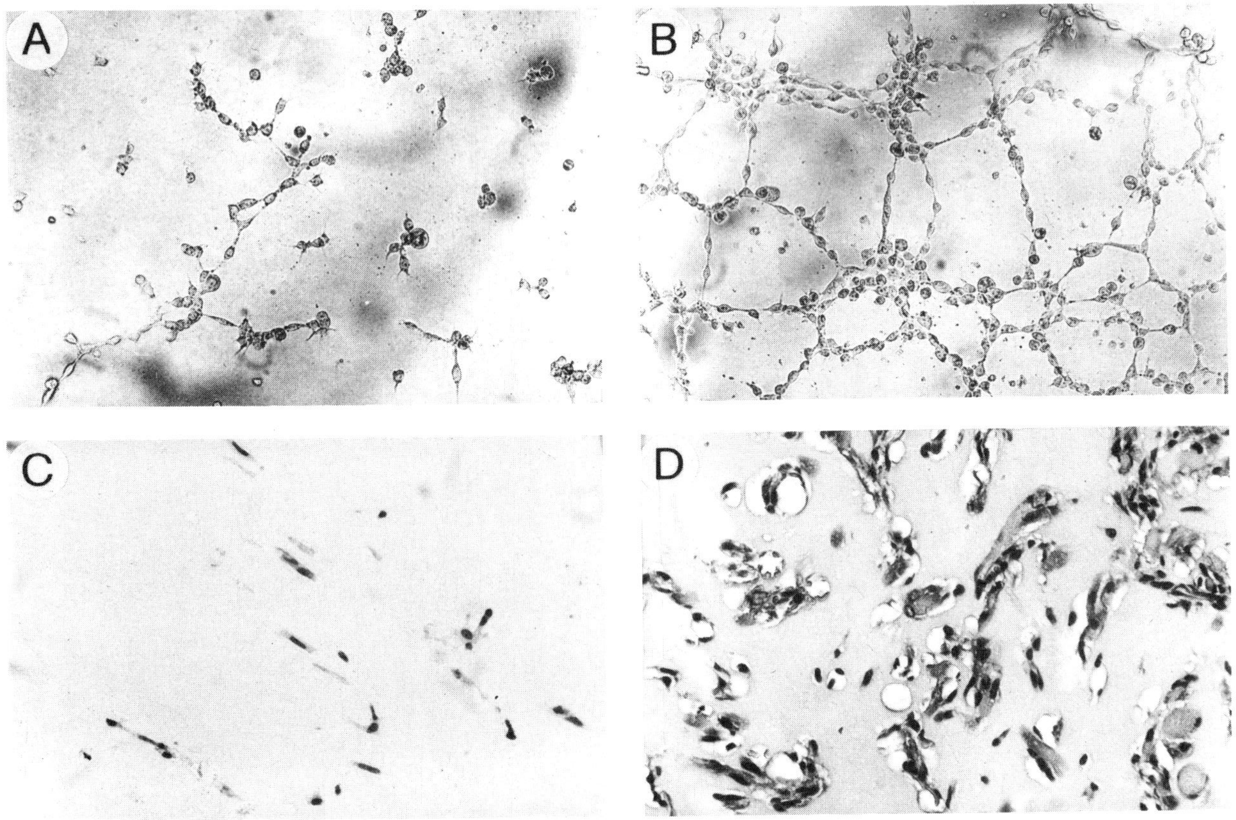

Figure 6. EA.hy926 endothelial cells seeded on Matrigel and incubated for 6 h with (A) 0.1% bovine serum albumin in DMEM (negative control), and (B) this medium 1:1 (vol:vol) diluted with conditioned medium of bone marrow plasma cells of a patient with active multiple myeloma. Endothelial cell morphogenesis is in (B). x100. Hematoxylin and Eosin stained sections of Matrigel plugs soaked with (C) the medium negative control alone or (D) 1:1 added with the myeloma plasma cell conditioned medium. Solid or canalized, reciprocally anastomosed capillaries are observed in (D), whereas not organized endothelial cells in (C). x250.

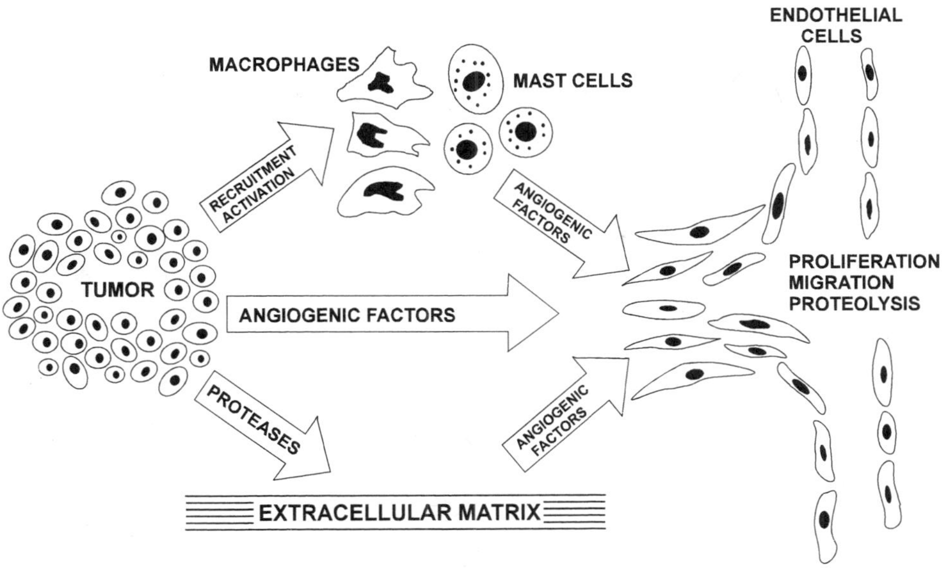

Figure 7. Direct and indirect ways of angiogenesis induction by a tumor.

3. Mobilization of growth factors (e.g., bFGF) and differentiating factors (e.g., TGF-β) from the extracellular matrix stores by proteinases secreted by tumor cells, as in physiologic angiogenesis due to endothelium proteinases (16).
4. Down-regulation of specific genes inhibiting endothelial cell growth (21). Normal cells secrete thrombospondin, an angiogenesis-inhibiting protein down-regulated during tumorigenesis (20). The neoplastic transformation prevents the synthesis of protein p53 and parallels the non-expression of thrombospondin. Thus, protein p53 would appear to inhibit angiogenesis by regulating thrombospondin synthesis.

6. POSSIBLE REGULATION OF ANGIOGENESIS IN MULTIPLE MYELOMA

The close association between angiogenesis and *active* MM indicates that this is the vascular phase of plasma cell tumors, and thus the counterpart to the vascular tumor implants of the rabbit iris and of locally invasive and metastatic solid tumors. Conversely, MGUS and *non-active* MM represent the avascular phase, and correspond to tumor spheroids, to tumor implants of the rabbit eye anterior chamber or to *in situ* tumors. Since most patients with active MM have a microvessel area ≥2% and LI ≥1%, a 2% "vascular bone marrow threshold" seems to be required for this phase and rapid tumor growth. Angiogenesis correlates with LI% but not with plasmacytosis, which mostly measures the differentiation, non-growing compartment (11).

Overall, these findings suggest that, like solid tumor cells, highly proliferating but not slowly proliferating nor differentiated MM plasma cells possess an angiogenic capability that could be expressed by the release of a variety of factors as follows (Figure 8): a) recruitment and activation of the bone marrow microenvironment to release IL-6, IL-8, G-CSF, GM-CSF, TNF-α (22); b) extracellular matrix proteolysis with bFGF and TGF-β

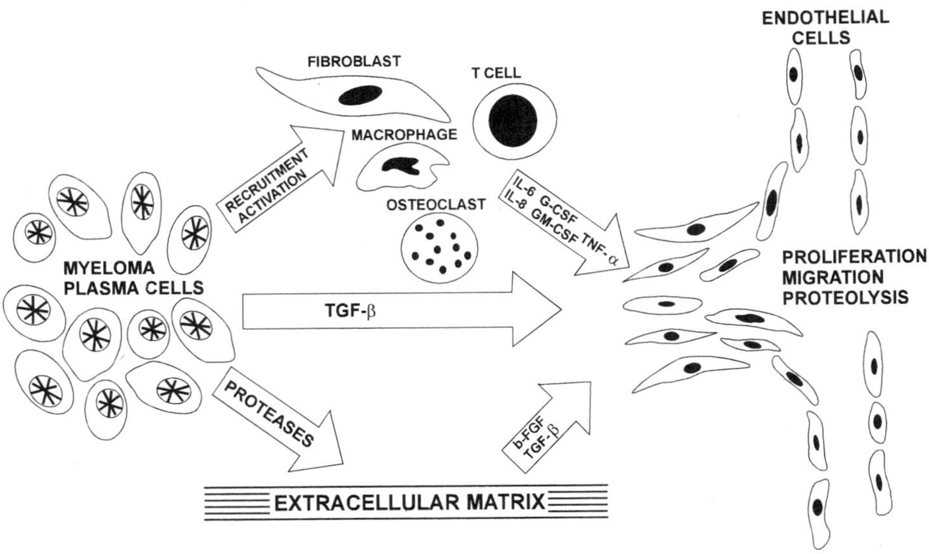

Figure 8. Direct and indirect hypothetic ways of angiogenesis induction by multiple myeloma plasma cells.

release; c) secretion of TGF-β (22). It should be noted that IL-6, IL-8 and GM-CSF are mostly secreted in the active MM (23) where angiogenesis is found. Because in turn angiogenesis favours plasma cell growth, it could thus complete a positive loop (24). The progression of MGUS and non-active MM to active MM could take place when plasma cells become able to induce angiogenesis as described, resulting in formation of new vessels that themselves promote progression. We have provided evidence of similar loops in non-Hodgkin's lymphomas of B-cell (25) and T-cell (26) lineage.

7. BONE MARROW ANGIOGENESIS AS A POSSIBLE PROGNOSTIC MARKER IN MULTIPLE MYELOMA

Mean survival is shorter in patients with LI ≥1% (15 months) than in those with LI <1% (40 months), irrespective of the cell mass (11). According to the Gompertzian growth, MM with elevated LI% is still far from the steady state, since its mass is in the exponential portion of the growth curve. Patients rapidly respond to induction cytostatic treatment ("early responders"), but their response is short-lived and followed by an equally rapid relapse due to massive recruitment of G0 plasma cells, and hence by shorter overall survival. Since LI% refers to the whole myelomatous population—not to GF alone—even very small variations (e.g., by 1%) really denote substantial changes in GF proliferative activity, which must be taken into account when advancing a prognosis.

Our study suggests that the microvessel area and the LI% are closely associated with the MM active phase and are mutually correlated. A disease in a given steady state (MGUS, non-active MM) can thus be supposed at risk of progression towards the subsequent larger-mass steady state (active MM) if the bone marrow shows angiogenesis. On the logistic regression analysis, the risk is greater the larger the microvessel area (3.9 times higher for each 1% increment), and the LI (for each 0.6% increment) (Figure 9) (13). Microvessel area variations are therefore less restricted than those of LI% as a risk

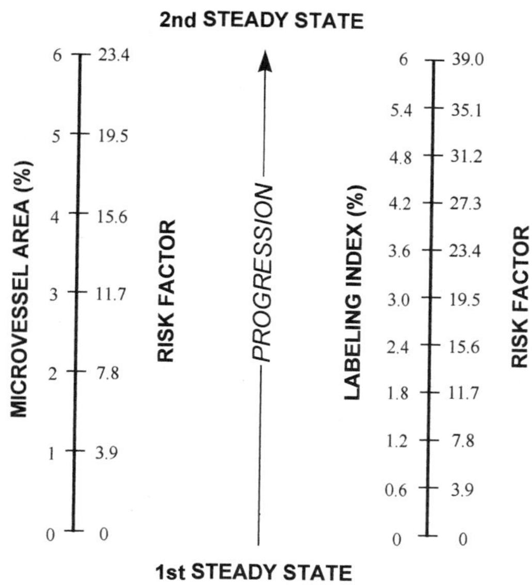

Figure 9. The risk of progression from the first steady state, i.e., MGUS or non-active myeloma, to the second steady state, i.e., active myeloma, is higher (by a 3.9-fold increase of the risk factor) the larger the microvessel area (by 1% increase) and the LI (by 0.6% increase).

assessment parameter and could be a useful guide to prognosis, just as LI% is applied in plasma cell proliferative diseases. Obviously, the prognostic significance of microvessel area warrants further assessment in longitudinal studies, as it has been carried out in patients with solid tumors (27).

8. FUTURE DIRECTIONS

Further investigation is needed of the mechanisms whereby MM cells induce angiogenesis. In MM, cytokines with angiogenic activity have already been identified. Our next step will be to assess the mechanisms responsible for their release, and then identify the MM cell systems triggering recruitment and activation of inflammatory cells (through chemokines?).

Hopefully, the continued investigation on angiogenesis will yield useful prognostic information. MGUS, or else non-active MM with angiogenic phenotype, or developing such phenotype during follow-up, could then be considered to be at risk of progression and in need of more frequent check-ups.

Study of angiogenesis could clarify the mechanism(s) of intravasion of myeloma cells and their dissemination. A further benefit could be the creation of anti-angiogenesis protocols for the treatment of MM characterized by excess angiogenesis. Proteinase inhibitors, antiangiogenic factor antibodies, antiangiogenic compounds or other approaches still under investigation or being clinically tested could prove useful (28).

ACKNOWLEDGMENTS

These studies were supported in part by the Finalized Project Clinical Applications of Oncology Research (Grant 92.02269.PF39) of the Italian Research Council, Rome, and by the Associazione Italiana per la Ricerca sul Cancro (A.I.R.C., Project Diagnosis and Prognosis in Clinical Oncology), Milan, Italy.

REFERENCES

1. Folkman J.: Angiogenesis in cancer, vascular, rheumathoid and other disease. Nature Med., 1: 27–31, 1995.
2. Williams S.: Angiogenesis in three-dimensional cultures. Lab. Invest., 69: 491–493, 1993.
3. Ribatti D., Vacca A., Roncali L., Dammacco F.: Angiogenesis under normal and pathological conditions. Haematologica, 76: 311–320, 1991.
4. Sutherland R.M., McCredie J.A., Inch W.R.: Growth of multicell spheroids in tissue culture as a model of nodular carcinomas. J. Natl. Cancer Inst., 46: 113–117, 1971.
5. Gimbrone M.A. Jr., Leapman S., Cotran R.S., Folkman J.: Tumor dormancy *in vivo* by prevention of neovascularization. J. Exp. Med., 136: 261–267, 1972.
6. Folkman J.: What is the evidence that tumors are angiogenesis dependent? J. Natl. Cancer Inst., 82: 4–6, 1990.
7. Ellis L.M., Fidler I.J.: Angiogenesis and metastasis. Eur J. Cancer, 32A: 2451–2460, 1996.
8. Holmgren L., O'Reilly M.S., Folkman J.: Dormancy of micrometastasis: balanced proliferation and apoptosis in the presence of angiogenesis suppression. Nature Med., 1: 149–153, 1995.
9. Naik P.N., Karrim J., Hanahan D.: Variation in apoptosis during multi-stage tumorigenesis: down-modulation contributes to tumor progression from angiogenic progenitors. Genes & Dev., 13: 1847–1857, 1996.
10. Billadeau D., Ahmann G., Greipp P., Van Ness B.: The bone marrow of multiple myeloma patients contains B cell populations at different stages of differentiation that are clonally related to malignant plasma cells. J. Exp. Med., 178: 1023–1031, 1993.
11. Durie B.G.M.: Staging and kinetics of multiple myeloma. *In*: P.H. Wiernik, G.P. Canellos, R.A. Kyle, C.A. Schiffer (eds.), Neoplastic Diseases of the Blood, Vol. I, 2nd Ed., Churchill Livingstone, New York, 1991, pp. 439–451.
12. Salmon S.E., Seligmann M.: B-cell neoplasia in man. Lancet, ii: 1230–1233, 1974.
13. Vacca A., Ribatti D., Roncali L., Ranieri G., Serio G., Silvestris F., Dammacco F.: Bone marrow angiogenesis and progression in multiple myeloma. Br. J. Haematol., 87: 503–508, 1994.
14. Vacca A., Di Loreto M., Ribatti D., Di Stefano R., Gadaleta-Caldarola G., Iodice G., Caloro D., Dammacco F.: Bone marrow of patients with active multiple myeloma: angiogenesis and plasma cell adhesion molecules LFA-1, VLA-4, LAM-1 and CD44. Am. J. Hematol., 50: 9–14, 1995.
15. Vacca A., Di Stefano R., Frassanito A., Iodice G., Dammacco F.: A disturbance of the IL-2/IL-2 receptor system parallels the activity of multiple myeloma. Clin. Exp. Immunol., 84: 429–434, 1991.
16. Mignatti P., Rifkin D.B.: Biology and biochemistry of proteinases in tumor invasion. Physiological Rev., 73: 161–195, 1993.
17. Van Wart H.E., Birkedal-Hansen H.: The cysteine switch: a principle of regulation of metalloproteinase gene family. Proc. Natl. Acad. Sci. USA, 85: 5578–5582, 1990.
18. Pepper M.S., Mandriota S.J., Vassalli J.D., Orci L., Montesano R.: Angiogenesis-regulating cytokines: activities and interactions. *In*: V. Günthert, W. Birchmeier (eds.), Current Topics in Microbiology and Immunology, Vol. 213/II: Attempts to Understand Metastasis Formation II, pp. 31–67, Berlin: Springer-Verlag, 1996.
19. Sozzani S., Locati M., Allavena P., Van Damme J., Mantovani A.: Chemokines: a superfamily of chemotactic cytokines. Int. J. Clin. Lab. Res., 25: 69–82, 1996.
20. Polverini P.F.: How the extracellular matrix and macrophages contribute to angiogenesis-dependent diseases. Eur. J. Cancer, 32A: 2430–2437, 1996.
21. Stellmach V., Volpert O.V., Crawford S.E., Lawler J., Hynes R.O., Bouck N.: Tumor suppressor genes and angiogenesis: the role of TP53 in fibroblasts. Eur. J. Cancer, 32A: 2394–2400, 1996.
22. Gregoretti M.G., Gottardi D., Ghia P., Bergui L., Merico F., Bertero M.T., Novarino A., Marchisio P.C., Caligaris-Cappio F.: Bone marrow microenvironment/B cell interactions in multiple myeloma. *In*: F. Dammacco, B. Barlogie (eds.), Multiple Myeloma and Related Disorders. Ares Serono Symposia Publ.; Challenges of Modern Medicine, Vol. 4, pp.1–10, Rome: Christengraf, 1994.
23. Merico F., Bergui L., Gregoretti M.G., Ghia P., Aimo G., Lindley I.J.D., Caligaris-Cappio F.: Cytokines involved in the progression of multiple myeloma. Clin. Exp. Immunol., 92: 27–31, 1993.
24. Vacca A., Ribatti D., Roncali L., Dammacco F.: Angiogenesis in B-cell lymphoproliferative diseases. Biological and clinical studies. Leuk. Lymphoma, 20: 27–38, 1995.
25. Vacca A., Ribatti D., Fanelli M., Costantino F., Nico B., Di Stefano R., Serio G., Dammacco F.: Expression of tenascin is related to histologic malignancy and angiogenesis in B-cell non-Hodgkin's lymphomas. Leuk. Lymphoma, 22: 473–481, 1996.
26. Vacca A., Moretti S., Ribatti D., Pellegrino A., Pimpinelli N., Bianchi B., Bonifazi E., Ria R., Serio G., Dammacco F.: Progression of mycosis fungoides is associated with changes in angiogenesis and expression of the matrix metalloproteinases 2 and 9. Eur. J. Cancer, 1997 (in press).
27. Weidner N.: Intratumor microvessel density as a prognostic factor in cancer. Am. J. Pathol., 147: 9–19, 1995.
28. Folkman J.: Fighting cancer by attacking its blood supply. Scientific American, 275: 150–154, 1996.

26

CALCIUM METABOLISM IN THE ELDERLY

Ligia J. Dominguez, Roberta Ruggero, Dario Bruno, Girolamo Catalano, Domenica A. La Milia, and Mario Barbagallo*

Division of Geriatrics
Istituto di Medicina Interna e Geriatria
Università degli Studi di Palermo
Palermo, Italy

INTRODUCTION

Mineral homeostasis represents one of the multiple areas at risk in the elder population. This includes the ion calcium, which is the most abundant inorganic element in the human body and an essential key for many physiologic processes (1).

The critical role of calcium was first delineated 100 years ago when Ringer described the importance of calcium on cardiac contraction (2). At present, numerous physiologic roles are recognized for this ion (Table 1). In bone, calcium is important for the structural integrity of the skeleton, which serves as a reservoir of calcium ion for other physiologic functions. Calcium is a critical factor in several life-defining biochemical processes, such as the coupling between excitation and contraction in muscular tissue, the coagulation cascade, the permeability of plasma membranes to sodium ions, therefore cellular excitability, and the release of cellular secretory products. Calcium serves in several second messenger systems, including cAMP and phosphatidylinositol cell signaling systems, and it itself can serve as a key intracellular messenger (1,3). Considering all these important physiologic roles, calcium metabolism modifications associated with aging may affect the entire economy and represent one of the most threatening factors to be considered in the care of the elderly organism.

Since most of calcium in the body is content in the bone, calcium and bone metabolism systems are highly integrated. Both systems are perturbed by aging. In terms of homeostasis, the alterations of calcium metabolism (such as decreased intake, intestinal absorption and renal conservation) are counteracted by the reservoir properties of bone at the expense of bone loss, leading to inadequate mechanical support, increased fragility of the skeleton, and a consequent increased occurrence of fractures (4,5).

In this review, we describe the anatomical and functional components of calcium and bone metabolism and the behavior of this highly integrated systems during aging.

* Correspondence to: Prof. Mario Barbagallo, Associate Professor of Geriatrics, Università degli Studi di Palermo, Via F. Scaduto 6/c, 90144 Palermo, Italy. Tel: (091) 6552885; fax: (091) 6552890; e-mail: mabar@unipa.it.

Recent Advances in Geriatrics, edited by Barbagallo, Licata, and Sowers.
Plenum Press, New York, 1998.

Table 1. Physiologic roles of calcium

Intracellular level	Cellular membrane
• Regulation of cAMP-dependent reactions	• Regulation of permeability
• Regulation of ATP hydrolysis	• Electrical properties (depolarization = excitability)
• Regulation of phosphorylation reactions	• Elasticity
• Coupling factor in muscular contraction	• Tight junctions and desmosomes
• Release of hormones and neurotransmitters	Extracellular level
• Cellular enzymatic activation	• Enzymatic activation
• Regulation of the cellular response to hormones	• Calcification (bone and other tissues)
	• Coagulation cascade
	• Fertility (sperm activity)

CALCIUM HOMEOSTASIS

A normal adult contains approximately 1000 g of calcium, of which 99% resides in the bone, hence constituting an important calcium depot as well as preserving the structural integrity of the skeleton. This compartment represents a dynamic storage of calcium, since the ion is continually and freely exchanged under the influence of several calciotropic hormones (Fig. 1). The remaining 1% of total body calcium is in the extracellular fluid (ECF). Because calcium is so important to so many physiologic processes, its concentration in the ECF and intracellular milieu is rigorously controlled (1,3).

The elevated gradient between intra- and extracellular compartments (approximately 100 nM and 1 mM respectively) is necessary to maintain the cellular responsiveness to diverse extracellular stimuli. This difference in calcium concentration is maintained by the concerted effects of a variety of transport mechanisms operating at various subcellular levels (6,7) (Fig. 2). Calcium enters the cell via voltage-dependent and receptor dependent channels; and leaves the cell through the operation of a magnesium-dependent calcium-ATPase and a sodium-calcium exchanger. Uptake of calcium by intracellular organelles such as the mitochondria and the endoplasmic reticulum also helps maintain a low cytoplasmatic calcium level. Calcium enters the mitochondria via a calcium uniporter and the endoplasmic reticulum via a distinct calcium-ATPase, from the one located in the plasma

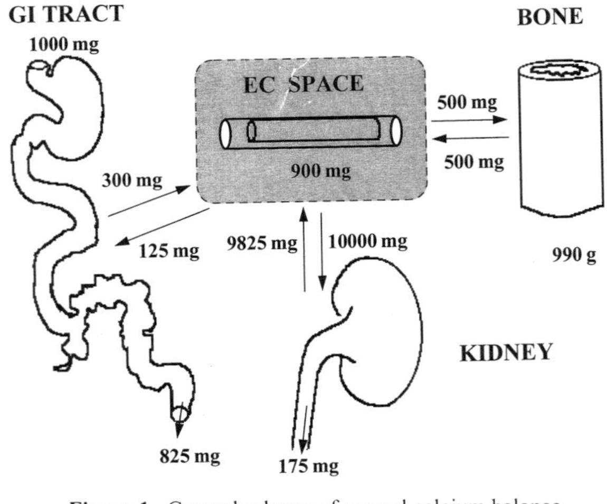

Figure 1. General scheme of normal calcium balance.

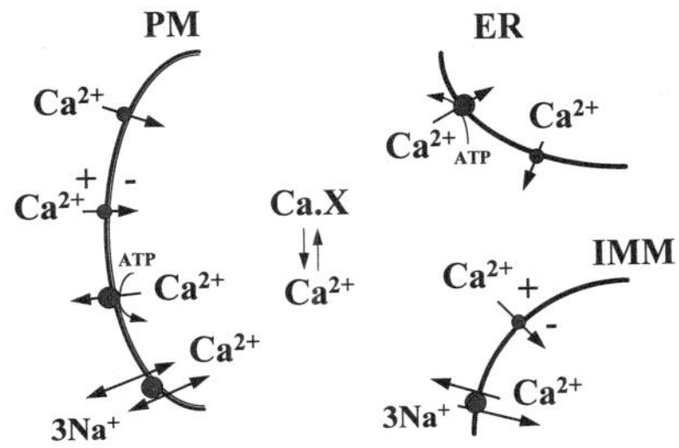

Figure 2. Major pathways for the transport of calcium across cellular membranes. PM = plasma membrane; 1 = steady calcium influx; 2 = voltage dependent calcium influx; 3 = plasma membrane calcium ATPase; 4 = plasma membrane sodium/calcium exchanger (direction depends on thermodynamic balance between sodium and calcium electrochemical potential gradients and vary with tissue and condition); ER = endoplasmic reticulum; 5. ER calcium ATPase; 6. second-messenger-activated calcium efflux; IMM = inner mitochondrial membrane; 7. mitochondrial calcium uniporter; 8. mitochondrial sodium/calcium exchange; Ca.X = calcium bound to cytosolic molecules.

membrane. Calcium leaves the mitochondria via a sodium-calcium exchanger and the endoplasmic reticulum via a constant efflux, which increases in the presence of inositol-1,4,5,-triphosphate (IP_3). (6,7)

REGULATION OF CALCIUM HOMEOSTASIS

Calcium homeostasis is regulated by complex and integrated mechanisms that modify calcium balance and bone mass (Fig. 1). Calcium balance is attained by concerted calcium fluxes through the gut, skeleton and kidney, the three major organs involved in normal serum calcium regulation. These fluxes are continually regulated by diverse hormonal stimulus, some directly related to calcium and phosphorus metabolism, such as PTH, vitamin D and calcitonin, which secretion is regulated by ionized seric calcium, therefore called calciotropic hormones. Other hormones, not regulated by calcium levels, hence not considered calciotropic, have also a considerable influence on calcium balance. These non-calciotropic hormones include sexual hormones, thyroid hormone, adrenal steroids and growth factors (Fig. 3). Other factors that may influence calcium balance include medicaments and physical activity (1,3,5,6).

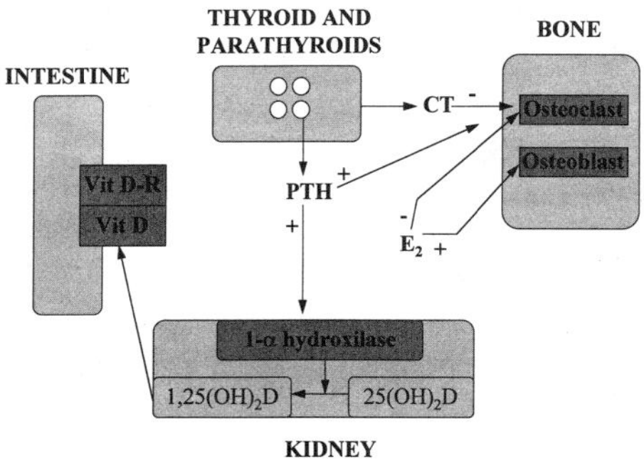

Figure 3. General scheme of calcium balance regulation. CT: calcitonin; PTH: parathyroid hormone; Vit D-R: vitamin D receptor; E2: estradiol.

Small Intestine

Intestinal absorption of calcium is the only source of this mineral for the body's needs. The amount of calcium absorbed is determined in part by the quantity present in the diet and the absorptive capacity of the intestine, regulated by 1,25 dihydroxyvitamin D. Dietary calcium is absorbed in the duodenum and superior portion of the jejunum. When dietary calcium is lower than 200 mg/day, the net intestinal absorption is zero, because approximately the same amount is secreted into the gastrointestinal tract lumen daily. Absorption fraction varies from 15 to 40% and involves both active transport and passive diffusion (8).

Bone

Calcium is continuously gained and lost from bone in a process called bone remodeling. Indeed, in the adult human-being in calcium equilibrium, studies with radioisotopes have demonstrated the existence of an extensive pool of continuous exchanges between the ECF and the skeleton (9) that is considered an essential dynamic storage of calcium in the body. In normal adults, bone resorption delivers approximately 200 to 600 mg/day of Ca into the ECF with an equivalent amount of bone formation.

Kidney

The kidney is the most important regulator of calcium excretion. Calcium is filtered at the glomerulus, reabsorbed at tubular level and only 1–3% of the glomerular filtered load is excreted in the urine. Calcium reabsorption in the proximal tubule is not controlled by calciotropic hormones but is coupled to sodium reabsorption. About 10% of the filtered calcium is delivered to the distal tubules, where it is controlled by parathyroid hormone (PTH), which acts increasing calcium reabsorption. Calcium excretion is also modify by other factors, such as sodium excretion, glomerular filtration rate and diuretic administration (1,3).

Parathyroid Hormone

The most important function of PTH, product of parathyroid glands, is to elevate seric calcium in response to hypocalcemia, stimulating the osteoclasts to reabsorb bone calcium, increasing calcium renal tubular reabsorption, and elevating intestinal absorption of dietary calcium by stimulating the renal synthesis of $1,25(OH)_2D_3$ (10). A deficient intake of calcium in the diet, even with only minimal reduction in ionized seric calcium, is able to stimulate the secretion of PTH. When bone or kidney cells are exposed to PTH, there is a rapid increase in intracellular cyclic AMP levels. In the kidney, this leads to a release of cyclic AMP into the tubular fluid, ultimately to be excreted in the urine. Urinary cyclic AMP can be directly measured and is a well-established marker of PTH bioactivity (10).

Vitamin D

Vitamin D is derived from the diet and from the conversion of the cholesterol metabolite 7-dehydrocholesterol to vitamin D by the action of ultraviolet light in the skin. Vitamin D needs of two hydroxylations to achieve its biological active form. In the liver, vitamin D is hydroxylated to yield 25-OHD, the major circulating form and an accurate indicator of body stores of this hormone. A second hydroxylation in position 1 occurs in the kidney, (favored by PTH), producing the active form of the hormone, $1,25(OH)_2D$.

The most important biological effect of the active metabolite 1,25$(OH)_2$D (calcitriol) is to increase calcium and phosphorus intestinal absorption and to promote calcium uptake by the bone. It increases calcium intestinal absorption by stimulating the production of a calcium-binding protein which is involved in active transport from the intestinal lumen, across the intestinal epithelial cell, and into the ECF (11).

Calcitonin

Calcitonin is a 32-amino acid peptide which is produced by the parafollicular C cells within the thyroid gland. It has a potent inhibitory action on osteoclasts and bone resorption. However, calcitonin's role in chronic calcium regulation is discussed, since in states of extreme calcitonin deficiency (total thyroidectomy) or excess (thyroid medullar carcinoma) there do not appear to be major abnormalities in regulation of serum calcium levels or skeletal disturbances (12).

Bone Mass

Human skeleton develops during childhood and adolescence and reaches a peak of bone mass around the age of 35 years. Since bone mass is one of the most important factors that determine fracture risk, an elevated bone mass at maturity is considered the best protection against bone mass loss that invariably accompanies aging. The accomplishment of an elevated peak of bone mass is determined by at least three groups of factors: genetic, nutritional-endocrine and mechanical. The bone mass that is acquired during development is mainly determined by genetic factors. However, an adequate calcium intake during growth is important in order to maintain a positive calcium balance that provide the means to reach the maximal genetic potential of bone mass peak (1,3).

ALTERATIONS OF CALCIUM METABOLISM IN THE ELDERLY

Aging is associated with several modifications of calcium metabolism (Table 2). Calcium intake, intestinal absorption and renal conservation, all tend to decrease with age (13,14). That favors the instauration of a negative calcium balance and a progressive state of calcium deficiency in the elderly subject. Indeed, the functional reserve of most organ systems necessary for normal calcium and bone homeostasis decreases with age. The elderly are less able to accommodate minor stresses (e.g. low dietary calcium) for which younger adults are able to fully compensate (e.g. through an increase in 1,25-dihydroxy vitamin D production and through renal calcium conservation). Alterations in calcium and bone metabolism are aggravated by illness and medicaments commonly used in old age that affect both systems. Bone calcium depot properties compensate the above deficits with an increase mobilization of calcium to the ECF which leads to a gradual reduction of bone mass, an increased bone fragility and an increase risk of fractures (4,5).

Table 2. Alterations of calcium metabolism associated with aging

• Decreased calcium intake	• Decreased renal conservation
• Decreased calcium absorption	• Increased bone turnover
• Increased serum levels of PTH	• Decreased physical activity
• Altered vitamin D status	• Increased intracellular calcium

Table 3. Optimal daily calcium intake according to NIH Consensus Conference

Age	mg/day
Neonates	
0-6 months	400
6 months to 1 year	600
Children	
1-5 years	800
6-10 years	800–1200
Adolescents	
11-24 years	1200–1500
Male adults	
25-65 years	1000
Elderly (>65 y)	1500
Female adults	
20-25 years	1000
Pregnant and nursing	1200–1500
Postmenopausal (>50 y)	1500
Elderly (>65 y)	1500

Alteration of Calcium Intake and Absorption

In the adult age after the bone peak mass is achieved, an adequate calcium intake is the amount of calcium enough to compensate the daily loss and thus to maintain an equilibrium in calcium balance. The Consensus Conference from the NIH has recently stated mean recommended calcium intake throughout the different life periods (Table 3) (15). In elderly men and women, an adequate calcium intake is of extreme importance. Indeed, the daily requirement is higher (1500 mg/day) than in the young individual, due to the modifications of calcium balance regulatory mechanisms, mentioned above.

In contrast to the NIH suggestions, several studies have demonstrated that dietary calcium content tends to be reduced in men as well as in women with advancing age (16,17). Calcium daily intake below 600 mg (about one third of the NIH recommendation) is common in old populations (15). Further, the already insufficient intake of food with high content of calcium, such as dairy products, are aggravated by the use of oligomineral drinking water in which the concentration of calcium is very low.

At present, the importance of an adequate calcium intake is evident throughout an individual's life time, in the young to warrant the achievement of the maximal potential bone mass peak, and in the elderly, to prevent the bone mass loss that invariably accompanies aging and/or menopause, and consequently to reduce the risk of fracture (18). In fact, in a recent meta-analysis Cummings et al. report a significant positive correlation between calcium intake and bone mass in women (19). Similar results were found by Kelly et al. additionally showing that this correlation was more evident in men that in women, perhaps because of a higher calcium intake in male subjects (20).

There is a progressive decline in calcium absorption efficiency (that is the percentage of the oral calcium load that is absorbed) after about 60 years of age, in part attributed to the age-related alterations in vitamin D status, discussed below. This decreased calcium absorption may be further aggravated in some elderly persons by diminished gastric acid production (which allows to maintain calcium in an ionized state, the only state of the element which is absorbed), and by the development of acquired lactase deficiency with aging with a consequent avoidance of dairy products (21,22).

Altered Vitamin D Status

Regarding the age-related changes in the vitamin D endocrine system, there is a linear decrease of plasma 25(OH)D and $1,25(OH)_2D$ levels between the ages of 65 and 90 (23,24). Several factors may contribute to the reduced levels of vitamin D metabolites and consequent decreased efficiency of calcium absorption mechanisms in advanced age (Table 4). This alteration is a consequence of either a relative vitamin D deficit in the diet of elderly population or a reduction in sunlight exposure. The reduction of 25(OH)D level is followed by a relative deficit of $1,25(OH)_2D$ secondary to a diminished capacity of renal hydroxylation of vitamin D, aggravated in women by the estrogen deficiency, and by a reduced responsiveness of renal 1-α-hydroxylase to circulating PTH (25). There is also evidence of a reduction on duodenal $1,25(OH)_2D$ receptor number and sensibility with age (26), which may contribute to a reduction in calcium-binding protein that in normal circumstances favors active calcium transport from the luminal duodenal surface to the blood stream.

Alterations of Ionized Calcium and PTH Levels

A reduction of total and ionized serum calcium with aging has been recognized by many (27,28,29) but not all authors (30). Reduction in total calcemia is partially attributable to the reduction of calcium-binding to plasmatic proteins, which are also reduced in the elderly (3). However, the reduction in ionized calcium body with aging is in accordance with the elevation of PTH levels reported by several authors (28,31–34). The possibility that this increase in PTH levels could reflect a reduced glomerular clearance or an increase primary secretion of the hormone is ruled out by studies showing that there is an age-related increase in nephrogenous cyclicAMP and a decrease in tubular maximum phosphate reabsorption, two parameters of increased PTH action (35,36).

Further, recent studies have confirmed the secondary nature of the increment of PTH level with age. As such, McKane et al. have reported that a high calcium intake maintained for 3 years in a group of elderly women was able to reduced PTH and deoxypyridinoline levels to comparable levels obtained in a control group of young individuals (37).

In contrast, calcitonin level is not modify in the elderly subject, although it has been suggested a reduced calcitoninic response to calcitoninopoietic stimulus in the aged population (38).

Decreased Renal Conservation

The fact that intestinal and urinary calcium losses are not reduced in the elderly despite the diminished calcium intake and the elevation of PTH secretion (that favors calcium renal reabsorption) is interpreted as an index of a reduced ability of the body to conserve calcium (13).

Table 4. Causes of vitamin D deficiency in elderly persons

- Deprivation of sunlight (northern latitudes)
- Diminished capacity of the skin to convert cholesterol to vitamin D
- Intestinal malabsorption of fat-soluble vitamin D
- Diminished dietary vitamin D intake by avoidance of vitamin D-supplemented dairy products
- Drug-induced increase in 25D hepatic degradation
- Production of 1.25D by the kidney (selective partial resistance to PTH)

Bone Turnover Modifications in the Elderly

In young normal individuals the remodeling cycle is very efficient: the amount of new bone formed is equal to that reabsorbed. With advancing age, osteoblast efficiency declines; the volume of resorbed bone is not completely replaced by an equivalent volume of new bone. Each remodeling cycle thus results in a small bone deficit. Age-related bone loss can be regarded as the consequence of the accumulated deficits of many incompletely filled resorption cavities. Any increase in remodeling activity, whether it be due to an increase in the activation rate of new bone remodeling units or an increase in the amount of bone resorbed per unit, will ultimately increase the rate of bone loss.

Several studies have clearly documented the age-related acceleration of bone remodeling activity by the elevation of urinary and seric levels of markers of bone neoformation such as total and bone-specific alkaline phosphatase (39–41) and osteocalcin (39,41,42) as well as of markers of bone resorption, such as urinary hydroxyproline and pyridinoline (43) tend to increase with age in both men and women, with and exacerbation in female subjects with menopause.

Age-related bone turnover acceleration is responsible for the prevalence of bone resorption over bone formation, and is also consistent with the above discussed increase in PTH levels which stimulates osteoclastic activity.

The potential physiopathologic importance of the incremented bone turnover in the reduction of bone mass in the elderly has been actually confirmed by several studies. Bone turnover level is closely correlated with bone mass loss velocity, calculated from repeated measurements of bone mineral content either vertebral or radial, i.e., the higher the bone turnover, the higher the annual velocity of bone mass reduction (44,45). According to Delmas, the combination of a single measurement of biochemical markers of bone formation and resorption, i.e. osteocalcin and urinary excretion of hydroxyprolin and dipyridinolin is enough to predict with accuracy the bone mass loss in the next two years after the measurement (45). Further, several studies suggest that bone turnover markers measurements in the elderly may be correlated with the fracture risk. As such, elevated levels of serum osteocalcin are associated with an increased risk of femoral fracture in the elderly (46) and an elevated urinary excretion of cross-links has been documented in patients with femoral fracture (47). Delmas has proposed that the measurement of bone turnover may be used as a marker of bone fragility (48).

Calcium Supplementation and Bone Mass

Numerous studies have evidenced that calcium supplements are able to reduce bone loss and to decrease fracture incidence (49,50). This effect is particularly evident in studies where women in the first five years after menopause were excluded, in whom calcium deficit and elevated PTH level are less important factors in the accelerated bone turnover than the fall in estrogen levels (49).

In the evaluation of calcium supplementation role it should be emphasized that an adequate calcium intake should not be considered a therapy for bone mass loss but an essential strategy for the maintenance of health in the elderly organism. In conditions of estrogen deficit, such as postmenopause and, further, in conditions in which bone mass is already reduced such as postmenopausal and senile osteoporosis, an adequate calcium intake may not be considered a substitute of estrogens or of a specific therapy, but should be associated with hormone replacement therapy and/or medicaments that reduce bone turnover and fracture risk (51,52).

Modifications of Intracellular Calcium in the Elderly

In contrast to the progressive bone loss and decrease in total body calcium, a gradual increment of calcium accumulation in vascular soft tissues and intracellular compartment is observed with aging (53,54). Recent studies from our group have demonstrated that in "normal" subjects the aging process is associated with an elevation in intracellular calcium levels (55,56). Concomitantly, vascular wall calcium content increases linearly with age (57). These alterations are indistinguishable from those present in essential hypertension, or in NIDDM independently of age (58).

Atherosclerosis may itself be related to altered vascular intracellular calcium homeostasis. Indeed, an increase of calcium influx into endothelial cells is associated with, and may be induced by an influx of plasma components (mainly LDL), and with enhanced release of chemotactic and growth factors that promote leukocyte and macrophage infiltration into the vessel wall and smooth muscle proliferation, thereby initiating the formation of the atherosclerotic lesion (59). Moreover, the accumulation of calcium may trigger the transition of the smooth muscle cell from a contractile state to a proliferative and synthetic state during which proliferation and migration to the media occur. Cholesterol-fed rabbits that develop atherosclerosis have increased calcium in their aortic wall cells and an increased calcium influx into the aortic smooth muscle cells (60). Indeed, cholesterol itself has been shown to increase calcium current and calcium influx in arterial smooth muscle cells (59). Aging and atherosclerosis are, thus, both characterized by a parallel accumulation of calcium and cholesterol in the arterial wall (60). This process is markedly accelerated in hypertension and diabetes, which interestingly are associated with these same ionic lesion prematurely, at all ages.

The elevated PTH levels observed in the elderly and discussed above, may favor a progressive shift of calcium from the skeleton to the soft tissue and from the extracellular to the intracellular compartment, in conjunction with the ionophore action of PTH, that stimulates calcium entrance into the cell (62). Elkeles proposed in the '50s the theory of "calcium shift" in the elderly, according to which the progressive bone calcium loss and its accumulation in vascular tissues, may be the cause of the elevated incidence of osteoporosis, hypertension and atherosclerosis in the elderly subject (63). Confirming the possible relevance of this hypothesis, we observed that an elevated bone turnover, measured by bone histomorphometry, is associated with a reduced bone mass in experimental hypertension (64).

CONCLUSIONS

The aging process is associated with numerous profound alterations in intra- and extracellular calcium homeostasis and with an accelerated bone turnover. Reduction of total body calcium and elevation of bone turnover are associated with a gradual reduction in bone mass, and with an increased skeleton fragility and fracture risk. An adequate calcium intake is a necessary condition for the health of the elderly organism, but cannot be considered an alternative to the specific therapy, to which it should be added when bone mass loss is established.

REFERENCES

1. West JB (Editor), Best and Taylor's physiological basis of medical practice. 12th edn. Hormonal regulation of mineral metabolism. Chapter 56. Williams and Wilkins, Baltimore, 1991.

2. Ringer S. A third contribution regarding the infusion of the inorganic constituents of the blood on the ventricular contraction. J Physiol 1883;22:2–5.
3. Passeri M, Pioli G, Pedrazzoni M, Girasole G, Passeri G. Le alterazioni senili dell'omeostasi del calcio e del fosforo. Giorn Geront 1991;39:327–339.
4. Garn SM, Rohmann CG, Wagner B. Bone loss is a general phenomenon in man. Fed Proc 1967; 26: 1729–1736.
5. Newton-John HF, Morgan HD. The loss of bone with age, osteoporosis and fractures. Clin Orthop 1970;71:229–252.
6. Nicholls DG. Intracellular calcium homeostasis. Br Med Bull 1986;42:353–358.
7. Borle AB. Control, modulation and regulation of cell calcium. Rev Physiol Biochem Pharmacol 1981; 90: 13–153.
8. Sheikh MS, Ramirez A, Emmett M, Santa Ana C, Schiller LR, Fordtran JS. Role of vitamin D-dependent and vitamin D-independent mechanisms in absorption of food calcium. J Clin Invest 1988;81:126–132.
9. Staub JF, Tracqui P, Lansson S, Milhaud G, Perault-Staub AM. A physiological view of in vivo calcium dynamics: the regulation of a non linear self organised system. Bone 1989;10:77–86.
10. Martin KJ, Hruska KA, Freitag JJ, Klahr S, Slatopolsky E. The peripheral metabolism of parathyroid hormone. N Engl J Med 1979;301:1092–1098.
11. Reichel H, Koeffler HP, Norman AW. The role of the vitamin D endocrine system in health and disease. N Engl J Med 1989;320:980–991.
12. Austin LA, Heath H III. Calcitonin-Physiology and pathophysiology. N Engl J Med 1981; 304:269.
13. Heaney RP, Recker RR, Stegman MR, Moy AJ. Calcium absorption in women: relationship to calcium intake, estrogen status, and age. J Bone Miner Res 1989;4:469–475.
14. Heaney RP. Nutritional factors in bone health. in: Osteoporosis: Etiology, Diagnosis and Management. Riggs BL, and Melton LJ III editors. Raven Press NY, NY., 1988, pp359–372.
15. NIH Consensus Development Panel on Optimal Calcium Intake. Optimal Calcium Intake. JAMA 1994;272:1942–1948.
16. Nordin BEC. Calcium balance and calcium requirements in spinal osteoporosis. Am J Clin Nutr 1962;10:384–390.
17. Riggs BL, Wahner HW, Melton LJ III, Richelson LS, Judd HL, O'Fallon M. Dietary calcium intake and rates of bone loss in women. J Clin Invest 1987;80:979–982.
18. Heaney RP. Effect of calcium on skeletal development, bone loss and risk of fractures. Am J Med 1991;91(suppl.5B):23S-27S.
19. Cummings RG. Calcium intake and bone mass: a quantitative review of the evidence. Calc Tissue Int 1990;47:194–201.
20. Kelly PJ, Pocock NA, Sambrook PN, Eismann JA. Dietary calcium, sex hormones, and bone mineral density in men. Br Med J 1990;300:1361–1364.
21. Recker RR. Calcium absorption and achlorhydria. N Engl J Med 1985;313:70.
22. Newcomer AD et al. Lactase deficiency: Prevalence in osteoporosis. Ann Intern Med 1978;89;218.
23. Slovik DM, Adams KS. Neer RM, Holick MF, Potts JT Jr. Deficient production of 1,25-dihydroxyvitamin D in eldely osteoporotic patients. N Engl J Med 1981;305:372–374.
24. Baker MR, Peacok M, Nordin BEC. The decline in vitamin D status with age. Age Ageing 1980; 9: 249–252.
25. Fujisawa Y, Kida K, Matsuda H. Role of change in vitamin D metabolism with age in calcium and phosphorus metabolism in normal human subjects. J Clin Endocrinol Metab 1984;59:719–726.
26. Ebeling PR. Evidence of an age-related decrease in intestinal responsiveness to vitamin D: Relationship between serum 1,25-dihydroxyvitamin D_3 and intestinal vitamin D receptor concentrations in normal women. J Clin Endocrinol Met 1992;75:176.
27. Lindgarde F. Potentiometric determination of serum ionized calcium in anormal human population. Clin Chim 1972;40:477–482.
28. Orwoll ES, Meier DE. Alterations in calcium, vitamin D and parathyroid hormone physiology in normal men with aging; relationship to the developent of senile osteopenia. J Clin Endocr Metab 1986; 63: 1262–1269.
29. Sherman SS, Hollis BW, Tobin JD. Vitamin D status and related parameters in a healthy population: the effect of age, sex and season. J Clin Endocrinol Metab 1990; 71:405–413.
30. Kotowicz MA, Melton LJ III, Cedel SL, O'Fallon WM, Riggs BL. Effect of age on variables relating to calcium and phosphorus metabolism in women. J Bone Min Res 1990;5:345–52.
31. Gallagher JC, Riggs BL, Jerpbak CM. The effect of age on serum immunoreactive parathyroid hormone in normal and osteoporotic women. J Lab Clin Med 1980;95:372–385.

32. Marcus R, Madvig P, Young G. Age-related changes in parathyroid hormone and parathyroid hormone action in normal humans. J Clin Endocr Metab 1984;58:223–230.
33. Epstein S, Bryce G, Hinman JW, Miller ON, Riggs BL, Hui SL, Johnston CC Jr. The influence of age on bone mineral regulating hormones. Bone 1986;7:421–425.
34. Insogna KL et al. Effect of age on serum immunoreactive parathyroid hormone and its biological effects. J Clin Endocrinol Metab 1981;53:1072.
35. Young G, Marcus R, Minkoff JR, Kim LY, Segre GV. Age-related rise in parathyroid hormone in man: The use of intact and midmolecule antisera to distinguish hormone secretion from retention. J Bone Min Res 1987;2:367–374.
36. Forero MS, Klein RF, Nessenson RA, Nelson K, Heath H 3d, Arnaud CD, Riggs BL. Effect of age on circulating immunoreactive and bioactive parathyroid hormone levels in women. J Bone Min Res 1987; 2: 363–366.
37. McKane WR, Khosla S, Egan KS, Robins SP, Burritt MF, Riggs BL. Role of calcium intake in modulating age-related increases in parathyroid function and bone resorption. J Clin Endocrinol & Met 1996; 81: 1699–1703.
38. Palummeri E, Cervellin G, Pedrazzoni M, Di Ruvo R, Butturini L, Provvedini D, Barbagallo M, Bonati PA, Carbognani A. Evidenze di un coinvolgimento dell'asse calcitonina-enterormoni nella patogenesi dell'osteoporosi senile. In Scritti in onore di Ugo Butturini, Tipolitografia Benedettina Editrice, Parma, 1985,pp291–300.
39. Schiele F., Henny J., Hitz S., Peticlerc C., Gueguen R., Siest G. Total, bone and liver alkaline phosphatase in plasma:Biological variation and reference limits. Clin Chem 1983;23:634–641.
40. Eastell R., Delmas PD, Hodgson SF, Eriksen EF, Mann KG, Riggs BL. Bone formation ratein older normal women: concurrent assessment with bone histomorphometry, calcium kinetics, and bioogical markers. J Clin Endoc Metab 1988;67:741–748.
41. Garnero P, Delmas PD. Assessment of the serum levels of bone alkaline phosphatase with a new immunoradiometric assay in patients with metabolic bone disease. J Clin Endocrinol Metab 1993;77:1046–1053.
42. Epstein S, Poser J, McClintock R, Johnston CC, Brycs G, Hui S. Differences in serum bone Gla protein with age and sex. Lancet 1984;ii:118–120.
43. Delmas PD, Stenner D, Wahner HW, Mann KG, Riggs BL. Increase in serum bone gamma-carboxyglutamic acid protein with aging in women. J Clin Invest 1983;71:1316–1321.
44. Kamel S, Brazier M, Neri V, Picard C, SamsonL, Desmet G, Sebert JL. Multiple molecular forms of pyridinolines cross-links excreted in human urine evaluated by chromatographic and immunoassay methods. J Bone Min Res 1995;10:1385–1392.
45. Johansen J, Riss BJ, Delmas PD et al: Plasma BGP. An indicator of spontaneous bone loss and effect of estrogen treatment in postmenopausal women. Eur J Clin Invest 1988;18:191–195.
46. Uebellhart D, Schlemmer A, Johansen Gineyts E., Christiansen C, Delmas PD. Effect of menopauseand hormone replacement therapy on the urinary excretion of pyridinium crosslinks. J Clin Endocrinol Metab 1991;72:367–373.
47. Szulc P, Chapui MC, Meunier PJ, Delmas PD. Serum undercarboxylated osteocalcin is a marker of the risk of hip fracture in elderly women. J Clin Invest 1993;91:1769–1774.
48. Alekson K, Vergnaud P., Gineyts E, Delmas PD. Increased bone resorption and decreased bone formation in elderly women with hip fracture. Bone Miner 1992;17(S1):184.
49. Delmas PD. Biochemical markers of bone turnover I: Theoreticalconsideration and clinical use in osteoporosis. Am J Med 1993;95(suppl.5A):11S-16S.
50. Chapui MC, Arlot ME, Dubouef F, et al. Vitamin D3 and calcium to prevent hip fracture in elderly women. N Engl J Med 1992;327:1637–1642.
51. Reid IR, Ames RW, Evans MC, Gamble GD, Sharpe SJ. Effect of calcium supplementation on bone loss in postmenopausal women. N Engl J Med 1993;328:460–464.
52. Riggs BL, Melton LJ. The prevention and treatment of osteoporosis. N Engl J Med 1992;327:620–627.
53. Liberman UA, Weiss SR, Broll J, Minne HW, Quan H, Bell NH, et al. Effect of oral alendronate on bone mineral density and the incidence of fractures in postmenopausal women. N Engl J Med 1995; 333: 1437–1443.
54. Fujita T. Aging and calcium. Mineral Electrolyte Metab 1986;12:149–156.
55. Barbagallo M, Dominguez LJ, Putignano E, Barbagallo Sangiorgi G, Resnick LM. Effect of aging on intracellular divalent cation metabolism: a link to the increased incidence of hypertension and non insulin-dependent diabetes mellitus in the elderly? Arch Gerontol Geriatr 1996;suppl 5:233–238.
56. Barbagallo M., Gupta R.K., Resnick L.M. Effect of aging on cellular divalent cations: Relation to hypertension and diabetes. J Invest Medicine 1995;43(suppl 2):300A.

57. Lansing AI, Alex M, Rosenthal TB. Calcium and elastin in human atherosclerosis. J Geront 1973; 5: 112–117.
58. Resnick LM, Gupta RK, Bhargava KK, Gruespan H, Alderman MH, Laragh JH. Cellular ions in hypertension, diabetes, and obesity: A nuclear magnetic spectroscopic study. Hypertension 1991;17:951–957.
59. Orimo H, Ouchi Y. The role of calcium and magnesium in the development of atherosclerosis. Experimental and clinical evidence. Ann NY Acad Sci 1990;598:444–457.
60. Sen L, Biasecky RA, Smith E, Smith TW, Colucci W. Cholesterol increases the L-type voltage-sensitive calcium channel current in arterial smooth muscle cells. Circ Res 1992;71:1008–1014.
61. Fleckenstein A, Frey M, Zorn S, Fleckenstein-Grun G. Experimental basis of long term therapy of arterial hypertension with calcium antagonists. Am J Cardiol 1985;56:3H-14H.
62. Schleiffer R, Berthelot A, Gairard A. Action of parathyroid extract on arterial blood pressure and on contraction and 45Ca exchange in isolated aorta in the rat. Eur J Pharmacol 1979;58:163–168.
63. Elkeles A. A comparative radiological study of calcified atheromas in males and females over 50 years of age. Lancet 1957;ii:714–715.
64. Barbagallo M, Quaini F, Baroni MC, Barbagallo CM, Boiardi L, Arlunno B, Passeri G, Delsignore R, Passeri M. Histological evidence of increased bone turnover in spontaneously hypertensive rats. Cardioscience 1991;2:15–17.

THE EPIDEMIOLOGY OF OSTEOPOROSIS

Leonardo Sartori

Istituto di Medicina Interna
Università degli Studi di Padova
Padova, Italy

The definition of osteoporosis as a "systemic skeletal disease, characterized by low bone mass and microarchitectural deterioration of bone tissue, with a consequent increase in bone fragility and susceptibility to fracture" imply a direct relationship between bone loss and fracture incidence. Being very difficult to have extensive and reliable data on the prevalence of bone loss, osteoporosis-associated fractures have been used as a parameter to estimate the prevalence of the disease as well as comparing data from different geographic areas.

The relationship between *bone mass* and fracture incidence is indeed very strong. Environmental and life-style factors are acknowledged important determinants of bone density; yet these and other identified predictors account for only 20 to 35% of the total variance in bone mass which appears to be mainly under genetic control. Bone loss is likely to be the single most important risk factor for fracture, and a 2.4–3.0-fold increase in risk for every S.D. decrease of bone mass has been described[1]. Nevertheless, while bone loss at a specific site is the limiting condition to define a fracture as osteoporotic, the prevalence of osteopenia in a specific population is higher than the prevalence of the corresponding fractures.

Recently, the World Health Organisation has indicated specific bone density threshold values to distinguish among normal bone status, osteopenia, osteoporosis and established osteoporosis. Applying these criteria, a consistent percentage of the United States white women would be defined as osteopenic (T-score between −1 and −2.5 S.D.) already at the age of 30, and the percentage of osteoporotic defined women would increase from 15 to 20%, 40 and 70% for every decade after 50 years of age[2]. Extrapolating these percentages to the Italian population, more than 3 million of Italian women would be classified as osteoporotic. We should however be very cautious in using these strict criteria since bone loss is known to vary greatly from one site to another, and the fracture risk will thus change accordingly to the number and type of sites examined.

It should also be taken into account that not all fractures are related to the loss of bone and other variables, such as type and entity of the trauma, may have a role in fracture outcome. Beside that, comorbidity, a common event in the elderly patients, can further complicate the frame[3]. *Falls*, another important cofactor in fracture onset, also increase

Recent Advances in Geriatrics, edited by Barbagallo, Licata, and Sowers.
Plenum Press, New York, 1998.

with age, particularly in whites females. One-third of community-dwelling older adults and 50% the nursing homes residents will fall each year[4]. In the U.S.A., the rate of post-menopausal women experiencing at least one fall/year increases from 1/5 in the 60–64 years old group to 1/3 in the 80–84 years old group[5]. Although only 1% of falls leads to a fracture of the hip, fractures alone account for 30–40% of fall injuries among the elderly[6]. Even when they do not result in major injury, falls may have long-term health consequences for the elderly and fear of falling *per se* can lead to decreased independence and mobility[7].

Femoral fractures represent the single most important factor in determining the social and economic costs of osteoporosis. Nowadays 1,660,000 hip fractures are estimated to occur world-wide, with a related cost of some 23 billion dollars[8]. The impact of these fractures can be fearful: 12–30% of the patients will die within one year from the diagnosis, and 25–30% of the survivors will lose their self-sufficiency.

Age- and sex-adjusted incidence rates of hip fracture are higher in Caucasians but, within single racial or ethnic groups, environmental factors (latitude, diet, physical activity, etc.) can induce substantial differences[9]. In Europe, hip fracture incidence appears to be higher in Scandinavia, intermediate in central Europe and lower in the Mediterranean countries[10]. Racial and ethnic differences with respect to the female:male ratio are also reported[11]. As far as Italy is concerned, the MEDOS study found 1,437 hip fractures (81% in women) among 847,508 subjects 50 years of age and older, while the incidence rate increased with age up to 1,155/100,000 in the 85+ years group[12].

An increase in age-adjusted hip fracture incidence over time has been described, with rates still growing in Australia, Finland, Hong Kong, and the United Kingdom but levelling off in some parts of the Great Britain, Sweden and the United States[13]. In Italy hip fracture incidence has shown a steady increase until 1990, with a subsequent tendency to level off but for the oldest old age-group.

A 5 to 40% excess mortality due to hip fracture has been reported by different Authors[14–19]. Noteworthy, this increase in mortality occurs within 6 months after the fracture, diminishes with time and is higher in males then females[20,21]. However, most of the deaths attributed to hip fracture are related to the presence of a serious coexisting illness rather than the fracture management *per se*[22]. In Italy, census data from the '80s have demonstrated a 7,235-fold increase in mortality due to hip fracture between the 35–39 years and the 90+ years of age groups while in the Veneto region, 12 months after the fracture the survival rates were 87% and 74% in females and in males, respectively[23,24].

Compared to fractures of the hip, *vertebral fractures* are more difficult to assess (only 17% of these fractures are associated with a substantial trauma) and, consequently, data are relatively scanty. Recent papers suggest that only a third of all vertebral deformities come to medical attention, with an hospitalization rate of 2–8%[13,25]. In the U.S.A. the prevalence of vertebral fractures increases with age in both sexes reaching an incidence of 64.3% in the 90+ years group, and an overall female to male ratio of 1.9[26]. At the age of 50, 65 and 80 years a white women has 18%, 28% and 32% probability of vertebral fracture occurrence. Half of the estimated 1,300,000 osteoporotic fractures per year in the U.S.A. are thought to be vertebral, with an annual incidence in white women (18/1,000 person/year) much higher than that of femoral fractures (6.2/1,000/year)[27].

In the short term, as compared to fractures of the hip, vertebral fractures do not seem to induce any significant increase in mortality however, 5 years after fracture diagnosis, the estimated survival (61%) is significantly less than predicted (76%), leading to a long term overall mortality quite similar to hip fracture[28]. The conspicuous length of time from fracture diagnosis to death do not allow an outright explanation for the increases in mortality attributed to vertebral fractures, though comorbidity appears to play a major role[29].

Less than 20% of *distal forearm fractures* are admitted to the hospital and, as for vertebral fractures, hospital discharge data cannot represent reliable means to evaluate epidemiological parameters. Interestingly, the incidence of distal forearm fractures increases steadily in post-menopausal women up to the age of 65, but levels off from then on. No specific trend in the incidence of distal forearm fracture is seen in men. In distal forearm fractures, mortality do not appears to be significantly different from controls[30].

In the U.S.A., at the age of 50, the lifetime risk of fracture in white women has been estimated to be 17.5%, 15.6%, 16% for hip, vertebral and distal forearm fractures respectively, with corresponding values of 6%, 5%, and 2.5% in white men[2]. However, fractures of proximal humerus, pelvis and tibia are also considered to be osteoporosis-related. In fact, like other osteoporosis-associated fractures, they show a prevalence in the female population and a characteristic increase with age.

Eighty percent of *proximal humerus* fractures are seen after the age of 35 with a 12 and 3 fold increase, in females and males respectively, from the 35–44 years to the 80+ years of age groups. The female to male ratio is approximately 3:1[31]. In 3/4 of the cases proximal humerus fractures occur in frail patients after a minimal trauma[32]. Humerus fracture incidence has also shown an increase over time[33]. Census data from Italy demonstrated a 89-fold increase in mortality due to humerus fracture when comparing the 35–39 years to the 90+ years of age groups[23].

The incidence of *pelvis* fracture increases 14- and 16-fold, in women and men respectively, from the 35–44 years to the 85+ years of age groups. The vast majority of single breaks of the pelvis bones appears to be related to moderate trauma[34]. In Italy, mortality due to pelvis fracture showed a 566-fold increase from the 35–39 years to the 90+ years of age groups[23].

Though data for fractures of the *proximal tibia* are less exhaustive, among older individuals the majority of these fractures are definitely osteoporosis-related[35]. The mortality data from the Italian census showed a 94-fold increase in death due to tibia fracture when comparing the 35–39 years group to the 90+ years of age group[23].

Though important, mortality is not the only *social burden* related to osteoporosis. The consequences of osteoporosis-associated fractures, beside increasing the length of hospital admissions and delaying the functional recovery, represent a major threat to life quality and self-sufficiency. In Italy, between 1980 and 1992, in patients over 50 years of age an average of 4752, 18985, 22646, 67320, and 19102 hospital discharges/year for fracture of the pelvis, humerus, distal forearm, femur, and tibia-fibula were recorded respectively. The corresponding numbers of hospitalization days/year were 68986, 201615, 15830, 1518327, and 226002[36].

In the MEDOS study, 14.4% of the patients developed acute complications (decubitus ulcers, thrombosis, embolisms, pulmonary and urinary infections) after an hip fracture event[12]. Ten years after a vertebral fracture-diagnosis, the prevalence of chronic back pain and the need of help in activities of daily living are twice as much as those of non-fractured controls.

A computer simulation on 10,000 women 50 years of age and older showed a 54% lifetime risk of osteoporosis-associated fractures (18% hip, 35% vertebral, and 17% distal forearm), with 13% of these patients undergoing a significant worsening of their functional status exemplified by 7% loss of self-sufficiency and 8% institutionalisation requirement (26% and 50% respectively when only hip fractures were taken into account)[37]

Evaluating pure economic costs of osteoporotic fractures is rather difficult since social and cultural approaches to the disease vary greatly from one country to the other. In Sweden for example, 46% of hip fracture costs are accounted to rehabilitation, while in the U.S.A. hospital admissions (63%) and institutionalisation (28%) represent the major contributors[38].

However, when looking at these data, two tightly related demographic events should be taken into account: the unprecedented number of postmenopausal women and the dramatic growth of the elderly population. In the world there are nowadays nearly 500 million women aged 50 years or older, and people over 65 years of age will increase from 323 million in 1992 to 1,555 million by the year 2050, when some 6,260,000 hip fractures are expected to occur world-wide, at an estimated cost of 87 billion dollars![39,40]

REFERENCES

1. Kanis J. A., Pitt F.A. Epidemiology of Osteoporosis. Bone, 13: S7-S15, 1992.
2. Melton III L. J., Chrischilles E.A , Cooper C., et al. How many women have osteoporosis? J. Bone Miner. Res., 7: 1005–1010, 1992.
3. Sernbo I., Gullberg B., Johnell O. Hip Fracture in Malmö over Three Decades. Bone, 14: S19-S22, 1993.
4. Rubenstein L. Z., Robbins A. S., Shulman B. L. et al. Falls and instability in the elderly. J. Am. Geriatr. Soc. 36: 226–278, 1988.
5. Nevitt M. C. and Cummings S. R., and the Study of Osteoporotic Fractures Research Group. Type of fall and risk of hip and wrist fractures: the study of osteoporotic fractures. J. Am. Geriatric Soc. 41: 1226–1234, 1993.
6. Sattin R. W., Humber D. A. L., DeVito C. A., et al. The incidence of fall injury events among the elderly in a defined population. Am. J. Epidemiol., 131: 1028–1037, 1990.
7. Tinetti M. E., Mendes de Leon C. F., Doucette J. T., et al. Fear of falling and fall-relates efficacy in relationship to functioning among community-living elders. J. Gerontol., 46: M140-M147, 1994.
8. Randell A., Sambrook P. N., Nguyen T. V., Lapsley H., Jones G., Kelly P. J., Eisman J. A.: Direct clinical and welfare costs of osteoporotic fractures in elderly men and women. Osteoporosis Int., 5: 427–432, 1995.
9. Maggi S., Kelsey J., Litvak J., et al. Incidence of hip fractures in the elderly: a cross-national analysis. Osteoporosis Int., 1: 232–241, 1991.
10. Johnell O., Gullberg B., Allander A., et al. The apparent incidence of hip fracture in Europe: a study of national register sources. Osteoporosis Int., 2: 298–302, 1992.
11. Bauer R. L. Ethnic differences in hip fracture: a reduced incidence in Mexican Americans. Am J. Epidemiol., 127: 145–149, 1988.
12. Mazzuoli G. F., Gennari C., Passeri M., et al. Incidence of hip fracture in Italy: an Italian survey. Osteoporosis Int., 1: S8-S9, 1993.
13. Cooper C., Melton II L. J. Magnitude and impact of osteoporosis and fractures. Osteoporosis, Marcus R, Feldman D., and Kelsey J. eds., Academic Press, San Diego, U.S.A.: 419–434, 1996.
14. Cummings S.R., Kelsey J.L., Newitt M.C., et al. Epidemiology of osteoporotic fractures. Epidemiol. Rev., 7: 178–200, 1985.
15. Lewinnek G., Kelsey J., White A., et al. The significance and comparative analysis of the epidemiology of hip fractures. Clin. Orthop., 152: 35–42, 1980.
16. Miller C. W. Survival and ambulation following hip fracture. J. Bone Joint Surg. (Am), 60: 930–934, 1978.
17. Pemberton J. Are hip fractures underestimated as a cause of death? The influence of coroners and pathologists on the death rate. Community Med., 10: 87–88, 1988.
18. Sartori L. Rilievi epidemiologici ed importanza sociale dell'osteoporosi. I bisfosfonati nella pratica clinica: acquisizioni e prospettive. M. Passeri and S. Adami eds., Edizioni ETS, Pisa: 175–195, 1994.
19. Weiss N. S., Liff J. M., Ure C. L , et al. Mortality following hip fracture. J. Chronic Dis., 12: 879–882, 1983.
20. White B. L., Fisher W. D., Laurin C. A. Rate of mortality for elderly patients after fracture of the hip in the 1980's. J. Bone Joint Surg., 69-A: 1335–1339, 1987.
21. Sexson S. B., and Lehner J. T. Factors affecting hip fracture mortality. J. Orthop. Trauma, 1: 298–305, 1988.
22. Poór G., Jacobsen S. J., and Melton III L. J. Mortality following hip fracture. Facts Res. Gerontol. 7: 91–109, 1994.

23. Crepaldi G., Sartori L., D'Angelo A., et al. La mortalità per frattura in Italia: caratteri generali ed aspetti regionali. Basle, October 24–25 1989: Masson: 15–18, 1989.
24. Sartori L., Barbieri F.. Aspetti epidemiologici e costo sociale dell'osteoporosi in Italia. Osteoporosis News 1(4): 1–9, 1991.
25. Kanis J. A., McCloskey E. V. Epidemiology of vertebral osteoporosis. Bone, 13: S1-S10, 1992.
26. Cooper C., Atkinson E. J., O'Fallon W. M., et al. Incidence of clinically diagnosed vertebral fractures: a population-based study in Rochester, Minnesota, 1985–1989. J. Bone Miner. Res., 7: 221–227, 1992.
27. Melton III L. J., Lane A. W., Cooper C., et al. Prevalence and incidence of vertebral deformities. Osteoporosis Int., 3: 113–119, 1993.
28. Cooper C., O'Neill T., Silman A., on behalf of the European Vertebral Osteoporosis Study Group. The epidemiology of vertebral fractures. Bone, 14: S89-S97, 1993.
29. Johansson C., Gärdsell P., Mellstrom D., et al. Bone mineral measurement is a predictor of survival. Bone Miner., 17(Suppl. 1): 166, 1992.
30. Cooper C., Atkinson E. J., Jacobsen S. J., et al. Population-based study of survival after osteoporotic fractures. Am. J. Epidemiol., 137(9): 1001–1005, 1993.
31. Rose S. H., Melton III L. J., Morrey B. F., et al. Epidemiologic features of humeral fractures. Clin. Orthop., 168: 24–30, 1982.
32. Kelsey J. L., Browner W. S., Seeley M. C., et al. Risk factors for fractures of the distal forearm and proximal humerus. Am. J. Epidemiol., 135: 477–489, 1992.
33. Bengnér U., Johnell O., Redlund-Johnell I. Epidemiology of ankle fractures 1950 and 1980: increasing incidence in elderly women. Acta Orthop. Scand., 57: 35–37, 1986.
34. Melton III L. J., Sampson J. M., Morrey B. F., et al. Epidemiologic features of pelvic fractures. Clin. Orthop., 155: 43–47, 1981.
35. Foltin E. Bone loss and forms of tibial condylar fracture. Arch. Orthop. Trauma Surg., 106: 341–348, 1987.
36. Sartori L., Busato F., Pizzardini M., Barbieri F., and Crepaldi G. Epidemiology of osteporotic fractures in Italy: 1980–1992. Osteoporosis Int. 6: S130, 1996.
37. Chrischilles E. A., Butler C. D., Davis C. S., et al. A model of lifetime osteoporosis impact. Arch. Intern. Med., 151: 2026–2032., 1991.
38. Ray N. F., Chan J. K., Thamer M., et al. Medical expenditures for the treatment of osteoporotic fractures in the United States in 1995: report from the National Osteoporosis Foundation. J. Bone Miner. Res., 12: 24–35, 1997.
39. Sartori L., and Crepaldi G. Osteoporosis treatment: focusing the target. Aging Clin. Exp. Res., 8: 219–220, 1996.
40. Melton III L. J. Hip fractures: a world-wide problem today and tomorrow. Bone, 14: S1-S8, 1993.

28

DIAGNOSIS OF OSTEOPOROSIS

Giovanni Passeri

Institute of Internal Medicine
Policlinico, University of Padova
Via Giustiniani 2
35128 Padova, Italy

Osteoporosis is a condition characterized by skeletal fragility; in recent years this disease has gained relevance both at the clinical and socio-economical level particularly in the elderly, in view of the increasing risk of fracturative events that is directly linked to the status of the skeletal apparatus.

Many factors contribute to elevate the risk of a fracture. A low pick bone mass reached at the age of 30 predisposes for a lower and insufficient bone mass in the post-menopause and in the elderly, and this leads to skeletal fragility and dramatically increment of fractures. About 1/3 of caucasian women are facing osteoporosis, and a large number of these will face a fracture during their life. After the menopause, we can document an accelerated bone loss, that causes excessive bone mass loss, skeletal fragility and increased risk of further fractures, especially after the age of 70. The most frequent sites of fractures are, after the menopause, vertebrae, wrists, and ribs, while in the elderly hip fractures are those that are seriously jeopardizing self-sufficiency (1).

In the elderly, many important risk factors for bone fractures, other then and together with low bone mass, are present. Impaired stability, high risk of falls, reduced protective responses, due to a less efficient skeletal-muscular apparatus, are dramatically increasing the risk of osteoporotic fractures.

Therefore, it is important an early diagnosis of osteoporosis in order to start as soon as possible all the preventive, pharmacological, physiotherapeutic and environmental measures, that are allowing a significant reduction of osteoporotic fractures risk (2).

The diagnosis of osteoporosis has to be considered as a group of clinical, instrumental and biochemical elements in order to fully take care of the patient. This concept is important mainly for 2 reasons: first of all, there is the widespread habit of taking into consideration mostly to the bone mass measurements and second, each one of the three above mentioned parts of a correct diagnostic approach, by itself, is not sufficient to reach a well-constructed diagnosis and to discriminate between an involutional or a secondary cause of bone loss.

In fact, the first goal in the diagnosis of osteoporosis, is to identify primary and involutional form of bone loss (both post-menopausal and senile), that are accounting for around 90% of the osteoporosis, and to differentiate them from secondary osteoporosis. It

Recent Advances in Geriatrics, edited by Barbagallo, Licata, and Sowers.
Plenum Press, New York, 1998.

is well-known that many times, low bone mass or a spontaneous fracture can be the first evident clinical sign of an endocrine or bone marrow or neoplastic disorder, as well as connective or gastrointestinal diseases, chronic obstructive pulmonary insufficiency, alcoholism and inappropriate and excessive prescription of bone damaging drugs (Table 1).

A detailed clinical history together with a careful physical examination are mandatory, and will help to underline risk factors for osteopenia that are known to predispose to osteoporosis. Race as well as familiarity, low calcium intake and inappropriate dietary habits, insufficient exercise, late menarche, parity, lactation, age of menopause, smoking, abuse of alcohol and drugs, and excessive use of prescribed pharmacological aids are all factors that must be taken into account in the evaluation of patients with any osteopenic situation. All the previous pathological events or long periods of immobilization in the past, must be carefully considered because they can explain, for example, the low pick bone mass reached by a patient. During the conversation with the patient, it is possible also to explain them that the tedious and continuous pain is very often of arthritis origin, and that osteoporosis and osteoarthritis are 2 very well distinct problems, often coexisting.

The physical aspect of the patient is also very informative: it is well known that women with a tall stature and thin aspect, clear, thin and transparent skin, poor muscular apparatus and low muscle strength are exposed to a higher risk of reaching the fracture threshold than women of short stature, strong structure, dark skin, good muscular apparatus and a moderate quantity of fat to protect the hip in the event of a fall. It is also important to mention that fat tissue is a reservoir of estrogens.

In some cases an excess of lumbar kyphosis is very suggestive of vertebral crushes, and this clinical presentation is often sufficient, by itself to put diagnosis of osteoporotic fractures, in the absence of any important traumatic event.

In the past ten years the bone densitometric evaluation apparatus' have improved dramatically (3). We can, nowadays, measure bone mass in a very careful and reliable

Table 1. Primary and secondary osteoporosis

Primary osteoporosis	
• Post-menopausal and senile (involutional)	
• Juvenile	
• Idiopatic	
Secondary osteoporosis	
• Endocrine diseases	• Neoplastic disorders
Hypogonadism	Multiple myeloma
Ovarian agenesis	Systemic mastocytosis
Hyperadrenocorticism	Carcinoma
Hyperthyroidism	
Hyperparathyroidism	• Connective tissue diseases
Hypothyroidism	Osteogenesi imperfecta
Hypoparathyroidism	Homocystinuria
Acromegaly	Marfan's syndrome
	Enlers Danlos syndrome
• G.I. diseases	
Gastrectomy	• Miscellaneous causes
Malabsorption	Immobilization
Starvation	Chronic obstructive pulmonary diseases and acidosis
Anorexia	Alcoholism and heroin
Chronic obstructive jaundice	Heparin and other bone-damaging drugs
Primary biliary cirrhosis	Rheumatological causes

way, although the perfect densitometric evaluation is not available yet. In fact, the ideal densitometric evaluation should have, together, all the following characteristic. Reliability is the first goal, with high accuracy and precision, short scanning time and repeatability. A good densitometric examination should analyse both trabecular and cortical sites by scanning different bone sites and predict fracture risk. It should also expose the patient to the lowest radiation dose possible. The ultimate goal should be a three dimensional, volumetric evaluation of the calcium content in a bone site. As today, no one of the actual densitometric apparatus meets all these characteristics, although some have been validated by experts, world-wide.

All the bone density evaluation systems are listed in Table 2. The oldest one is the standard X-ray of the vertebral spine and of the hip. This is still very important when it comes to estimate vertebral crush but has a very low sensitivity to detect reductions of calcium crystals. In fact, before a normal X-ray can detect a decrement of bone mass, more then 20% of it has been already lost.

Single photon absorptiometry (SPA) and dual photon absorptiometry (DPA) have been widely used in the '80s. They were utilizing radioactive sources, such as iodine, gadolinium or americium. These machines had some inconvenience: their maintenance was quite expensive because the radioactive source was warding out in general after about one year, and it had to be appropriately disposed and replaced by a new and expensive one.

Nowadays, the most used systems are Single X-Ray absorptiometry (SXA) and Dual X-Ray absorptiometry (DXA), that are considered the most accurate and reliable bone mass measures by the international institutions of scientists in the field of osteoporosis (EFFO, National Osteoporosis foundation) (3,4). During the Consensus Development Conference held in Amsterdam in 1996, it has been stated that "several studies have shown that bone mineral density (BMD) measured by SXA and DXA predicts subsequent fracture occurrence....However, recent data have shown that BMD measurements at the hip may be more predictive of hip fracture." Very reliable and sensitive are the "pencil beam" X-ray system, used in the last ten years. Recently, it has been introduced the fan bean X-ray system: the main characteristic are a quick execution time, and a good resolution and definition of images, very similar in quality to X-ray films. New technological improvements are allowing the morphometric analysis of the vertebral spine also in the lateral, that can substitute the traditional X-ray film of the spine. Therefore with the densitometer, during the same examination, we can obtain a measure of bone mineral content as well as a quite reliable morphometric image of this bone site. There is also to remember that new software systems are going to be available in the near future to obtain with this technique a better definition and a more detailed evaluation (5,6).

QCT, Quantitative Computerized Tomography, has also been proposed for the capability of evaluating directly the vertebral body, allowing the measurement of the trabecular

Table 2. Bone density evaluation

- X-rays
- Single photon absorptiometry (SPA)
- Dual photon absorptiometry (DPA)
- Single X-ray photon absorptiometry (SXA)
- Dual X-ray photon absorptiometry (DXA)
- Quantitative computerized scan (QCT)
- Peripheral quantitative computerized scan (pQCT)
- Quantitative ultrasound (QUS)
- Quantitative magnetic resonance (QMR)

part. A lot of disadvantages have to be mentioned in order to explain the scarce use of this technique: the high radiation dose for each exam, sub optimal precision and accuracy, the long scanning time as well as the cost of the machine and of the single exam. Better results have been obtained by employing a dual energy QCT (DEQCT). Peripheral QCT of the arm has been proposed: this machine has a good precision and accuracy, and expose the patient to a quite low radiation dose.

Quantitative Magnetic Resonance (QMR) is still an experimental technique, available only in very few research laboratories. It should allow a very detailed examination of the trabecular bone structure, almost at a microscopic level, giving also information about the elastic strength of the tissue. This method is expected to be very expensive, and it is not conceivable at the moment a widespread use for a daily diagnostic use.

Ultrasound evaluation has been intensively used at some appendicular sites (patella, os calcis, wrist, fingers). This system is very interesting because relatively inexpensive, and it does not expose the patient to any kind of radiations. Ultrasounds have not been internationally accepted: it is not defined, in fact, the correspondence with the DXA technique, and it is not clear yet what is the accuracy of this method, that is not analysing directly the bone mineral content, but probably the elastic module and, at large, the quality of bone tissue.

Laboratory diagnosis of osteoporosis can be faced as a multi-steps evaluation. Considering the increasing cost of health care in general, and the necessity of limiting the diagnostic expenses, especially in those countries with a state-provided health care system, it is reasonable to start with an initial and relatively inexpensive screening, in order to exclude any secondary form of osteoporosis. In over 85–90% of the cases, the initial evaluation, consisting of ESR, CBC, Protein electrophoresis, serum calcium and phosphate, Total alkaline phosphatase, serum creatinine, and 24-hours urine calcium, will result in the range of normality, allowing, together with the previously discussed physical and densitometric evaluations, to put diagnosis of involutional osteoporosis. Only when these tests will result abnormal, or in the presence of clinical doubts of secondary forms of osteoporosis, a more detailed biochemical screening is mandatory. Ionized calcium, PTH, sex and thyroid hormones, bone specific markers, 25-OH-D^3, intestinal calcium absorption test and bone biopsy are the mostly widely used tests for this reason.

Regarding the specific biochemical markers of bone turn-over, it has not been found yet a group of reliable and reproducible ones that can reflect, accurately, bone metabolism (7). A bone marker should be organ-specific, able to reflect the different phases of bone remodelling; once in the circulatory system or in the urine, it should have a long half-life, and be present either in the serum or in the urine without being metabolized. It should last unaltered, once drawn, for a long time span and the analytic method should be specific, sensitive, easily reproducible, and inexpensive. The cost of most of bone markers is unfortunately quite high, and not all the laboratories are enough experienced to perform routinely these tests (8).

Many new markers have been recently proposed, but it is clear that the ideal one is way far to come. The markers of bone remodelling are generally divided into formation and resorption ones (Table 3) (9). The choice of the markers must be guided by the clinical signs and it is very important, for the interpretation of the results, to know what kind of information's it can provide in face of any specific clinical suspect (10). Bone specific markers are instead very useful for monitoring a pharmacological approach, because they can provide informations regarding the therapeutical response of the single patient in relative short time (4–12 weeks), while it takes at list 12–18 months to see a real effect at the densitometric level (11,12).

Table 3. Markers of bone turn-over

Formation markers	Resorption markers
Serum markers of cellular activity	
Total alkaline phosphatase	Acid phosphatase tartrate-resistant
Bone-specific alkaline phosphatase	
Osteocalcin	
Serum markers of bone matrix	
Carboxy-terminal propetide of Type I procollagen	Carboxy-terminal telopeptide of Type I collagen
Urine markers of bone matrix	
	Hydroxyproline
	Hydroxylisine glycosides
	Pyridinium crosslinks
	Amino-terminal telopeptide of Type I collagen
	Carboxy-terminal telopeptide of Type I collagen

A complete diagnostic evaluation of a patient with the suspect of osteoporosis is a mandatory process that allows a correct preventive or therapeutical approach from the pathophysiological point of view. All these factors have to be considered in the idea of optimissing the resources, in order to prevent the real consequence of osteoporosis: the fracture.

REFERENCES

1. Cummings SR, Black DM, Nevitt MC et al: Bone density at various sites for prediction ofhip fractures. Lancet, 341:72–75, 1993.
2. Kanis A: Osteoporosis. Blackwell Science ed. Oxford, 1994.
3. Genant HK, Engelke K, Fuerst T et al: Noninvasive assessment of bone mineral and structure: State of the art. J Bone Min Res, 11: 707–730, 1996.
4. Genant HK, Grammp S, Gluer C et al: Universal standardization for dual X-ray absorptiometry: patient and phantom cross calibration results. J Bone Miner Res, 9:1503–1514, 1994.
5. Wahner HW, Fogelman I: The evaluation of osteoporosis: Dual energy X-ray absorptiometry in clinical practice. Martin Dunitz ed., London 1994.
6. Miller PD, Bonnick SL, Rosen CJ: Clinical utility of bone mass measurement in adults: Consensus of an international panel. Seminar Arthr Rheum, 25:361–372, 1996.
7. Delmas P D: Biochemical markers of bone turnover. J Bone Min Res, 8 (suppl. 2): S549-S555,1993.
8. Demers LM, Kleerekoper M:. Recent advances in biochemical markers of bone turnover. Clin Chem, 40: 1994–1995, 1994.
9. Eriksen EF, Brixen K, Charles P: New markers of bone metabolism:clinical use in metabolic bone disease. Eur J Endocrinol, 132: 251–263, 1995.
10. Price CP, Thompson PW: The role of biochemical tests in the screening and monitoring of osteoporosis. Ann Clin Biochem, 2: 244–260, 1995.
11. Calvo MS, Eyre DR, Gundberg CM:. Molecular basis and clinical application of biological markers of bone turnover. Endocr Rev, 17: 333–368, 1996.
12. Riggs BL, Melton LJ III, O'Fallon WM: Drug therapy for vertebral fractures in osteoporosis: evidence that decreases in bone turnover and increases in bone mass both determine antifracture efficacy. Bone, 18: S179-S201, 1996.

29

NEW TRENDS IN THE TREATMENT OF OSTEOPOROSIS

Mario Barbagallo,[1] Ligia J. Dominguez,[1] Giuseppe Barbagallo-Sangiorgi,[1] and Mario Passeri[2]

[1]Division of Geriatrics
Istituto di Medicina Interna e Geriatria
University of Palermo
[2]Istituto di Clinica Medica Generale e Terapia Medica
University of Parma

INTRODUCTION

Osteoporosis is "a systemic disease characterized by a reduction in bone mass and a microarchitectonic alteration of the skeleton, with a consequent increase in skeleton fragility and susceptibility to fractures", as defined by the last Consensus Development Conference[1]. With this definition, the alteration in skeletal structure, which is not yet easy to evaluate, becomes an important factor determining the risk of fracture of the osteoporotic patient, in addition to the bone mass, which to certain limit can be easily evaluated. This is an aspect that may create some problems at the time of taking a decision on how to proceed with a subject with decreased bone mass. Currently, the measurement of the quantity of bone present constitutes the basis to support any therapeutical decision[2]. The quantification of bone mass may be performed with DEXA, TAC or ultrasound, although this last method has not been yet adequately standardized.

When bone mass is low (conventionally indicated as a decrease of one standard deviation respect to the bone mass peak achieved during adulthood), it is necessary to recommend adequate daily habits (diet, exercise, sun exposure), particularly in old ages. After 65–70 years of age, an increased proportion of subjects are below this limit, with virtually all subjects affected in old age. Therefore, it is of extreme importance to avoid the possibility of falling during this life period.

One may ask whether this is the moment to associate a pharmacological therapy that limit the bone mass loss or at least decreases the bone loss rate. Although it is generally accepted that before 65 years of age the "fracture threshold" of 2.5 standard deviations below the bone mass peak is the limit under which a pharmacological therapy should be initiated, there are still some questions that remain unanswered. Is it pertinent to administrate medicaments before 65 years of age when the bone mass is not lower than 2.5 standard deviations? And after 65–70 years, who should receive pharmacological ther-

Recent Advances in Geriatrics, edited by Barbagallo, Licata, and Sowers.
Plenum Press, New York, 1998.

apy considering the fact that as age progresses, there is a physiological bone loss that leads to values not only below 1, but also below 2.5 standard deviations of the bone peak mass during adulthood? Regarding the first question, the pharmacological therapy in this case is preventive and the decision to initiate it should be taken after evaluation of the patient's general condition and the bone loss rate, assessed by repeated densitometric studies as well as with measurements of bone turnover biochemical markers. Regarding the second question, the single case should be considered with evaluation of associated pathologies (frequently seen), of the biochemical markers behavior and emphasizing on the prevision of fractures during the remaining life, the so called "life time risk". This risk is delineated by a threshold line that lies approximately one standard deviation below the mean bone mass values for the different ages. In other words, the decision of a pharmacological intervention should be always the result of an individualized thinking process and not only the consequence of the result of a single exam.

BONE TURNOVER

Bone tissue is continually formed and reabsorbed by opposite processes tightly connected in time and space, resulting in bone remodeling[3,4]. In the adult skeleton these two processes are in equilibrium and take place inside the BMU which contains cells with resorption function (osteoclasts) and cells with neo-formation functions (osteoblasts). Thus, inside each BMU, bone is first reabsorbed by the osteoclasts and the cavity left by this resorption is then filled up with new tissue formed by the osteoblasts.

In both, trabecular and compact bone, the remodeling processes entail cellular events that take place at the bone surface. This surface is larger in the trabecular bone, consequently and despite it represents only 20% of total bone mass, as much as 80% of bone turnover occurs in this type of bone. As a result of the high surface/volume ratio characteristic of trabecular bone, the alterations in bone turnover and subsequent decrease in bone mass are first manifested in sites with a larger proportion of trabecular bone, such as the vertebrae.

While during development the bone balance is positive, as age progresses, and even more in osteoporotic patients, the cavities formed by osteoclasts are not completely filled up. Then, the sum of these mini-deficits determines the progressive bone loss. The more elevated is bone turnover, the higher is the number of these mini-deficits and the resulting bone mass loss. Recent studies have demonstrated that the level of bone turnover is directly related to the bone mass and to the architectonic efficiency of bone[5,6]. In fact, a high turnover is associated with reduced bone mass, increased bone fragility, and increase incidence of fractures[7].

At present, it is possible to evaluate bone turnover with enough sensitivity and accuracy through the measurement of biochemical markers of bone formation and resorption. Among the markers of bone neo-formation, the most sensitive are osteocalcin, total and bone alkaline phosphatase, and collagen I propeptide. Respect to bone resorption, urinary excretion of pyridinoline and deoxypyridinoline, released during collagen I degradation in the process of bone resorption, have been demonstrated to be more sensitive when compared to conventional markers such as urinary hydroxyproline[8].

From a therapeutical point of view, the study of bone turnover is extremely useful since it consent, together with bone mass measurement: 1) to identify subjects with a high turnover even in the presence of a normal or slightly reduced bone mass, that presumably will loose bone mass prematurely; 2) to identify subjects with high turnover among osteopenic and osteoporotic patients, who may need a specific therapy; 3) to follow up the effects of therapy.

MODIFICATIONS OF BONE TURNOVER IN THE ELDERLY

The aging process is associated with acceleration of bone remodeling. In fact, several studies have documented elevated levels of total and bone-specific alkaline phosphatase[9–11] and serum osteocalcin[10,12–14], as well as urinary hydroxyproline and pyridinoline[15]. All these markers tend to increase with age in both men and women, with an acceleration after the menopause in women. The acceleration of bone remodeling with age results in a prevalence of bone destruction respect to bone formation in the elderly, that may be worsen by the age-dependent increase in circulating levels of parathyroid hormone, that is a known stimulator of osteoclastic activity[16,17].

Levels of bone turnover biochemical markers are tightly connected with the velocity of bone loss, evaluated by repeated measurements of both radial and vertebral bone mineral content[18,19]. Furthermore, elevated levels of osteocalcin in elderly has been shown to be correlated to the risk of femoral fracture[20] and conversely, patients with femoral fracture have higher levels of urinary crosslinks[21]. Delmas proposed that the evaluation of bone turnover may be used as a predictor of bone fragility[22].

PREVENTION

The prevention of bone loss remain the first goal in the therapy of osteoporosis, since it is more appropriate to attempt a prevention of bone mass loss instead of stopping an already established process and/or to rebuild an already lost tissue, particularly if structural damage is already present.

Preventive measures include dietary and physical activity recommendations, avoiding risk factors that may favor bone loss. An adequate calcium intake (from 1 g/day in the healthy adult to 1.5 g/day in postmenopausal women and in the elderly), a reduced intake of protein and fiber, regular physical activity, stop smoking and limit alcohol consumption, and particular attention to the eventual use of drugs that may negatively affect bone mass (cortisone, antiepileptics, heparin, loop diuretics, etc.) are all recommended for the achievement and maintenance of an optimal bone mass (Table 1).

Particular relevance deserves an adequate calcium intake, especially in the elderly, in whom the recommended daily amount of calcium in the diet is higher than in the young person (1.5 g/day) considering the age-related alterations of calcium balance regulation[23]. Further, the intake of dairy products tend to decrease with age in men and women[24,25]. The calcium deficiency is aggravated by a decreased intestinal absorption of calcium, secon-

Table 1. Non-pharmacological measures in the prevention of osteoporosis

• Diet with adequate calcium intake and low meat and fiber content
• Exercise
• Limit smoking and alcohol consumption
• Adequate sun exposure
• Limit, when possible, the use of medicaments with negative effects on calcium balance (cortisone, antiepileptics, heparin, loop diuretics, etc.)

dary to alterations in vitamin D metabolism associated with aging[26–28], that result in a relative deficit of the active metabolite.

It is at present increasingly evident the importance of an adequate calcium intake in the prevention of bone loss associated with aging and/or menopause and in the reduction of risk fracture[29]. A recent meta-analysis has reported a close positive relation between calcium intake and bone mass [30,31]. In the elderly, administration of vitamin D should be considered when necessary to correct the deficit of this hormone.

PHARMACOLOGIC THERAPY OF OSTEOPOROSIS

After an adequate clinical evaluation of the single patient, if the addition of a pharmacologic therapy is required, the clinician has several possibilities of intervention. An increasing number of medicaments are being used for the treatment of osteoporosis (Table 2). While there are several agents that act decreasing bone turnover and inhibiting bone deconstruction, only few of them act stimulating bone formation.

The goal of a therapeutical intervention should not be only to increase bone mass, but also to promote the formation of an architectonically and qualitatively valid bone, thus able to prevent the occurrence of osteoporotic fractures, such as vertebral, femoral and distal radius fractures. The two phenomena (increase of bone mass and reduction of fracture risk), despite being tightly correlated (a reduction of an standard deviation in bone mass is associated with a twofold increase in the risk of fracture), are not completely equivalent. For example, in the elderly the factor age is an independent risk for the occurrence of fracture, i.e. for the same bone mass the risk of fracture increases with age[32].

The new agents used in the treatment of osteoporosis should demonstrate not only to increase bone mineral density, but also to be efficacious in decreasing the incidence of fractures. While all medicaments currently used have demonstrated an effective improvement in bone mass or at least arrest the bone loss, it is more difficult to document the effects of treatment on the incidence of fractures. To obtain this type of information, large studies are needed, with a sufficiently long follow up period.

Estrogen or estrogen-progesterone replacement therapy even long after the menopause, is able to prevent postmenopausal bone loss until the treatment is maintained[33–35]. Estrogens act through inhibition of the production of interleukines (particularly IL-6) and other local factors that stimulate the proliferation and activity of osteoclasts[36–38]. Epidemiological data indicate that the risk of vertebral, hip and Colles fractures may be reduced as much as 50% with hormone replacement therapy, no matter when the therapy has begun including a relatively long period after the menopause[39,40]. Estrogen replacement therapy is also useful because reduces the characteristic symptoms of climacteric years and it has demonstrate favorable effects on ischemic heart disease and blood pressure.

Hormone replacement therapy may be administered by different routes: oral, parenteral and transdermic. This therapy is not yet widely used because of the uncertain effects

Table 2. Drugs used in the treatment of osteoporosis

Inhibitors of bone resorption	Stimulators of bone formation	Drugs with uncertain effects
Estrogens ± progestins	Fluoride	Vitamin D and derivatives
Bisfosfonates	Parathyroid hormone	Anabolic steroids
Calcitonin		Ipriflavone
Calcium		

on the risk of breast cancer and other unknown metabolic effects. Although, the risk of endometrial cancer is virtually eliminated with the concomitant administration of progestins, the fear of unknown risks and the fact that it should be maintained for at least 10 years after the menopause, renders its use still limited. In addition, hormone replacement therapy can not be proposed for use in men and in individuals older than 65 years. An attractive alternative to estrogens are compounds with agonist-antagonist effects on the estrogen receptor (tamoxifen, raloxifen), which may have an estrogen-like action (agonist) on bone estrogen receptors, without the negative side effects.

The therapy with bisphosphonates has been tested in some epidemiological studies, not yet enough for an absolute and unquestionable statistic judgment, but sufficiently indicative of the beneficial effect not only in the increment of bone mass, but also in the reduction of fracture risk. Bisphosphonates belong to a family of compounds analogous to inorganic pyrophosphate, that binds with high affinity to hydroxyapatite crystals, and remain bound to the skeleton for long periods of time[41]. These agents are potent inhibitors of bone resorption, may be administered per os, but have a low intestinal absorption that may be further reduced by the use of chelating agents present in the diet (particularly calcium), therefore they should be taken in fasting conditions and long before food ingestion. The relative potency of each compound depends on the nature of the lateral chain[42]. In two controlled studies, with small samples, it has been demonstrated that the administration of etidronate is able to reduce the incidence of fractures, particularly in the group of patients with severe osteoporosis[43,44]. Among the most recent bisphosphonates (third generation), the one examined in extensive studies is alendronate, which has a potency of one thousand fold respect to etidronate, consenting an effective inhibition of bone resorption mediated by osteoclasts, without inhibition of bone mineralization[45].

Alendronate has been demonstrated to produce a significant and rapid decrease of bone turnover, with reduction in circulating levels of biochemical markers of bone resorption (deoxypyridinoline) and formation (osteocalcin and bone alkaline phosphatase)[46–48]. The effects of 3-year treatment with alendronate on bone mineral density have been recently reported in 994 women with postmenopausal osteoporosis. This is the largest study of its type that confirms the efficacy of therapy with the drug. Women in treatment with alendronate have shown a significant and progressive increment in bone mineral density in all the skeletal sites studied. After 3-year therapy, the group treated with 10 mg alendronate exhibited an increment in bone mineral density of 8.8% at vertebral sites, 5.9% in the femoral neck, 7.8% at the femoral trochanter and an increase of 2.5% in total body calcium. Concurrently with these changes, there was a correspondent reduction of 48% in the number of women with a vertebral fracture (3.2 vs. 6.2% of controls). Additionally, there was a reduction in the progression of vertebral deformity and height loss in the alendronate-treated group compared to the placebo-treated group. Also the incidence of fractures in sites different from the vertebrae was significantly inferior in the subjects treated with the bisphosphonate[49].

Calcitonin is a peptide hormone that can not be administered per os because of its degradation by gastric secretion, therefore must be given by injection or nasal spray. It has a very potent inhibitory action of osteoclast activity in vitro, and is able to prevent postmenopausal bone loss, particularly at vertebral level[50]. The effect of calcitonin is higher in subjects with elevated bone turnover[51]. It has been reported that calcitonin at adequate doses and by injection is able to increase bone mass, effect that is maintained at least during the first year of treatment[52]. The analgesic properties of calcitonin have expanded its use. Controlled studies directed to examine the effects of calcitonin on the incidence of fractures have not included enough number of patients to conclude that the positive effects observed with calcitonin therapy are definitive[53,54].

Several studies have reported that calcium supplementation is followed by a reduction in bone loss and incidence of fractures[55,56]. This effect is particularly evident in studies where women in the first five years after menopause have been excluded, in whom calcium deficit is a secondary factor respect to the fall in estrogen levels[55]. In the evaluation of calcium role, it should be emphasize that an adequate calcium intake may not replace a specific therapy when this is indicated, but should be considered a primary element in the preservation of health in the elderly. An adequate calcium intake should be added to an specific therapy when indicated.

Ipriflavone is a synthetic molecule derived from flavonoids, which can be used per os and in some experimental studies has been demonstrated to inhibit osteoclastic activity and to stimulate osteoblastic activity[57]. Effects on bone mass *in vivo* have been examined but are not yet available in regards to the effects on fracture occurrence.

While the list of drugs that inhibit bone resorption is numerous, the agents that increase bone formation, currently commercial are fluoride and anabolic hormones. The other agent included in Table 2, is parathyroid hormone that is still in experimental phase.

Fluoride salts effectively increase bone mass, particularly at trabecular level, but their effects on fracture risk are still discussed[58,59]. This controversy is possibly due to the fact that fluoride salts increases bone formation but the quality of this bone is not architectonically valid and/or these agents induced and altered bone mineralization. The therapy with fluoride at doses of 50–75 mg/day may be followed by side effects, such as lower limbs pain syndrome, often secondary to microfractures, and gastric pain[60]. However, a new fluoride compound, with slow release formula that consents the use of a lower dose (25 mg) in association with calcium, has been recently studied in a group of 99 patients followed for 4 years. In these patients, an increment in bone mass at vertebral level (+4.8% per year) and a reduction in the occurrence of new fractures (relative risk 0.3) without remarkable side effects was demonstrated after therapy[61]. It is still discussed whether the positive effect on trabecular bone is not associated with a reduction in cortical bone.

Anabolic steroids have been proposed in the treatment of osteoporosis considering their stimulatory effects on bone neo-formation through a mechanism not clear at present. Some studies have demonstrated that nandrolone decanoate, the most frequently used agent with anabolic action comparable to testosterone, is 2–3 times less effective than testosterone respect to the effects on bone mineral content, but the consequences on fracture incidence are not yet available[62,63]. It is not yet known whether these agents indeed stimulate bone neo-formation or whether they act in an analogous manner with estrogens and androgens, by inhibition of bone resorption. Their use is limited due to the variable ratio of the anabolic/androgenic action, that may result in important side effects such as virilization in women and feminization in men (secondary to gonadothropin inhibition).

Vitamin D has been also proposed as treatment in osteoporosis. In western countries, the elderly particularly the institutionalized subjects, are often affected of vitamin D deficiency. Circulating levels of 25(OH)D^3, the precursor of the biologically active form of vitamin D, tend to decrease with age[27]. These alterations are the consequence of diets poor on vitamin D as well as a decreased sun exposure. Small doses of vitamin D are recommended for the correction of this deficits in the elderly, that will increase calcium absorption and eventually improve latent mineralization defects. Conversely, high doses of vitamin D in the treatment of osteoporosis are matter of controversy, and the effects on fracture incidence are dubious[55,64]. It is also unclear the specific effect of calcitriol on bone mass, because there are studies demonstrating an increase in bone mineral density of 1–2%/year, but it is not clear if this effects are secondary to the correction of a underlying mineralization defect (osteomalacia). In old institutionalized women a reduction in the incidence of fractures have been reported after treatment with vitamin D and calcium[55,65].

Other agents for the treatment of osteoporosis are currently under study. Parathyroid hormone stimulates bone neo-formation as well as bone turnover[66,67]. Its active fragment 1–34 given by injection has been shown to increase bone mass at trabecular level. However, the efficacy of parathyroid hormone in the treatment of osteoporosis is not determined. It has been suggested that some "growth factors" such as growth hormone and IGF-I may have a role in osteoporosis therapy in the future, but clinical data are not available at the present [67].

CONCLUSIONS

In summary, all patients with osteoporosis or at risk to develop it, with or without fracture, should receive a daily calcium supplement, making sure that they are not vitamin D deficient. The specific pharmacologic therapy when indicated according to an adequate clinical evaluation, recommend estrogens as the first choice, followed by bisphosphonates and calcitonin. We recommend a basal measurement of biochemical turnover markers with a control after 4–6 weeks to evaluate the modifications of these parameters after therapy. Bone mineral density should be measured before starting treatment and after 12 months of therapy.

It is very important to intervene the earliest possible with non-pharmacological measures and, when necessary, with pharmacological therapy, before an important decrease in bone mass is established. The pharmacological therapy should always be associated with adequate life style modifications, including dietary recommendations, exercise and in the elderly, the prevention of falls.

REFERENCES

1. Consensus Development Conference. Prophylaxis and treatment of osteoporosis. Am J Med, 1993;94:646–650.
2. Barbagallo M, Passeri M. Diagnostica strumentale della osteoporosi. Terapia Moderna, 1989;3:181–184.
3. Parfitt AM. Quantum concept of bone remodeling and turnover: Implications for the pathogenesis of osteoporosis. Calc Tissue Int 1979;28:1–5.
4. Manolagas SC, Jilka RL. Mechanisms of disease: bone marrow, cytokines and bone remodeling. Emerging insights into the pathophysiology of osteoporosis. N Engl J Med 1995, 332:305–311.
5. Riis BJ. Biochemical markers of bone turnover in diagnosis and assessment of therapy. Am J Med 1991;91(suppl.5B):64S-68S.
6. Garnero P, Hauser E, Chapui MC, et al. Can markers (MK) of bone turnover predict hip fractures (FX) in elderly women? J.Bone Min Res 1995;10(suppl1):S140.
7. Barbagallo M. Valore degli indici di turnover osseo nell'osteoporosi. Giorn.Gerontol 1989;37:255–264.
8. Uebellart D, Gineyts E, Chapui MC, Delmas PD. Urinary excretion of pyridinium crosslinks: a new marker of bone resorption in metabolic bone disease. Bone Miner 1990;8:87–96.
9. Schiele F, Henny J, Hitz S, Peticlerc C, Gueguen R, Siest G. Total, bone and liver alkaline phosphatase in plasma: Biological variation and reference limits. Clin.Chem 1983;23:634–641.
10. Eastell R, Delmas PD, Hodgson SF, Eriksen EF, Mann KG, Riggs BL. Bone formation rate in older normal women: concurrent assessment with bone histomorphometry, calcium kinetics, and biological markers. J Clin Endocrinol Metab 1988;67:741–748.
11. Garnero P, Delmas PD. Assessment of the serum levels of bone alkaline phosphatase with a new immunoradiometric assay in patients with metabolic bone disease. J Clin Endocrinol Metab 1993;77:1046–1053.
12. Epstein S, Poser J, McClintock R, Johnston CC, Brycs G, Hui S. Differences in serum bone Gla protein with age and sex. Lancet 1984;ii:118–120.

13. Delmas PD, Stenner D, Wahner HW, Mann KG, Riggs BL. Increase in serum bone gamma-carboxyglutamic acid protein with aging in women. J Clin Invest 1983;71:1316–1321.
14. Pedrazzoni M, Ciotti G, Davoli L, Barbagallo M, et al. Variazioni dell'osteocalcina sierica con l'età in soggetti normali. Giorn Gerontol 1988;36:419–424.
15. Kamel S, Brazier M, Neri V, et al. Multiple molecular forms of pyridinolines cross-links excreted in human urine evaluated by chromatographic and immunoassay methods. J Bone Min Res 1995;10:1385–1392.
16. Gallagher JC, Riggs BL, Jerpbak CM. The effect of age on serum immunoreactive parathyroid hormone in normal and osteoporotic women. J Lab Clin Med 1980;95:372–385.
17. Marcus R, Madvig P, Young G. Age-related changes in parathyroid hormone and parathyroid hormone action in normal humans. J Clin Endocrinol Metab 1984;58:223–230.
18. Johansen J, Riss BJ, Delmas PD, et al. Plasma BGP: an indicator of spontaneous bone loss and effect of estrogen treatment in postmenopausal women. Eur J Clin Invest 1988;18:191–195.
19. Uebellhart D, Schlemmer A, Johansen Gineyts E., Christiansen C, Delmas PD. Effect of menopause and hormone replacement therapy on the urinary excretion of pyridinium cross-links. J Clin Endocrinol Metab 1991;72:367–373.
20. Szulc P, Chapui MC, Meunier PJ, Delmas PD. Serum undercarboxylated osteocalcin is a marker of the risk of hip fracture in elderly women. J Clin Invest 1993;91:1769–1774.
21. Alekson K, Vergnaud P., Gineyts E, Delmas PD. Increased bone resorption and decreased bone formation in elderly women with hip fracture. Bone Miner 1992;17(S1):184.
22. Delmas PD. Biochemical markers of bone turnover I: Theoretical consideration and clinical use in osteoporosis. Am J Med 1993;95(suppl.5A):11S-16S.
23. NIH Consensus Development Panel on Optimal Calcium Intake. Optimal Calcium Intake. JAMA 1994;272:1942–1948.
24. Nordin BEC. Calcium balance and calcium requirements in spinal osteoporosis. Am J Clin Nutr 1962;10:384–390.
25. Riggs BL, Wahner HW, Melton LJ III, Richelson LS, Judd HL, O'Fallon M. Dietary calcium intake and rates of bone loss in women. J Clin Invest 1987;80:979–982.
26. Heaney RP, Recker RR, Stegman MR, Moy AJ. Calcium absorption in women: relationship to calcium intake, estrogen status, and age. J Bone Miner Res 1989;4:469–475.
27. Baker MR, Peacok M, Nordin BEC. The decline in vitamin D status with age. Age Ageing 1980;9:249–252.
28. Orwoll ES, Meier DE. Alterations in calcium, vitamin D and parathyroid hormone physiology in normal men with aging; relationship to the developent of senile osteopenia. J Clin Endocrinol Metab 1986;63:1262–1269.
29. Heaney RP. Effect of calcium on skeletal development, bone loss and risk of fractures. Am J Med 1991;91(suppl.5B):23S-27S.
30. Cummings RG. Calcium intake and bone mass: a quantitative review of the evidence. Calc Tissue Int 1990;47:194–201.
31. Kelly PJ, Pocock NA, Sambrook PN, Eismann JA. Dietary calcium, sex hormones, and bone mineral density in men. Br Med J 1990;300:1361–1364.
32. Hui SL, Siemends CW, Johnston CC. Age and bone mass as predictors of fracture in a prospective study. J Clin Invest 1988;81:1804–1809.
33. Lindsay R, Hart DM, Forrest C, Baird C. Prevention of spinal osteoporosis in oophorectomized women. Lancet 1980;ii:1151–1154.
34. Riggs BL, Melton LJ. The prevention and treatment of osteoporosis. N Engl J Med 1992;327:620–627.
35. Barbagallo M, Carbognani A, Palummeri E, et al. The comparative effect of ovarian sex steroids administration on bone mineral status in oophorectomized rats. Bone 1989;10:113–116.
36. Girasole G, Jilka RL, Passeri G, et al. 17-beta estradiol inhibits interleukin-6 production by bone marrow-derived stromal cells and osteoblasts in vitro: a potential mechanism for the antiosteoporotic effect of estrogen. J Clin Invest 1992;89:883–891.
37. Jilka RL, Hangoc G, Girasole G, et al. Increased osteoclast development after estrogen loss: mediation by interleukin 6. Science 1992;257:88–91.
38. Passeri G, Girasole G, Jilka RL, Manolagas SC. Increased interleukin-6 production by murine bone marrow and bone cells after estrogen withdrawal. Endocrinology 1993;133:822–828.
39. Ettinger B, Genant HG, Cann CE. Long term estrogen therapy prevents bone loss and fracture. Ann Int Med 1985;102:319–324.
40. Kiel DP, Felson HT, Anderson JJ, et al. Hip fracture and the use of estrogens in postmenopausal women: the Framingham Study. N Engl J Med 1987;317:1169–1174.

41. Fleisch H. Bisphosphonates: pharmacology and use in the treatment of tumor-induced hypercalcemia and metastatic bone disease. Drugs 1991;42:919–944.
42. Shinoda H, Adamek G, Felik R, Fleisch H, Schenk R, Hagan P. Structure-activity relationship of various bisphosphonates. Calcif Tissue Int 1983;35:87–99.
43. Storm T, Thamsborg G, Steiniche T, et al. Effect of intermittent cyclical etidronate therapy on bone mass and fracture rate in women with postmenopausal osteoporosis. N Engl J Med 1990;322:1256–1271.
44. Watts NB, Harris ST, Genant HG , et al. Intermittent cyclical etidronate treatment of postmenopausal osteoporosis. N Engl J Med 1990;323:73–79.
45. Schenk R, Eggli P, Fleisch H, Rosini S. Quantitative morphometric evaluation of the inhibitory activity of new aminobisphoshonates on bone resorption in the rat. Calc Tissue Int 1986;38:342–349.
46. Passeri M, Baroni MC, Pedrazzoni M, Pioli G, Barbagallo M, Costi D, Biondi M, Girasole G, Arlunno B, Palummeri E. Intermittent treatment with intravenous 4-amino-1-hydroxybytilidene-1–1-bisphosphonate (AHBUBP) in the therapy of postmenopausal osteoporosis. Bone Miner 1991;15:237–238.
47. Chestnut CH, McClung MR, Ensrud KE, et al. Alendronate treatment of the postmenopausal osteoporotic woman: effect of multiple dosages on bone mass and bone remodeling. Am J Med 1995;99:144–152.
48. Adami S, Passeri M, Ortolani S, et al. Effects of oral alendronate and intranasal calcitonin on bone mass and biochemical markers of bone turnover in postmenopausal women with osteoporosis. Bone 1995;17: 383–390.
49. Liberman UA, Weiss SR, Broll J, et al. Effect of oral alendronate on bone mineral density and the incidence of fractures in postmenopausal women. N Engl J Med 1995;333:1437–1443.
50. Overgaard K, Riis BJ, Christiansen C, et al. Effect of calcitonin given intranasally on early postmenopausal bone loss. Br Med J 1989;299:477–479.
51. Avioli LV. Heterogeneity of osteoporotic syndromes and the response to calcitonin therapy. Calcif Tissue Int 1991;49(suppl.2):S16-S19.
52. Passeri M, Palummeri E, Barbagallo M, et al. La sequenza calcitriolo-calcitonina nella terapia della osteoporosi. Minerva Endocrinol 1989;14:57–62.
53. Burckardt P, Burnard B. The effect of treatment with calcitonin on vertebral fracture rates in established osteoporosis. Osteoporos Int 1993;3:24–30.
54. Overgaard K, Hansen MA, Jensen SB, Christiansen C. Effect of salcatonin given intranasally on bone mass and fracture rates in established osteoporosis: a dose-response study. Br Med J 1992;305:556–561.
55. Chapui MC, Arlot ME, Dubouef F, et al. Vitamin D3 and calcium to prevent hip fracture in elderly women. N Engl J Med 1992;327:1637–1642.
56. Reid IR, Ames RW, Evans MC, Gamble GD, Sharpe SJ. Effect of calcium supplementation on bone loss in postmenopausal women. N Engl J Med 1993;328:460–464.
57. Bonucci E, Ballanti P, Martelli A, et al. Ipriflavone inhibits osteoclastic differentiation in parathyroid transplanted parietal bone of rats. Calcif Tissue Int 1992;50:314–319.
58. Riggs BL, Hodgson SF, O'Fallon WM, et al. Fluoride treatment in osteoporotic women: effect on fracture rate in a 4-year controlled clinical trial. N Engl J Med 1990;322:802–809.
59. Hedlund LR, Gallagher JC. Increased incidences of fractures in osteoporotic patients treated with sodium fluoride. J Bone Min Res 1989;4:223–225.
60. Riggs BL. Treatment of osteoporosis with sodium fluoride or parathyroid hormone. Am J Med 1991;91(suppl 5B):37S-41S.
61. Pak CYC, Khashayar S, Adams-Huet B, Piziak V, Peterson RD, Poindexter JR. Slow-release sodium fluoride in the management of postmenopausal osteoporosis. Ann Int Med 1995;123:401–408.
62. Johansen JS, Hassager C, Podephant J. Treatment of postmenopausal osteoporosis. Is the anabolic steroid nandrolone decanoate a candidate? Bone Miner 1989;6:77–86.
63. Need AG, Chatterton BE, Walker CJ, Steiner TA, Horowitz M, Nordin BEC. Comparison of calcium, calcitriol, ovarian hormones and nandrolone in the treatment of osteoporosis. Maturitas 1986;8:275–280.
64. Tilyard MW, Spears GFS, Thompson J, Dovey S. Treatment of postmenopausal osteoporosis with calcitriol or calcium. N Engl J Med 1992;326:357–361.
65. Chapui MC, Arlot ME, Delmas PD, Meunier PJ. Effect of calcium and cholecalciferol treatment for three years on hip fractures in elderly women. Br Med J 1994;308:1081–1082.
66. Neer R, Slovik D, Daly M, Lo C, Potts J, Nussbaum S. Treatment of postmenopausal osteoporosis with daily parathyroid hormone plus calcitriol. In "Osteoporosis 1990", Christiansen C, Overgaard K eds. Osteopress Aps, Copenhagen, 1990:pp.1314–1317.
67. Mundy GR. Calcium Homeostasis: Hypercalcemia and hypocalcemia, 2nd ed. Martin Dunitz, London, 1990.

30

UPDATE ON ITALIAN CENTENARIANS

Italian Multicentric Study on Centenarians

L. Motta, R. Rapisarda, S. Sangiorgi, G. Receputo, and F. B. Tomasello*†

The prolongation of survival in the industrialised nations is indubitably the most important demographic reality of the end of this millennium [1]. The aging of the population is correlated with two factors, i.e. the reduction in the birth and death rates [2]. The progressive increase in the number of elderly subjects has prolonged survival to 100 years of age and over, and this is one of the most important issues in modern gerontology research.

This study focuses on a nationwide survey of centenarians [3–6]. The first poll of Italian centenarians was conducted in 1993 and involved numerous university departments of geriatrics and gerontology (Bari, Bologna, Brescia, Catania, Catanzaro, Florence, Genoa, Milan 1,2, Modena 1,2, Naples, Palermo, Parma, Perugia, Rome, Sienna, Turin, Trieste 1,2) which formed a consortium called the Italian Multicentric Study on Centenarians co-ordinated by the Department of Internal Medicine and Geriatrics, University of Catania. The census furnished a reliable projection of the number of centenarians in Italy on 31/12/1993 and estimated about 4,000 centenarians, with a mean density of 70.25 centenarians per 1,000,000 inhabitants, prevalently in North Italy (Table 1). This figure is one of the highest in Europe [7].

The study aims were to endeavour to understand the underlying reasons determining longevity and to reveal the socioeconomic, genetic, clinical, and biological characteristics of centenarians.

The study group adopted a computerized case sheet to compile information on:

- recent and remote familial and case history
- diet and pharmacological treatment
- physical examination
- laboratory tests
- evaluation scales.

Three hundred and eighty two of the 1,162 centenarians polled were randomly selected and studied [8].

* The participants in the Multicentric Study are listed in the Appendix

† Address for correspondence: Luciano Motta M.D., Ph.D. Institute of Internal Medicine and Geriatrics, Cannizzaro Hospital, Via Messina, 829, 95126 Catania, Italy

Recent Advances in Geriatrics, edited by Barbagallo, Licata, and Sowers.
Plenum Press, New York, 1998.

Table 1. Distribution of centenarians throughout Italy

	December 31, 1993		June 30, 1996	
	Population	Centenarians per million inhabitants	Population	Centenarians per million inhabitants
North (4 centers)	208	83.5	267	100
Center (3 centers)	161	50	62	87
South (3 centers)	215	44	255	46
Total	584	55	584*	65.5

*does not include Pavia.

Data on the socioeconomic situation of the centenarians [9] revealed that 79% of them were females and 21% males, 81% had limited schooling, 54.5% lived in urban areas, 77.9% lived in their own homes with their children and/or relatives, 84.7% were widows/widowers. Familial history of longevity was evident (75.96±16.92 years).

Remote case history showed that 37.6% of the subjects studied had had an infectious disease: malaria (19.3%), typhus (18.1%), pneumonia (23.7%), pulmonary TBC (1.4%). Only 1 case of smallpox and 1 of plague were recorded. In addition, the subjects reported an elevated frequency of cold syndromes.

Recent case history showed that 30.1% of the centenarians were affected by cardiopathies (of haemodynamic (44%) rather than ischemic (5.3%) and arrhythmic nature (11.1%); 64.5% were normotensive, 24% was hypertensive (mean systolic and diastolic pressure being 176.4±25.3 and 91.4±9.6 mmHg, respectively); and that 88.3% took hypotensive drugs. Acute cerebral vascular disease was present in 7.8%, dementia in 11.6%, Parkinson's disease in 1.2%, and signs of peripheral arteriopathy were observed in 9.7% of the subjects. The most common gastrointestinal disorders were dyspepsia (30%), haemorrhoids (18.3%), bile stones mainly in females (13.3% in females versus 1.4% in males). Constipation was frequent (49.7%), as were urinary incontinence (22.3% in females and 10.3% in males) and nocturia (21.8% in males versus 12% in females).

Endocrine disorders included goiter (3.8%), hypothyroidism (2%) and hyperthyroidism (1.9%), almost exclusively in females. Also diabetes was more common in females. Mean age at onset and mean duration of diabetes were 94 years and 9.3 years, respectively. Onset had occurred before 70 years of age only in 2 females (mean 62.5 years), whereas it had onset about 50 years previously in the only male diabetic.

Laboratory tests (Tables 2, 3) revealed that the centenarians' haematological parameters were within the normal reference range for the healthy adult population. Hb concentration and red blood cell count were low, but within the normal range. Albuminaemia was relatively low and there was an increase in all the globulin fractions. Azotaemia and uricaemia concentrations were also slightly above normal range.

US revealed that the liver was often reduced in size, had an irregular margin and non homogeneous structure. Gall bladder US showed a reduction in size and the frequent presence of gallstones in the gall bladder and hepatic bile duct. In addition the calibre of the latter was increased.

Information on drug consumption was collected during interviews and revealed daily intake of 2.5±1.1 drugs/day (median 2) which is lower than reported for European or American elderly subjects (2–4.8). The most commonly used drugs were myocardiocinetics (40.3%), antihypertensives (21.3%), vasoactive drugs (19.3%) psyco-active drugs (19%), diuretics (17.7%), antithrombotics (9.9%), nitroderivates (4.9%), corticosteroids

Table 2. Haemocitometric examination of centenarians by sex

Parameters	No.	Total	F	M	Reference values
Haemoglobin	199	12.4 ± 1.7	12.4 ± 1.8	12.5 ± 1.7*	12–16 F / 14–18 M
Haemathocrit, %	199	40 ± 22	40 ± 25	39 ± 5	36–46 F / 38–47 M
Red blood cell count, 10^{12}/L	199	4.1 ± 0.6	4.1 ± 0.7	4.2 ± 0.6*	4.2–5.4 F / 4.5–6.3 M
MCV, f/L	199	92 ± 9	91 ± 8	93 ± 9	82–98
Leukocyte count, 10^9/L	199	6.3 ± 2.0	6.1 ± 1.9	7.0 ± 2.5	4.0–10.0
Polymophonuclear count, %	199	61 ± 13	60 ± 13	63 ± 13	50–65
Lymphocyte count, %	199	28 ± 11	29 ± 11	27 ± 11	20–35
Platelets, 10^6/L	199	209 ± 71	212 ± 72	197 ± 66	130–400

*indicates values outside reference intervals.

(2.9%), non steroid antiinflammatory drugs (NSAD) (2.2%) and laxatives (1.9%). The incidence of adverse drug reaction (ADR) was 13.4%.

Autopsy was performed in 141 centenarians and revealed that the most common disease was cardiopathy (57%), followed by respiratory (50.35%) and cerebrovascular diseases (34.7%) and neoplasias (16.3%).

Not all the data collected in the Italian Multicentric Study on Centenarians can be included herein. However, it must be underlined that sera and DNA from over 200 centenarians have been used to create data banks that will enable us to verify pathogenic hypothesis.

The contrast between the elevated number of "healthy centenarians" and the elevated mortality rate over a short time span is interesting.

Although centenarians age, they retain satisfactory homeostatic mechanisms. Their functional reserves reduce progressively, and survival is genetically determined and influ-

Table 3. Clinical chemistry data of centenarians by sex

Parameters	No.	Total	F	M	Reference values
Urea, mg/dl	233	49 ± 22	46 ± 20	58 ± 25*	18–50
GOT, U/L	212	21 ± 10	19 ± 10	21 ± 10	0–37
GPT, U/L	212	12 ± 8	11 ± 8	13 ± 7	0–40
ALP, U/L	200	198 ± 141	195 ± 137	210 ± 156	98–279
Glucose, mg/dl	252	89 ± 24	88 ± 25	91 ± 20	70–110
Cholesterol, mg/dl	257	182 ± 39	185 ± 40*	170 ± 33	<200
HDL, mg/dl	166	60 ± 40	64 ± 44*	48 ± 18	45–60 F / 40–50 M
Triglycerides, mg/dl	257	114 ± 50	120 ± 51	96 ± 40	<180
Uric acid, mg/dl	233	5.9 ± 4.0	6.0 ± 3.5*	7.1 ± 6.0*	2.4–5.6 F / 3.4–7.0 M
Total protein, g/dl	199	6.9 ± 0.7	7.0 ± 0.9	6.9 ± 0.7	6–8
A/G	199	1.3 ± 1.5	1.4 ± 1.7	1.2 ± 0.3	1.3–2.1
Electrophoresis albumin, %	199	53 ± 6	53 ± 7*	52 ± 6*	62–70
α1-globulin, %	199	3.3 ± 0.9	3.3 ± 1.1	3.3 ± 0.8	2.1–3.3
α2-globulin, %	199	10.5 ± 2.3	10.1 ± 2.2	10.6 ± 2.4	4.7–8.3
β-globulin, %	199	12.0 ± 2.6	11.9 ± 2.0	12.5 ± 3.0	4.6–8.3
γ-globulin, %	199	19.3 ± 5.4	19.1 ± 5.4*	20.7 ± 5.2*	11.4–17.8
Serum sodium, mmol/L	176	140 ± 4	140 ± 4	141 ± 5	135–145
Serum potassium, mmol/L	176	4.8 ± 2.5	4.9 ± 2.8	4.4 ± 0.4	3.5–5.0
Serum calcium, mmol/L	176	8.1 ± 5.9	8.4 ± 6.4	6.6 ± 2.4	8.1–10.4
TSH, mU/L	54	1.6 ± 0.9	1.6 ± 0.9	1.6 ± 0.9	0.25–3.1
Serum iron, mcg/dl	150	71 ± 26	71 ± 26	66 ± 25	60–120 F / 70–140 M
Ferritin, ng/ml	65	113 ± 115	105 ± 95	150 ± 182	15–300

*indicates values outside the reference intervals.

enced by environmental and socioeconomic factors. There are no losses, negative aspects or deterioration. The ageing process is very complicated and is characterized by changing, complex states of balance. Indubitably, the detection of genes and life styles capable of protecting subjects from tumours, cardiovascular, metabolic diseases and dementia, could help us to understand the biological basis of longevity.

The rise in the number of centenarians worldwide is related to the reduction of negative factors (poor hygiene, infectious diseases, poor nutrition, socioenvironmental situations) and the increment of positive factors (improved sociosanitary care, nutrition and hygiene, drastic reduction in morbidity, etc.). Death is often caused by accidents, such as a fall or sudden cold, which upset the centenarians' precarious balance.

Comparison of our data with those obtained by the ILSA [10] study conducted on a sample of 5,632 male and female subjects between 65 and 85 years revealed an exceptional health status profile in centenarians compared with the elderly. In fact, the incidence of all the diseases studied was lower in centenarians than in the elderly (hypertension 24% versus 65%; Parkinson's disease 1.2% versus 2.6%; thyroid disorders 7.7% versus 13.2%). The results on diabetes mellitus were noteworthy. The ILSA study reported a prevalence of 13.6%, while our study revealed a prevalence of 5.5%. Moreover, onset of diabetes in centenarians was very late (> 90 years) and did not determine complications. This finding showed that long term diabetes jeopardizes longevity. The data on dementia were also interesting. Our study on centenarians reported an incidence of 11.6% which was twice that observed in the ILSA study (5.1%), revealing that involutive cerebral processes do not affect survival.

In conclusion, our data revealed that the majority of Italian centenarians are "healthy", present a lower incidence of clinical manifestations, consume fewer drugs than the younger age classes, and live in a good environment (with the family in healthy conditions). Thus, centenarians can age with dignity and retain a good level of self-sufficiency.

A second census was conducted in 1996 (Table 4) by 22 University departments (all the afore-mentioned ones except Genoa and Trieste, plus Florence 2, Messina, Pavia and Rome 2). The projection estimated a total of about 5,000 centenarians in Italy on 30/6/1996, an increase by about 19% compared with the previous 1993 poll. An investigation on Sicil-

Table 4. Increase in number of Italian centenarians between 1993 and 1996

	December 31, 1993			June 30, 1996		
Center	Centenarians	Population	Centenarians per million inhabitants	Centenarians	Population	Centenarians per million inhabitants
Bologna	74	539,452	137	76	905,838	84 ↓
Catania	86	1,356,511	63	117*	1,957,389	60 ↓
Catanzaro	83	2,070,600	40	87	2,073,485	42 ↑
Modena	38	602,644	63	66	450,000	147 ↑
Napoli	46	1,500,000	31	51	1,500,000	34 ↑
Parma	36	402,000	90	38	390,000	97 ↑
Perugia	16	151,890	105	13	152,379	85 ↓
Roma	119	2,791,354	42	24	321,670	75 ↑
Siena	26	249,935	104	25	241,690	103 ↓
Torino	60	946,135	63	87	921,363	94 ↑
Total	584	10,610,521	55	584**	8,913,814	65
Increase: 19%						

*Catania + Messina; **does not include Pavia center which recorded 47 centenarians / 488, 257 inhabitants.

Table 5. Mortality rate in Sicilian centenarians from January 1, 1994 to June 30, 1996

Town	Centenarians (1993)	Deaths	Mortality rate (%)
Agrigento	5	2	40
Caltanissetta	4	2	50
Catania	36	32	88
Enna	9	7	77
Palermo	44	32	73
Ragusa	11	11	100
Siracusa	10	8	80
Trapani	6	6	100
Total	125	100	80

ian centenarians (Table 5) showed a high mortality rate (80%), mean age at death being 102.5 years, and confirmed the extremely rapid demographic turnover in centenarians.

The 1996 census has paved the way for the second part of the study on centenarians. At present, after sampling and recruiting the population each study center is collecting data using the same case sheet. Data on centenarians, over 60 year old controls, centenarians' siblings and homogeneous for age controls, and any centenarians surveyed in 1993 and still alive, are being acquired for longitudinal and transversal studies. We hope that results of the second phase of the study will match the significant and encouraging scientific findings furnished by the 1993 census.

REFERENCES

1. United Nations : World Population Prospects 1990. New York, 1991.
2. Antonini FM., Mannucci M. : A cosa servono i centenari per i gerontologi? Giorn. Geront. 1991; 39 : 525–32.
3. Maggi S., Bush T: Aspetti demografici in geriatria. Geriatrics 1988 ; 10: 9–17.
4. Antonini FM., Zingales LD., Cariani G : Invecchiamento della popolazione. In : Nicita M. (ed) : Geriatria oggi. Cosenza : Bios, 1987 : 3–25.
5. Annuario Statistico Italiano ISTAT, 1993.
6. Golini A. : Longevità e durata della vita : un approccio statistico-demografico. Giorn. Gerontol. 1991 ; 39 : 135–44
7. Campana F., Ettorre E., Marigliano V : Epidemiologia della longevità. In : Invecchiamento e longevità. Roma ; CESI., 1995 ; 85.
8. I centenari in Italia : aspetti epidemiologici e clinico-biologici. Italian Multicentric Study on Centenarians. Lettura al 96° Congresso della Società Italiana di Medicina Interna. (Roma, 12–15 ottobre 1995). Editore Luigi Pozzi.
9. Epidemiological and socioeconomic aspects of Italian centenarians. The Italian Multicentric Study on Centenarians. Archives of Gerontology and Geriatric, 1997 (in press).
10. Amaducci L., Scarlato G : Salute e malattie degli anziani : risultati a confronto. L' indagine ILSA. Congresso Nazionale " La salute degli anziani in Italia". CNR-Progetto finalizzato invecchiamento - ISTAT. Roma 21–22 marzo 1993.

APPENDIX

Twenty-one University Centers collaborated in the Italian Multicentric Study on Centenarians. This report was made possible by their enthusiastic cooperation in preparing the case sheets, recording the series and data processing. The success of the Italian

Multicentric Study on Centenarians must be shared equally among all the members of study centers.

A. Capurso, F. Resta, A. D'Amelio, Institute of Geriatrics, University of Bari
A. Gaddi, S. D'Addato, C. Galletti, Department of Gerontology, University of Bologna
M. Trabucchi, S. Boffelli, R. Rozzini, Geriatric Research Group, Brescia
L. Motta, R. Rapisarda, G. Receputo, Department of Internal Medicine and Geriatrics, University of Catania
R. Mattace, M. Motta, L. Pansini, Department of Experimental and Clinical Medicine, University of Catanzaro
G. Masotti, N. Marchionni, E. Petruzzi, Institute of Gerontology and Geriatrics, University of Florence
S. Bertolini, M. Agretti, P. Costelli, Department of Internal Medicine, University of Genoa
D. Mari, F. Duca, P. Ferrazzi, Department of Internal Medicine, University of Milan
E. Bosi, M. Manzoni, F.B. Tomasello, Scientific Institute Ospedale S. Raffaele, University of Milan
G. Salvioli, M.V. Baldelli, M. Neri, Department of Geriatrics, University of Modena
C. Franceschi, A. Cossarizza, D. Monti, Department of Biomedic Sciences, University of Modena
M. Varricchio, A. Gambardella, G. Paolisso, Department of Gerontology and Geriatrics, University of Naples
G. Baggio, M. Dalla Vestrà, S. Donazzan, Institute of Internal Medicine, University of Padova
G. Barbagallo Sangiorgi, M. Barbagallo, G. Fradà, Institute of Internal Medicine and Geriatrics, University of Palermo
M. Passeri, F. Fagnoni, P. Sansoni, Institute of Clinical Medicine, University of Parma
U. Senin, A. Cherubini, M.C. Polidori, Institute of Gerontology and Geriatrics, University of Perugia
V. Marigliano, C. Bauco, M. Cacciafesta, Institute of Gerontology and Geriatrics, University La Sapienza, Rome
S. Forconi, M. Guerrini, S. Boschi, Institute of Semeiotics and Geriatrics, University of Siena
F. Fabris, G. Cappa, E. Ferrario, Institute of Geriatrics, University of Turin
L. Giarelli, F. Cavalieri, G. Stanta, Institute of Anatomopathology, University of Trieste

31

CENTENARIANS IN WESTERN SICILY

Data and Characteristics

G. Fradà, R. Pollina, E. Pupella, G. Mangiacavallo, S. Chessari, and M. Palazzo

Institute of Internal Medicine and Geriatrics
University of Palermo

INTRODUCTION

Progressive aging of general population recorded in Italy has caused an increase of the number of centenarians. Such high age is often associated with failure of many psychic and physical functions, and centenarians are therefore often not independent (partially or completely) and require particular care.

Such a trend is found also in Sicily, where increased number of centenarians is quite evident and involves all aforementioned problems. These centenarians were born in Sicily and spent most of their lives in this region: they therefore afford a quite particular picture of the condition of aged people, in that it reflects a pyramidal family structure still prevailing in Sicily. The heritage of a traditional, mostly rural culture, not yet replaced by a more modern urban culture, in which family relationships and the role of the aged within the family are less valued.

MATERIALS AND METHODS

Psychometric tests were performed on a group of 58 centenarians (average age: 101.4 ± 1.9 years, ranging from 100 to 109) including 40 women and 18 men, living in various large and small towns in western Sicily.

Psychometric evaluation was based on some widely used psycho-diagnostic tests such as the Index of Independence in Activity Daily Living (ADL), concerning the ability to perform daily living activities (eating, washing, dressing, going to the bathroom, moving independently, continence) (1), and Instrumental Activities of Daily Living Scale (IADL), allowing evaluation of independence in using the telephone, shopping, preparing meals, looking after the household, and laundry, using means of transportation, being responsible of drug use, and the ability of handling money (2).

Recent Advances in Geriatrics, edited by Barbagallo, Licata, and Sowers.
Plenum Press, New York, 1998.

MMSE (Mini Mental State Examination) affords a reliable evaluation of the most important cognitive functions. It is easy to perform, it requires only 5 to 10 minutes and includes 11 items. It is aimed at evaluating some cognitive components, such as temporo-spatial orientation, attention, calculating ability (7 tests), short-term and long-term memory, language (oral and written), construction activity. Scoring ranges from 0 to 30.

GDS (Geriatric Depression Scale) for the evaluation of affective tone includes 30 items; scoring ranges from 0 to 30. Scores from 0 to 10 correspond to no depression; scores from 11 to 20 correspond to moderate depression; scores from 21 to 30 to severe depression (4).

Relatives' Stress Scale (RSS) (5) was used to evaluate stress in relatives living with and caring for centenarians. The Italian version used includes 15 items, while scoring ranges from 0 to 60. Scores from 0 to 15 correspond to no stress at all light stress; scores from 15 to 30 to moderate stress and scores from 30 to severe stress.

Educational level of centenarians was found to be quite low: 14 of them were illiterate, 4 had attended only the 1st class (elementary school), 4 had attained the 2nd class, 8 the 3rd class, 5 the 4th class, 13 had finished the 5th class, 7 had finished high school, and only one had achieved a university degree. 36 of our centenarians were living with their children, who looked after them, 5 were living in homes for the elderly, 6 were living with relatives, and 11 in their own home, but were looked after by relatives or by private personnel.

RESULTS

Functional ability in centenarians was quite impaired: ADL showed 41 of these subjects to be quite dependent, while 17 were independent. IADL showed that only one of four centenarians was independent, while 12 were partially independent and 45 completely dependent.

MMSE was performed on 40 out of 58 subjects (28 women, 12 men). In 18 subjects this test could not be performed because of severe sensorial failures, such as confusional state and/or moderate-to-severe mental deterioration. Average MMSE score was 19.1 ± 5.7, ranging from 6 to 30.

GDS was performed on 31 out of 58 subjects and an average score of 5.06 ± 4.27 ranging from 0 to 16 was obtained, which corresponds to practically no depression. 38 relatives of our centenarians underwent RSS and an average score of 13.1 ± 11.4 was obtained, which corresponds to moderate stress.

COMMENTS

Functional disability is quite common in aged people and its occurrence grows more and more frequent with age. ADL scores are conceived according to a progressive scale, from simpler functions, such as using the bathroom and eating, to the more complex ones, such as dressing and walking. ADL standard scores are useful for describing the patients' starting conditions and for setting the goals that may be attained by aged subjects with severe disabilities, particularly in rehabilitation programs.

ADL proves quite useful for identifying the patients needs and for planning regular daily assistance at home or at an institution. IADL scores (2) can be used to test abilities of a higher level. The usefulness of performing ADL and IADL together consists in the possibility of identifying particularly impaired functions in individual patients. Tests are now available which take into account the time required to answer questions, or to perform tasks, and they proved sensitive and useful (6,7). Other, more recent, mobility tests yield better information as to the risk of falls than does a standard physical test (8). Almost all our centenarians showed remarkable functional failures, as was evident from standard tests in starring conditions, and we therefore gave up performing further tests in our centenarians.

Moreover, such tests might be not well accepted by centenarians themselves, and particularly by their relatives, who considered time tests as feasible (standing up from a chair or armchair, taking a few steps without help, using the telephone) the time required to perform such tasks was found to be actually longer, this confirming functional limitation, which appeared in most cases to be due to the subjects no longer being used to walk without help.

Indeed we found out that relatives do all they can—and even more—for their centenarians, before it is necessary or even if it is not necessary, and we deemed that requiring them to behave differently would not be appreciated.

Mean value of MMSE in 40 of our centenarians was 19.1 ± 5.5 which is lower than scores obtained from younger people. A certain deterioration of cognitive functions is a frequent finding in aged subjects. Folstein et al. suggested that scores lower than 24 should be considered as indicating failure in this field. Thus, old age correlates to lower MMSE scores (Folstein et al., 1985; Nelson et al., 1986; Bleeker et al., 1988; Evans et al., 1993) (9–12). Other authors however, showed that old age "per se" is not the cause of lower MMSE scores. Hearing and visual loss do lower MMSE scores, but not significantly (Heeren et al., 1990) (13). Still other authors found that low MMSE scores could remain stable over a long period of time or could improve on the next control, thus excluding that demential condition was the only factor responsible of low MMSE scores Johansson et al., 1992) (14).

Results from a meta-analysis of data from previous epidemiological studies suggest that incidence of senile dementia increases exponentially at the beginning of old age but that such rate decreases starting with 80–84 years and is 0 at 95 years, when it is found in 40% of cases (15). Grimby and Berg (16) carried out a 6-year-study and found that among stress events taking place within this period (the subjects' own diseases, or their relatives' diseases, the consorts or a child's death, the death of other relatives or of friends, separation from children, change of residence) only doleful events concerning the consort or children caused lower performance in cognitive tests (more evident in men), which anyway proved to be quite low in all subjects. They also suggested that a subject's performance in cognitive functions tests might be influenced by other factors, such as education, sensorial failures and the like. Such factors should be taken into account when evaluating scores obtained from centenarians. If we consider 24 as cut-off value between normal and mentally deteriorated subjects, only 32.5% of our centenarians would prove normal, and this does correspond to the actual situation. Villardita too (17) suggests that 24 should not be considered as a reliable cut-off value, since some data show that aged subjects with low schooling but without dementia could attain scores not higher than 24, while patients with higher education and with low grade dementia may obtain scores up to 27 MMSE. It is therefore thought to involve about 40% error and Magni et al. (18) suggested to correct MMSE scores according to age and education.

Valente et al. (19) and Scurti et al. (20) proposed therefore to consider 19 as cut-off value: MMSE would thus keep its 100% sensitivity and 95% specificity and could hence be still considered as valid. Using 19 as cut-off value, 57.5% centenarians would prove to be normal: 23 of them obtained scores above 19, while 17 obtained scores lower than 19, due to sensorium deficiencies and to slight-to-moderate mental deterioration. It should also be recalled that most of our centenarians had a low schooling due to social and environmental conditions prevailing in Sicily when they were young. At the beginning of the twentieth century attending school was a luxury, particularly in the rural setting to which most of our centenarians belong. Moreover most of our centenarians show now some degree of sensorial deficiencies exerting a negative effect on test performance.

In the present study percentage of centenarians with normal cognitive functions proved to be higher than that found in the Italian Multicenter Study of centenarians (21) based on a more numerous sample and reporting that 44.5% of centenarians scored above 19 in MMSE. In the course of our study, however, it was impossible to perform MMSE in 18 out of 58 cases due to severe sensorial failures and moderate-to-severe mental deterioration. A correct evaluation of the actual incidence of mental deterioration in our group of centenarians is therefore impossible. Mean GDS scores obtained from our centenarians proved to be quite low, and even 16—the score obtained from 2 of our subjects—should be considered as corresponding to only slight depression. Such low values are quite surprising if we consider that our centenarians are usually not independent. Our data should be considered with some criticism, since GDS could not be performed in 27 out of our 58 cases, due to severe hearing loss, mental confusion, moderate-to-severe dementia, or—in a few cases—to difficulties arising from the subjects' environment. Our observations are also not in agreement with common findings in geriatrics. The incidence of depression was shown to be about 10–15% in subjects aged over 65 and to increase with age, due also to environmental and economic factors, to the presence of physical diseases-particularly if the latter are invalidating ones-and to psychic diseases. Data obtained from the Italian Multicenter Study on Centenarians confirm our opinion: infact 54.8% of centenarians were shown to be exempt of depression, 36% scored just above minimal depression threshold, while 9.1% showed signs of clinically relevant depression. Our centenarians, however, some of whom had been included in IMSC, failed to show any depressive condition. Such disagreement may be ascribed to the fact that IMSC includes centenarians from several parts of Italy. Our data, which refer only to subjects living in Western Sicily, are therefore considered together with those obtained from centenarians living in other regions of Italy, where family life and environmental conditions are quite different. It should also be recalled that particularly in the rural districts of our Region most aged people still take part in family life, i.e. live with their children, or live in their own home and are taken care of with much love and respect by their relatives. Five of our centenarians were living in homes for the elderly and they were lovingly looked after by the one personnel and their relatives visited them very often. Such circumstances certainly play an important role in averting depression, since centenarians are still well integrated and feel loved in their families or in homes for the elderly in spite of their own limitations. The presence of such physical limitations suggested to test the stress of relatives directly looking after centenarians. For this purpose we used a psychometric test devised by green (Great Britain) in 1982 in order to evaluate stress in family members personally looking after an elderly relative with dementia. We used the Italian version of this test, including 15 of its original items and excluding those concerning behavioral disorders, since the latter don't frequently occur in centenarians. Low average RSS scores obtained in present study are quite surprising but may be accounted for by the absence of mental deterioration in this group of centenarians and by the affectionate surrounding (hence the absence of depression), relatives being quite proud of having a centenarian in their family.

CONCLUSION

Results obtained from psychometric evaluation of a group of centenarians in western Sicily, as compared with those obtained from a larger number of centenarians living in other parts of Italy show that our centenarians do suffer from a similar number of diseases and function failures requiring treatment with a similar number of drugs, and from a similar degree of depression, i.e. minimal depression or no depression at all. Such circumstance may be tentatively ascribed to the affectionate care surrounding our centenarians, as shown also by the low degree of stress on the part of family members personally involved in taking care of centenarians. In our opinion living with the family and being surrounded by loving care is a factor that improves the quality of life in our centenarians.

REFERENCES

1. Rubenstein L.Z., Josephson K. R., Wieland G. D., English T. A., Sayre J.A., Kane R.L. Effectiveness of a Geriatric valuation unit: a randomized clinical trial. N. Engl. J. Med. 1984; 311:1664–7
2. Katz S., Ford A. B., Moscowitz R. W.,Jackson. V.A., Jaffee M. W. , Studies of illness in the aged: the index of ADL: a standardized measure of biological and psychosocial function. Jama 1963:185:914–9
3. Lawton M.T., Brody E.M., Assessment of older people: self mantaining and instrumental activities of daily living. Gerontologist 1969;9:179–86.
4. Folstein M.S.,Folstein S.E., McHugh P.R. Minimental state: a pratical method for rading the cognitive state of patients for the clinician. J. Psychiatr. Res. 1975;12:189–98.
5. Yesavage J.A., Brink T.L.,Rose L. et al. Development and Validation of Ageriatric Depression Screening Scale: A preliminary report. J. Psychiatr. Res. 1982; 17: 37–49.
6. Williams M.E., Hadler N.M., Earp J.A. manual ability as a marker of dependancy in geriatric woman. J. Chronic. Dis. 1982 35:115–226.
7. Williams M.E., Hornberger J.C. A quantitative method of identifying older persons at risk for increasing long term care services. J. Croni. Dis.1984; 37: 705–11.
8. Tinetti M.E., Ginter S.F. Identifying mobility dysfunction in elderly patients: standard neuromuscolar examination or direct assessment? Jama 1988; 259:1190–3.
9. Folstein M., Anthony J.C., Parhad I., Duffy B., Gruenberg E.M. The meaning cognitive impairment in the elderly J. Am. Ger. Soc. 1985; 4:228–35.
10. Nelson A., Fogel B.S., Faust D. Bedside cognitive screening instruments. A critucal assessment. J. Ner. Men.Dis.1987;2:73–83.
11. Evans D.A., Beckett L.A., Albert M.S., Hebert L.E., Sherr P. A., Fulkenstein H.H., Taylor J.O. Level of education and changes in cognitive function in a community population of older person. Ann. Epidemiol., 1993; 3:71–77.
12. Bleecker M.L., Bolla- Wilson K., Kawas C., Agnew J., Age specific norms for the mini- mental state exam. Neurology 1988; 38: 1565–68.
13. Heeren T.J., Lagaay A.M., Beek W.C.A., Rooymans H.G.M., Hijmans W.Reference values for the minimental state examination in octo and nonagerians. 1990 J. Am. Ger. Soc. 38: 1093–96.
14. Johansson B., Zarit S.H., Berg S.Changes in cognitive functioning of the oldest old. J. Gerontology 1992 47:2:75–80.
15. Johansson B., Berg S., The robustness of the terminal decline phoenomen: Longitudinal data from the digit-span memory test. J. Gerontology 1989, 44:184–86.
16. Ritchie K. Kildea D. Is senile dementia "age -related" or "ageing related"?- Evidence from meta-analysis of dementia prevalence in the oldest old. The Lancet, 1996, 8980:931.
17. Feher E.P., Mahurin R.K., Doody R.S., Cooke N., Sims J., Pirozzolo F. J. Establishing the limits of the mini-mental state. Arch. Neurol. 1992, 49:87–92.
18. Grimbly A., Berg S. Stressful life events and cognitive function in late life. Aging clin. Exp. Res. 1995, 7:35–39.
19. Villardita C. Diagnostica neuropsicologica:problematiche nell'anziano. Giorn. Geront. 1992, 40: 459–63.
20. Valente C., Maione P., Lippi A., Taiti P., Cavarzeran F., Rocca W.A., Amaducci L., Ravazzano A. Validazione del mini- mental state examination come strumento di screening per demenza in una popolazione italiana. Giorn. Geront. 1992 40: 161–65.

21. Scurti R., Pennese F., Palombo V., Cesauri O., Puddu G.M., Abate G. Validazione del mini-mental state in una popolazione geriatrica italiana. Giorn. Geront. 1993 41: 407–411.
22. Italian Multicentric Study on Centenarians, I centenari in Italia: aspetti epidemiologici e clinico-biologici. Lettura al 96° Congresso della S.I.M.I.-Roma 12–15 ottobre 1995.
23. Brandt J., Spencers M., Folstein M., The telephone interview for cognitive status. NNBM 1988 1:111–117
24. Del Lungo I., Bandinelli S., Benvenuti E., Cecchi F., Alunno S., Salani B., Benvenuti F., Ferrucci L., Baroni A., Lo screening del deterioramento cognitivo nelle persone anziane. Taratura di un test cognitivo verbale rispetto al MiniMental State, Giorn. Geront. 1997, (in press).
25. Pfeiffer E., A short portable mental status questionnaire for the assessment of organic brain deficit in elderly patient. J. Am. Geriatr. Soc. 1975, 23, 433–441.

CONTRIBUTORS

Abate G
Cattedra di Gerontologia e Geriatria
Università degli Studi di Chieti, Chieti

Acanfora D
Istituto di Medicina Interna, Cardiologia e Cardiologia Vascolare
Università Federico II di Napoli, Napoli

Afonso LC
Div of Endocrinology
Wayne State University Medical Center
Detroit, Michigan, USA

Alessi MA
Cattedra di Geriatria
Università degli Studi di Palermo, Palermo

Altobelli A
Cattedra di Gerontologia e Geriatria
Università degli Studi di Firenze, Firenze

Amato P
Istituto di Medicina Interna e Terapia
Università degli Studi di Palermo, Palermo

Annoni G
Cattedra di Gerontologia e Geriatria
Università degli Studi di Milano, Milano

Bakris GL
Rush Presbiterian/St. Luke's Medical Center
Chicago, Illinois, USA

Barbagallo M
Cattedra di Geriatria
Università degli Studi di Palermo, Palermo

Barbagallo Sangiorgi G
Istituto di Medicina Interna e Geriatria
Università degli Studi di Palermo, Palermo

Barbieri M
Dip. di Gerontologia, Geriatria e Malattie del Metabolismo
II Università di Napoli-Policlinico, Napoli

Benincà P
Cattedra di Gerontologia e Geriatria
Istituto di Medicina Interna
Università degli Studi di Padova, Padova

Bianchetti A
Geriatric Research Group, IRCCS "S. Giovanni di Dio"
Sacro Cuore Fatebenefratelli Hospital, Brescia

Bruno D
Cattedra di Geriatria
Università degli Studi di Palermo, Palermo

Bucca G
Cattedra di Gerontologia e Geriatria
Istituto di Clinica Medica I
Università degli Studi "La Sapienza," Roma

Bussolotto M
Cattedra di Gerontologia e Geriatria
Istituto di Medicina Interna
Università degli Studi di Padova, Padova

Cantini C
Cattedra di Gerontologia e Geriatria
Università degli Studi di Firenze, Firenze

Capurso A
Cattedra di Gerontologia e Geriatria
Università degli Studi di Bari, Bari

Capurso SA
Cattedra di Gerontologia e Geriatria
Università degli Studi di Bari, Bari

Caputo L
Cattedra di Gerontologia e Geriatria
Università degli Studi di Milano, Milano

Carbonin PU
Cattedra di Gerontologia e Geriatria
Istituto di Clinica Medica
Università Cattolica del Sacro Cuore, Roma

Castellani S
Cattedra di Gerontologia e Geriatria
Università degli Studi di Firenze, Firenze

Catalano G
Cattedra di Geriatria
Università degli Studi di Palermo, Palermo

Ceccon A
Cattedra di Gerontologia e Geriatria
Istituto di Medicina Interna
Università degli Studi di Padova, Padova

Cecioni I
Cattedra di Medicina Interna
Università degli Studi di Firenze, Firenze

Cherubini A
Istituto di Gerontologia e Geriatria
Policlinico Monteluce
Università degli Studi di Perugia, Perugia

Chessari S
Istituto di Medicina Interna e Geriatria
Università degli Studi di Palermo, Palermo

Coin A
Cattedra di Gerontologia e Geriatria
Istituto di Medicina Interna
Università degli Studi di Padova, Padova

Dammacco F
Istituto di Medicina Interna
Università degli Studi di Bari, Bari

Di Iorio A
Cattedra di Gerontologia e Geriatria
Università degli Studi di Chieti, Chieti

Di Minno G
Cattedra di Geriatria
Università degli Studi di Palermo, Palermo

Di Serio C
Cattedra di Gerontologia e Geriatria
Università degli Studi di Firenze, Firenze

Dominguez LJ
Istituto di Medicina Interna e Terapia
Università degli Studi di Palermo, Palermo

Durante M
Cattedra di Gerontologia e Geriatria
Istituto di Clinica Medica I
Università degli Studi "La Sapienza," Roma

Enzi G
Cattedra di Gerontologia e Geriatria
Istituto di Medicina Interna
Università degli Studi di Padova, Padova

Farrow SL
Div of Endocrinology
Wayne State University Medical Center
Detroit, Michigan, USA

Fradà G
Istituto di Medicina Interna e Geriatria
Università degli Studi di Palermo, Palermo

Furgi G
Istituto di Medicina Interna, Cardiologia e Cardiologia Vascolare
Università Federico II di Napoli, Napoli

Gambardella A
Dip. di Gerontologia, Geriatria e Malattie del Metabolismo
II Università di Napoli-Policlinico, Napoli

Gavras H
Boston University Medical School
Boston, Massachusetts, USA

Gavras I
Boston University Medical School
Boston, Massachusetts, USA

Geraci A
Istituto di Medicina Interna e Geriatria
Università degli Studi di Palermo, Palermo

Geroldi C
Geriatric Research Group, IRCCS "S. Giovanni di Dio"
Sacro Cuore Fatebenefratelli Hospital, Brescia

Ghiadoni L
Cattedra di Medicina Interna
Università degli Studi di Pisa, Pisa

Grandone E
Unità di Trombosi ed Aterosclerosi
IRRCS "Casa Sollievo della Sofferenza," S. Giovanni Rotondo

Granvillano L
Cattedra di Geriatria
Università degli Studi di Palermo, Palermo

Iannuzzi GL
Istituto di Medicina Interna, Cardiologia e Cardiologia Vascolare
Università Federico II di Napoli, Napoli

La Cava G
Cattedra di Gerontologia e Geriatria
Università degli Studi di Firenze, Firenze

La Milia DA
Cattedra di Geriatria
Università degli Studi di Palermo, Palermo

Licata A
Istituto di Medicina Interna e Terapia
Università degli Studi di Palermo, Palermo

Licata G
Istituto di Medicina Interna e Terapia
Università degli Studi di Palermo, Palermo

Makrilakis K
Rush Presbiterian/St. Luke's Medical Center
Chicago, Illinois, USA

Mancini FP
Istituto di Biochimica e Biotecnologie
Università degli Studi di Napoli, Napoli

Manduca S
Dip. di Gerontologia, Geriatria e Malattie del Metabolismo
II Università di Napoli-Policlinico, Napoli

Mangiacavallo G
Istituto di Medicina Interna e Geriatria
Università degli Studi di Palermo, Palermo

Manzella D
Dip. di Gerontologia, Geriatria e Malattie del Metabolismo
II Università di Napoli-Policlinico, Napoli

Margaglione M
Unità di Trombosi ed Aterosclerosi
IRRCS "Casa Sollievo della Sofferenza," S. Giovanni Rotondo

Marigliano V
Cattedra di Gerontologia e Geriatria
Istituto di Clinica Medica I
Università degli Studi "La Sapienza," Roma

Masotti G
Cattedra di Gerontologia e Geriatria
Università degli Studi di Firenze, Firenze

Mecocci P
Istituto di Gerontologia e Geriatria
Policlinico Monteluce
Università degli Studi di Perugia, Perugia

Minischetti M
Istituto di Medicina Interna
Università degli Studi di Bari, Bari

Modesti PA
Cattedra di Medicina Interna
Università degli Studi di Firenze, Firenze

Motta L
Cattedra di Gerontologia e Geriatria
Università degli Studi di Catania, Catania

Mussi C
Cattedra di Geriatria
Università degli Studi di Modena, Modena

Neri Serneri GG
Cattedra di Medicina Interna
Università degli Studi di Firenze, Firenze

Nocco ML
Cattedra di Gerontologia e Geriatria
Istituto di Clinica Medica I,
Università degli Studi "La Sapienza," Roma

Novo S
Istituto di Medicina Interna e Geriatria
Università degli Studi di Palermo, Palermo

Palazzo M
Istituto di Medicina Interna e Geriatria,
Università degli Studi di Palermo, Palermo

Paolisso G
Dip. di Gerontologia, Geriatria e Malattie del Metabolismo
II Università di Napoli-Policlinico, Napoli

Parrinello G
Istituto di Medicina Interna e Terapia
Università degli Studi di Palermo, Palermo

Passeri G
Cattedra di Medicina Interna
Università degli Studi di Padova, Padova

Passeri M
Istituto di Medicina Interna e Terapia
Università degli Studi di Parma, Parma

Paterna S
Istituto di Medicina Interna e Terapia
Università degli Studi di Palermo, Palermo

Pellegri M
Cattedra di Gerontologia e Geriatria
Università degli Studi di Firenze, Firenze

Pellegrino A
Istituto di Medicina Interna
Università degli Studi di Bari, Bari

Pernice C
Istituto di Medicina Interna e Geriatria
Università degli Studi di Palermo, Palermo

Petrella G
Dip. di Gerontologia, Geriatria e Malattie del Metabolismo
II Università di Napoli-Policlinico, Napoli

Piccirillo G
Cattedra di Gerontologia e Geriatria
Università degli Studi "La Sapienza," Roma

Picone G
Istituto di Medicina Interna, Cardiologia e Cardiologia Vascolare
Università Federico II di Napoli, Napoli

Pinto A
Istituto di Medicina Interna e Terapia
Università degli Studi di Palermo, Palermo

Polidori MC
Istituto di Gerontologia e Geriatria
Policlinico Monteluce
Università degli Studi di Perugia, Perugia

Pollice S
Istituto di Medicina Interna, Cardiologia e Cardiologia Vascolare
Università Federico II di Napoli, Napoli

Pollina R
Istituto di Medicina Interna e Geriatria
Università degli Studi di Palermo, Palermo

Pupella E
Istituto di Medicina Interna e Geriatria
Università degli Studi di Palermo, Palermo

Rajkumar V
Div of Endocrinology
Wayne State University Medical Center
Detroit, Michigan, USA

Rapisarda R
Cattedra di Gerontologia e Geriatria
Università degli Studi di Catania, Catania

Receputo G
Cattedra di Gerontologia e Geriatria
Università degli Studi di Catania, Catania

Remediani S
Cattedra di Gerontologia e Geriatria
Istituto di Clinica Medica I
Università degli Studi "La Sapienza," Roma

Rengo F
Istituto di Medicina Interna, Cardiologia e Cardiologia Vascolare
Università Federico II di Napoli, Napoli

Resnick LM
Div of Endocrinology
Wayne State University Medical Center
Detroit, Michigan, USA

Rizzo MR
Dip. di Gerontologia, Geriatria e Malattie del Metabolismo
II Università di Napoli-Policlinico, Napoli

Ruggero R
Cattedra di Geriatria,
Università degli Studi di Palermo, Palermo

Ryan A
Cattedra di Gerontologia e Geriatria
Università degli Studi di Milano, Milano

Salvetti A
Cattedra di Medicina Interna
Università degli Studi di Pisa, Pisa

Salvioli G
Cattedra di Geriatria
Università degli Studi di Modena, Modena

Sangiorgi S
Cattedra di Gerontologia e Geriatria
Università degli Studi di Catania, Catania

Santagada E
Cattedra di Gerontologia e Geriatria
Istituto di Clinica Medica I
Università degli Studi "La Sapienza," Roma

Sartori L
Cattedra di Medicina Interna
Università degli Studi di Padova, Padova

Senin U
Istituto di Gerontologia e Geriatria
Policlinico Monteluce
Università degli Studi di Perugia, Perugia

Sergi G
Cattedra di Gerontologia e Geriatria, Istituto di Medicina Interna
Università degli Studi di Padova, Padova

Sowers JR
Div of Endocrinology
Wayne State University Medical Center
Detroit, Michigan, USA

Steimberg J
Div of Endocrinology
Wayne State University Medical Center
Detroit, Michigan, USA

Taddei S
Cattedra di Medicina Interna
Università degli Studi di Pisa, Pisa

Tagliabue J
Cattedra di Gerontologia e Geriatria
Università degli Studi di Milano, Milano

Tagliamonte MR
Dip. di Gerontologia, Geriatria e Malattie del Metabolismo
II Università di Napoli-Policlinico, Napoli

Tarantini S
Cattedra di Gerontologia e Geriatria
Istituto di Clinica Medica I
Università degli Studi "La Sapienza," Roma

Tomasello FB
Cattedra di Gerontologia e Geriatria
Università degli Studi di Catania, Catania

Trabucchi M
Cattedra di NeuroPsicoFarmacologia
Università degli Studi "Tor Vergata," Roma

Troiano L
Istituto di Medicina Interna, Cardiologia e Cardiologia Vascolare
Università Federico II di Napoli, Napoli

Ungar A
Cattedra di Gerontologia e Geriatria
Università degli Studi di Firenze, Firenze

Vacca A
Istituto di Medicina Interna
Università degli Studi di Bari, Bari

Valenti G
Cattedra di Gerontologia e Geriatria
Università degli Studi di Parma, Parma

Vallotti B
Cattedra di Gerontologia e Geriatria
Università degli Studi di Firenze, Firenze

Varricchio G
Dip. di Gerontologia, Geriatria e Malattie del Metabolismo
II Università di Napoli-Policlinico, Napoli

Varricchio M
Dip. di Gerontologia, Geriatria e Malattie del Metabolismo
II Università di Napoli-Policlinico, Napoli

Vergani C
Cattedra di Gerontologia e Geriatria
Università degli Studi di Milano, Milano

Virdis A
Cattedra di Medicina Interna
Università degli Studi di Pisa, Pisa

Zito M
Cattedra di Gerontologia e Geriatria
Università degli Studi di Chieti, Chieti

AUTHOR INDEX